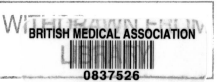

Ophthalmic Pathology

An illustrated guide
for clinicians

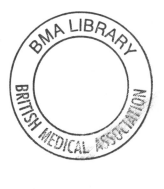

Ophthalmic Pathology

An illustrated guide for clinicians

K Weng Sehu

Tennent Institute of Ophthalmology, University of Glasgow, UK

William R Lee

Tennent Institute of Ophthalmology, University of Glasgow, UK

BMJ
Books

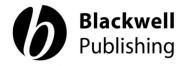

Blackwell
Publishing

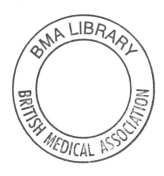

First published in 2005

Library of Congress Cataloging-in-Publication Data
Sehu, K. Weng
    Ophthalmic pathology: an illustrated guide for clinicians/K. Weng Sehu, William R. Lee
        p.;   cm.
    includes index.
    ISBN-13: 978 0 727917 79 9 (alk. paper)
    ISBN-10: 0 727917 79 X (alk. paper)
    1. Eye—Disease—Atlases   2. Eye—Diseases.
    [DNLM: 1. Eye Diseases—pathology—Atlases.] I. Lee, William R., 1932–   II. Title.
RE71.S44 2005
617.7—dc22
                                                                                        2005001742

A catalogue record for this title is available from the British Library

ISBN-13: 978 0 727917 79 9
ISBN-10: 0 727917 79 X

Set in Chennai, India by Newgen Imaging Systems (P) Ltd
Printed and bound in Haryana, India by Replika Press PVT Ltd.

Commissioning Editor: Mary Banks
Development Editor: Veronica Pock
Production Controller: Debbie Wyer

For further information on Blackwell Publishing, visit our website:
http://www.blackwellpublishing.com

The publisher's policy is to use permanent paper from mills that operate a sustainable forestry policy, and which has been manufactured from pulp processed using acid-free and elementary chlorine-free practices. Furthermore, the publisher ensures that the text paper and cover board used have met acceptable environmental accreditation standards.

Contents

Preface

Our original purpose in writing this book was to make available illustrations of the common pathological entities encountered in routine practice for junior colleagues who are undertaking postgraduate training. In so doing, we have attempted to provide an understanding of the basic processes involved in ophthalmic disease and thus this book should also be of interest to qualified ophthalmologists. Computer technology has advanced to such a level that it has enabled us to derive and modify images collected over a period of 40 years. A CD ROM has been created as it provides the highest quality annotated illustrations that are easily accessible with the additional facility to remove the annotations for self-testing. The electronic images allow viewing of screen illustrations at much higher magnifications than would be possible in a printed textbook. An illustrated text has also been prepared for portable convenience. Basic clinical and management sections have been added into each chapter to provide relevant background to the pathology presented. As a result, we hope that this book will also be of value to those pathologists with an interest in ophthalmic pathology by helping to bridge the gap between laboratory and clinical practice.

Weng Sehu
William Lee

ix

Acknowledgements

It is our pleasure to acknowledge the help and advice we have received from Dr Fiona Roberts, Dr Ridia Lim, Professor Peter McCluskey, and Dr Harald Schilling.

Dedication

To our respective families.

Chapter 1
Basics

In order to achieve a better understanding of disease processes occurring in different regions of the eye, this section describes the technology currently employed by the histopathologist in the examination of tissue specimens referred by ophthalmologists. It is important to be aware of the range of laboratory services locally available. When there is a suspicion of infection, the relevant specialist (bacteriologist/mycologist/virologist) should be consulted for advice concerning appropriate transport media and therapy. The value of an accurate and concise history cannot be overestimated and good collaboration will be rewarding to both clinicians and laboratory specialists.

Examination of the enucleated eye

A formalin-fixed enucleated globe bears little resemblance to the *in vivo* appearance due to opacification of the cornea, lens, vitreous, and retina. Previous intervention, for example removal of keratoplasty tissue, can produce secondary damage to the anterior segment tissues (Figure 1.1). In routine practice, it is unwise to try to cut across the lens because this produces damage to the anterior segment but occasionally a suitable illustration can be provided (Figure 1.2). By dividing the globe in the coronal plane, the pathologist has the advantage of examination of the lens and ciliary body from the posterior aspect (Figure 1.3) and the retina from the anterior aspect (Figure 1.4). For demonstration purposes, it is possible to divide the optic nerve and the lens (Figure 1.5). In general, the globe is divided above the optic nerve and at the edge of the cornea to avoid traumatic artefact to the main axial structures. After paraffin processing, the microtomist cuts into the centre of the eye. The orientation of the extraocular muscles on the posterior aspect of the globe allows the pathologist to identify the side from which the globe was enucleated (Figure 1.6). Orientation of the specimen is vital if the correct plane of cut is to be made.

Microscopic features

These are described wherever relevant to pathology in the corresponding chapters and are therefore only illustrated briefly in this chapter. The histological features of each of the following tissues are annotated in detail:
* cornea (Figure 1.7)
* chamber angle (Figure 1.8)
* iris (Figures 1.8, 1.9)
* ciliary body (Figures 1.8, 1.10, 1.11)
* lens (Figures 1.9, 1.11)
* retina and choroid (Figure 1.12)
* optic disc (Figure 1.13).

Features for identification of the age of a patient (in this case a child):
* thin Descemet's membrane
* "finger-like ciliary processes"
* intact, non-hyalinised ciliary muscle
* absence of proliferations in the pars plana epithelium
* absence of sub-RPE (retinal pigment epithelium) deposits (for example drusen).

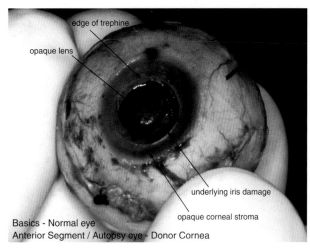

Figure 1.1

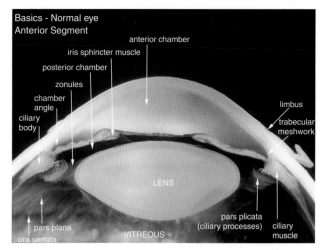

Figure 1.2

Figure 1.1 In the current litigious climate, the only normal autopsy material available for study will be that used for donor keratoplasty. In this example, formalin fixation accounts for opacification in the cornea and lens. Damage to the iris is the result of the trephine.

Figure 1.2 The anatomical features of the anterior segment are easily recognised. Note that formalin fixation leads to opacification of those tissues (cornea, lens, zonules, and vitreous) which are normally transparent.

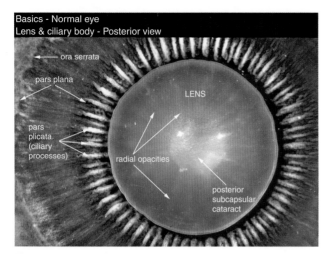

Figure 1.3

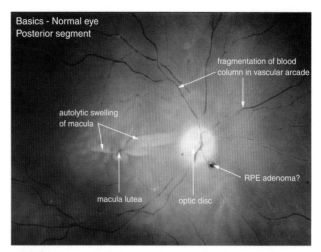

Figure 1.4

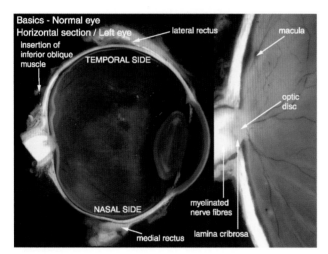

Figure 1.5

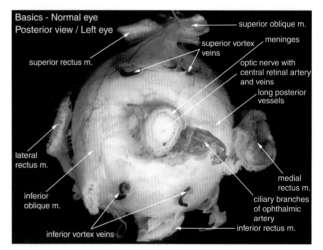

Figure 1.6

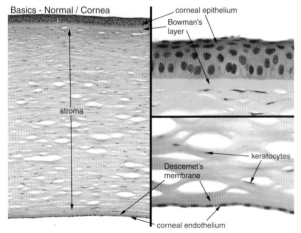

Figure 1.7

Figure 1.3 Dividing the eye in the coronal plane provides the opportunity to examine the ciliary body and lens in detail. In this case, there is a subcapsular cataract. The radial linear opacities in the lens substance are a common degenerative feature in the elderly globe. Note that in the pars plicata, there are ridges and troughs which explain the differing appearance of the ciliary processes in Figures 1.10 and 1.11.

Figure 1.4 In a globe removed at autopsy, there is often autolytic swelling of the macula due to delayed fixation. The opacification of the retina is the result of formalin fixation. After cessation of blood flow, the blood columns in the vessels tend to fragment ("cattle-trucking").

Figure 1.5 This normal globe is part of an exenteration and is fixed in gluteraldehyde. For demonstration purposes, the section passes through the centre of the optic nerve, the lens, and the pupil (left). The macula is located on the temporal side of the optic nerve, which is confirmed by the adjacent scleral insertion of the inferior oblique muscle. The distance from the optic nerve to the ora is greater on the temporal side than on the nasal side. A higher magnification of the posterior pole of the globe is shown on the right. Myelination of the axons in the optic nerve ends at the lamina cribrosa.

Figure 1.6 The orientation of the extraocular muscles in relation to the optic nerve reveals that this specimen is a left globe.

Figure 1.7 A full thickness section of the cornea (left) demonstrates the relative thinness of the epithelium and endothelium in relation to the stroma. Both cell layers are shown in higher magnification (upper right and lower right). Note the artefactual separation of the corneal lamellae.

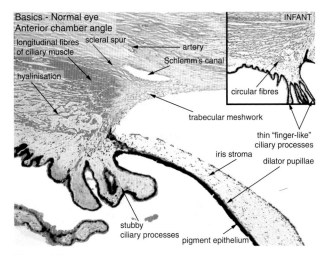

Basics - Normal eye
Anterior chamber angle

longitudinal fibres of ciliary muscle
scleral spur
hyalinisation
artery
Schlemm's canal
INFANT
circular fibres
trabecular meshwork
thin "finger-like" ciliary processes
iris stroma
dilator pupillae
stubby ciliary processes
pigment epithelium

Figure 1.8

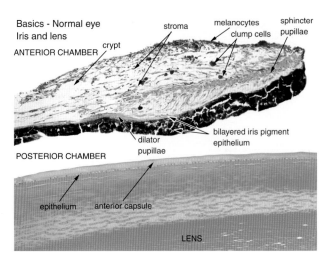

Basics - Normal eye
Iris and lens

ANTERIOR CHAMBER
crypt
stroma
melanocytes
clump cells
sphincter pupillae
bilayered iris pigment epithelium
dilator pupillae
POSTERIOR CHAMBER
epithelium
anterior capsule
LENS

Figure 1.9

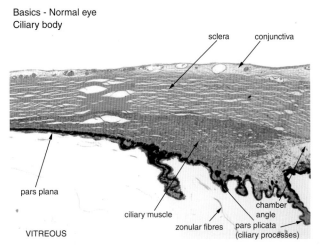

Basics - Normal eye
Ciliary body

sclera
conjunctiva
pars plana
ciliary muscle
zonular fibres
chamber angle
pars plicata (ciliary processes)
VITREOUS

Figure 1.10

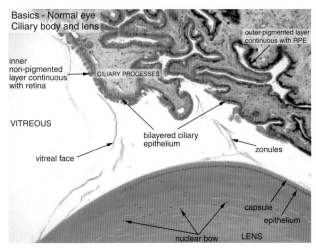

Basics - Normal eye
Ciliary body and lens

inner non-pigmented layer continuous with retina
CILIARY PROCESSES
outer pigmented layer continuous with RPE
VITREOUS
bilayered ciliary epithelium
zonules
vitreal face
capsule
epithelium
nuclear bow
LENS

Figure 1.11

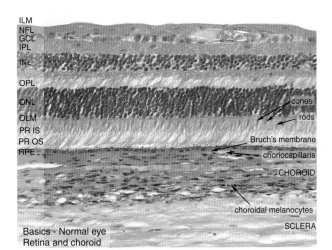

ILM
NFL
GCL
IPL
INL
OPL
ONL
OLM
PR IS
PR OS
RPE
cones
rods
Bruch's membrane
choriocapillaris
CHOROID
choroidal melanocytes
SCLERA
Basics - Normal eye
Retina and choroid

Figure 1.12

Figure 1.8 Hyalinisation and atrophy of the circular and oblique components of the ciliary muscle is a feature of ageing, but the longitudinal fibres inserting into the scleral spur persist. In an infant (inset), the components of the ciliary muscle are intact: note the thin ciliary processes.

Figure 1.9 In the pupillary portion of the iris, the sphincter pupillae is a prominent feature and the close relationship to the lens provides the opportunity to illustrate the anterior capsule and the epithelium of lens. The iris pigment epithelium terminates at the pupillary rim in the normal eye.

Figure 1.10 In this illustration of the normal ciliary body, the relative absence of hyalinisation in the ciliary muscle suggests the younger age of the patient. This section passes through one of the troughs in the pars plicata.

Figure 1.11 The ciliary processes are lined by a two-layered epithelium corresponding to the layers of the optic cup (see Chapter 6). The stroma of the ciliary processes contains blood vessels. The equator of the lens contains the nuclear bow. This section passes through a ridge in the pars plicata.

Figure 1.12 The normal histology of the retina, choroid, and sclera. ILM = inner limiting membrane, NFL = nerve fibre layer, GCL = ganglion cell layer, IPL = inner plexiform layer, INL = inner nuclear layer (bipolar cells), OPL = outer plexiform layer, ONL = outer nuclear layer (photoreceptor nuclei), PR = photoreceptors in inner segment (IS) and outer segment (OS) (cones have a distinctive pink inner segment), RPE = retinal pigment epithelium with underlying Bruch's membrane and choriocapillaris. The choroid contains blood vessels, nerves, fibroblasts, and melanocytes with branching processes. The sclera is avascular and contains scattered scleral fibroblasts.

Basic pathology definitions

The following text describes the histological appearance in basic pathological processes and serves only as an introduction. Additional illustrations are provided throughout the text.

Inflammation

For a detailed description of the functions of inflammatory cells, the reader is advised to consult specialised immunology texts. Inflammatory disease entities relevant to ophthalmic pathology are described in Chapter 8.

Cellular constituents

Polymorphonuclear leucocytes

Neutrophilic polymorphonuclear leucocytes
Acute purulent inflammation occurs after pathogenic organisms, particularly bacteria or fungi, are introduced into the ocular or orbital tissues. The predominant cell is the neutrophilic polymorphonuclear leucocyte (PMNL) which contains intracytoplasmic granules encasing lysosomal enzymes capable of destroying pathogenic organisms (Figure 1.14). The proteolytic enzymes are also destructive of normal tissues adding to the lytic enzymes secreted by pathogenic organisms.

Eosinophilic polymorphonuclear leucocytes
These possess intracytoplasmic granules which, with an appropriate stimulus from interleukin 6, release major basic protein and ribonuclease (Figure 1.15). These enzymes are often associated with reactions against protozoal parasites, such as *Toxocara canis*, but this response is disadvantageous in allergic conditions (for example vernal conjunctivitis) because release of enzymes leads to vasodilatation and oedema.

Mast cells

Mast cells are large mononuclear cells with intracytoplasmic pink granules (in an H&E stain) containing heparin, histamine, and prostaglandin (Figure 1.16). These cells are an important component of allergic reactions (for example vernal conjunctivitis).

Lymphocytes and plasma cells

Lymphocytes and plasma cells predominate in chronic inflammatory processes, particularly in autoimmune disorders. Both types of cells are small (Figure 1.17). Lymphocytes have a homogeneous nucleus and very little cytoplasm. Plasma cells are oval with a "cartwheel" or "clockface" nucleus, and a paranuclear clear area in the pink cytoplasm.

Granulomatous inflammatory reaction

The classic reaction is characterised by an infiltration of macrophages accompanied by lymphocytes and plasma cells. Macrophages frequently fuse to form multinucleate giant cells. Granulomatous inflammatory reactions occur during chronic infections by bacteria (for example *Mycobacteria* sp.) and fungi (for example *Aspergillus* sp.). Foreign material also stimulates a granulomatous reaction (Figure 1.18).

A granulomatous inflammatory reaction must be distinguished from granulation tissue which is formed by fibrovascular proliferation occurring as part of a healing response.

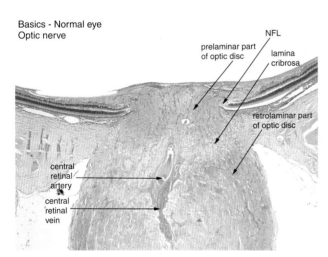

Figure 1.13

Figure 1.13 A longitudinal section through the optic nerve demonstrates the different components. The nerve fibre layer (NFL) is thickened at the edge of the disc. The prelaminar part contains non-myelinated axons which pass through the lamina cribrosa. In the retrolaminar part of the optic nerve, the axons are myelinated.

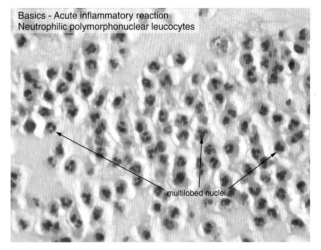

Figure 1.14

Figure 1.14 This illustration was taken from a pooled collection of polymorphonuclear leucocytes in the anterior chamber (hypopyon). These cells are recognised by their distinctive multilobed nuclei. The pink-staining material around the cells is plasma.

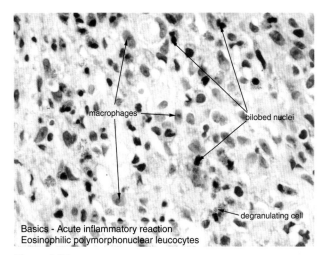

Basics - Acute inflammatory reaction
Eosinophilic polymorphonuclear leucocytes

Figure 1.15

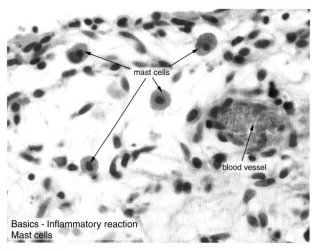

Basics - Inflammatory reaction
Mast cells

Figure 1.16

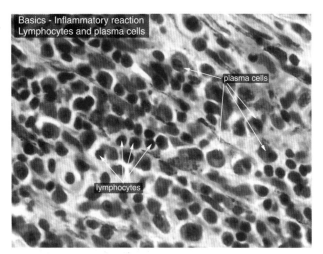

Basics - Inflammatory reaction
Lymphocytes and plasma cells

Figure 1.17

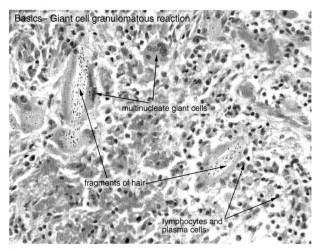

Basics - Giant cell granulomatous reaction

Figure 1.18

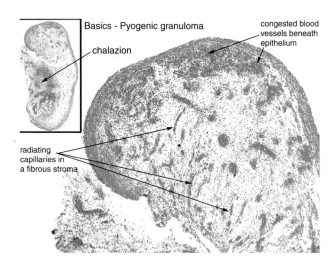

Basics - Pyogenic granuloma

Figure 1.19

Figure 1.15 Eosinophilic polymorphonuclear leucocytes (PMNLs) are often part of a reaction which contains macrophages. The eosinophils possess bilobed nuclei and bright red intracytoplasmic granules which are released into the tissue (degranulation). Macrophages have relatively larger oval nuclei and have a phagocytic function.

Figure 1.16 Mast cells are mononuclear cells and are larger than PMNLs. The red granules in the cytoplasm are characteristic. These cells are easily found in the normal iris stroma, as in this example.

Figure 1.17 This chronic inflammatory reaction in the choroid contains numerous lymphocytes and plasma cells. Note the clear area adjacent to the nucleus of the plasma cell.

Figure 1.18 Implantation of hair fragments into the conjunctiva induces a foreign body giant cell granulomatous reaction.

Figure 1.19 The term "pyogenic granuloma" is a misnomer as can be seen from this illustration: there is neither evidence of pus nor of a giant cell granulomatous reaction. The congested mass of tissue consists only of radiating blood vessels in loose fibrous connective tissue. A chalazion (see Chapter 2) is present beneath the pyogenic granuloma.

Pyogenic granuloma

Clinically this condition appears as a fleshy, granular, red mass over a pre-existing defect in the conjunctiva. Most commonly a pathologist will see a pyogenic granuloma over a chalazion (Figure 1.19) or over suture material in a muscle insertion after squint surgery.

Neoplasia

Knowledge of terminology used by pathologists is essential to a clinician in the interpretation of a pathological report.

Hypertrophy

An increase in the volume of tissue by enlargement of individual cells. While this is a common phenomenon in striated muscle following repetitive use (for example weight training), it is difficult to find a suitable example in ophthalmic pathology.

Hyperplasia

An increase in the volume of tissue due to the proliferation of cells (for example response of conjunctival epithelium or epidermis of the eyelid to an irritant – Figure 1.20).

Hyperkeratosis

Thickening of the keratin-containing layer in an epidermis (for example actinic keratosis – Figure 1.20).

Parakeratosis

Nuclear debris persists in a thickened keratin layer when the growth rate of the epithelium is accelerated (for example actinic keratosis – Figure 1.20).

Metaplasia

This is transformation of one cell type to another cell type (for example columnar epithelium of conjunctiva to stratified squamous in keratoconjunctivitis sicca). Two other forms of metaplasia of importance in ophthalmology are fibrous metaplasia of the retinal pigment epithelium (for example proliferative vitreoretinopathy following rhegmatogenous retinal detachment – see Chapter 10) and fibrous metaplasia of the lens epithelium (for example anterior subcapsular cataract – Figure 1.21).

Dysplasia

Irregular arrangement and loss of maturation of cells in an epithelium. The nuclei are irregular in size, shape, and chromatin distribution, and mitotic figures may be found in all levels. This can be regarded as a carcinoma-in-situ because the neoplastic cells have not penetrated the underlying basement membrane (Figure 1.22).

Mitotic figures

Mitotic division of cells involves the duplication of chromosomes and separation to form two daughter cells. A mitotic figure is most easily identified in metaphase when the nuclear material forms a broad line across the cell (Figure 1.22). Mitotic activity is a normal function of those cells which undergo "wear-and-tear" replacement (for example basal layer of epithelium). Pathologists attach great importance to the identification of mitotic figures, especially in neoplasias where an increase in mitotic activity reflects cell proliferation rates. Many examples of mitotic activity will be provided throughout this textbook to illustrate the varying appearances of the process.

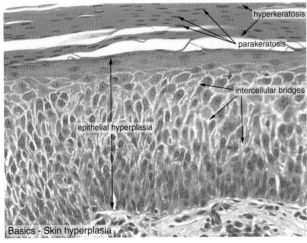

Figure 1.20

Figure 1.20 Sun damage to skin results in hyperplasia of the epidermis with excessive keratin formation (hyperkeratosis) and migration of epithelial cell nuclei into the surface keratin (parakeratosis). There is still maturation of the epidermal layers from basal to surface, which makes the distinction between hyperplasia and dysplasia (see Figure 1.22).

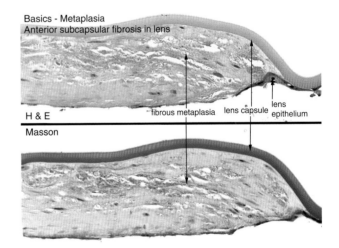

Figure 1.21

Figure 1.21 The formation of an anterior subcapsular fibrous plaque is one complication of anterior uveitis. The fibrous tissue staining green with the Masson stain (lower) is formed by metaplasia of lens epithelial cells to fibroblasts.

Atrophy

A decrease in size or number of cells. This process may be physiological or pathological. The lacrimal gland (see Chapter 5) becomes atrophic in later life (physiological) and the nerve fibre layer becomes atrophic in glaucoma (pathological).

Apoptosis

Apoptosis describes the programmed cell death which occurs in normal tissue (for example embryogenesis of the retina) and in disease. In the absence of inflammatory cell infiltration, individual cells undergoing apoptosis appear shrunken and the nuclei are fragmented (Figure 1.23). Programmed cell death is common in malignant tumours and explains the slow growth of basal cell carcinomas and uveal melanomas.

Necrosis

By comparison, in necrosis there is widespread cell death as observed in rapidly proliferating tumours such as retinoblastoma in which tumour growth exceeds the blood supply (see Chapter 11). When a population of cells dies simultaneously, the nuclei and cytoplasmic membranes disappear leaving a pale pink staining area of tissue in an H&E section.

Type of specimens

Pathological services are now used more frequently due to the importance of accountability, audit, and research.

The following types of specimen may be presented for pathological examination:
- eyelid (including lacrimal sac) – biopsy*
- conjunctiva – biopsy, impression cytology, and scrape
- cornea – lamellar or full thickness (penetrating keratoplasty), impression cytology, and scrape
- orbit (including lacrimal gland) – biopsy + exenteration
- optic nerve – biopsy or enucleation
- temporal artery biopsy
- globe – biopsy, evisceration, enucleation, exenteration
- aqueous and vitreous tap
- vitrectomy including membrane peeling
- subretinal membrane – excision.

Tissue preparation

Fixatives

Fixation is essential to good histopathology because excised tissue undergoes rapid autolysis and desiccation.

Formalin

This is the traditional universal fixative solution in ophthalmic pathology because it has prolonged chemical stability and is most appropriate for immunohistochemistry.

Gluteraldehyde

If scanning or transmission electron microscopy is required for diagnosis, gluteraldehyde fixation is essential. One advantage of this fixative is that the macroscopic appearances are closer to those observed *in vivo*, although it is less suitable for immunohistochemistry.

---

* The term "biopsy" refers to both partial removal (diagnostic) or total removal (excisional) of a suspicious mass. Fine needle biopsy is preferred in some centres to avoid unnecessary tissue damage.

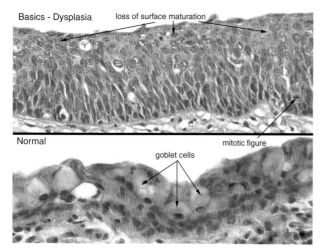

Figure 1.22

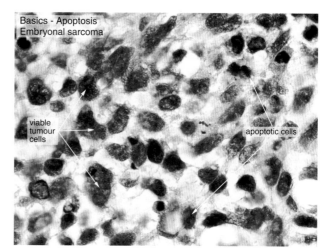

Figure 1.23

Figure 1.22 This is an example of metaplasia and dysplasia in the conjunctival epithelium (upper). The normal appearance is shown below for comparison. In the upper figure, the conjunctival epithelial cells have undergone metaplasia to squamous cells. Dysplasia is characterised by a failure of maturation in the cell population which exhibits the cytological characteristics of malignancy (e.g. marked variation in nuclear size and shape and mitotic figures located outside the basal layer). Although this is a premalignant change, there is no evidence of invasion into the underlying stroma and this change is classified as carcinoma-in-situ.

Figure 1.23 Programmed cell death in individual cells occurs in both physiological and pathological processes. In this orbital rhabdomyosarcoma, the apoptotic cells can be recognised by the small fragmented nuclei in comparison with large irregular nuclei of the viable cells.

Alcohol

Alcohol (for example gin) can be used for specimen fixation in countries where formalin is not available.

Preparation

Paraffin embedding

Currently, tissue is cut to provide histological preparations after it is embedded in paraffin wax. To achieve impregnation of the tissue by wax, it is necessary to remove water (ascending concentrations of alcohol) and lipid (xylene). The wax supports the tissue during sectioning (5–10 μm in thickness) and acts as an adhesive when the section is mounted on a glass slide. A reverse process takes place to remove the wax (xylene) and rehydrate the tissue (descending concentrations of alcohol) prior to tissue staining with water-soluble conventional stains or the application of immunohistochemistry.

Paraffin blocks and sections can be stored indefinitely.

Fresh/frozen sections

If an urgent diagnosis is required during a surgical procedure, the tissue can be rapidly frozen and sections cut on a freezing microtome. Section preparation is easier when the tissue is not fixed so the specimen should be transferred to the laboratory in saline or transport media.

Fresh tissue is also more suitable for the study of fat within cellular components (for example lipid keratopathy or sebaceous carcinoma) and for immunohistochemical studies in which a full exposure of antigenic epitopes is required.

For the best preservation of tissue, specially designed transport media (for example Michel's transport medium) should be used. Consultation with the pathologist is essential.

Plastic embedding

For transmission electron microscopy, it is necessary to embed tissue in hard plastic material (Araldite). Plastic material can be cut on a microtome to achieve the thin sections (0.05–0.06 μm) necessary for high-resolution imaging and are able to resist electron beam bombardment. Thin plastic sections (1 μm) are cut for light microscopy and stained with toluidine blue.

Macroscopic examination or specimen "grossing"

In ophthalmic pathology, specimens are often small and the initial examination requires magnification with a dissecting microscope. The specimen is measured and a description recorded before division into blocks for paraffin embedding. The methods for each tissue sample are described at the beginning of the relevant chapter. It is however appropriate to describe the methodology for the examination of a globe at this point.

Measurements

The maximum dimensions in the globe in the following sequence are measured using a calliper:

1 Antero-posterior (normal 24 mm).
2 Horizontal (normal 23.5 mm).
3 Vertical (normal 23 mm).

The following are examples of conditions that may alter the dimensions:

- Increase (25–30 mm): axial myopia, adult glaucomatous enlargement due to uveoscleral bulging (staphyloma formation) or buphthalmos resulting from infantile glaucoma.
- Decrease (15–18 mm): axial hypermetropia when the globe is shortened. Shrinkage (for example atrophia bulbi or phthisis bulbi) occurs after prolonged loss of pressure in the eye. Ocular hypotonia may be the consequence of inflammatory damage to the ciliary processes or to leakage of intraocular fluids through a defect in the corneoscleral envelope.

Transillumination

The shadow from a powerful light source behind the globe is used to locate intraocular masses.

Different cuts and terminology

The plane of section through an eye is extremely important in revealing the pathological features in a paraffin section. Cuts are carefully chosen to include all the pathological features and relationships in one plane of section.

In the horizontal plane, the paraffin sections should include the centre of the pupil, the lens, the macula, and the optic nerve (Figure 1.24). The temporal side of the eye is longer than the nasal side, so that a horizontal cut can be recognised in a section even when the retina and macula are atrophic. The inferior oblique muscle when present is useful to identify the posterior temporal sclera and overlies the macula.

The vertical plane is favoured for displaying surgery for glaucoma and cataract. However, in the case of a tumour or a foreign body, an oblique section may be required to cut across the feature of interest (Figure 1.25).

Anatomical location

For accurate clinical correlation, the ocular abnormalities should be described in their correct quadrants–referred to as superior, inferior, temporal, and nasal.

Calotte

The term "calotte" (French: "cap") is used for the two hemispheres which are cut from the globe before the central pupil-optic nerve block (PO block) is processed through paraffin. NB: This should not be confused with "culotte" (French: "knickers/panties")!

Stains for microscopy

Conventional histopathology

All of the conventional stains and the more sophisticated diagnostic techniques summarised in Tables 1.1 and 1.2 will be referred to in detail in subsequent chapters.

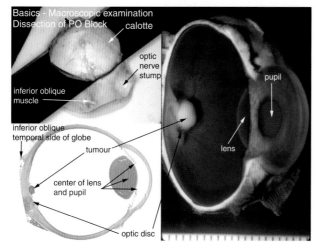

Figure 1.24

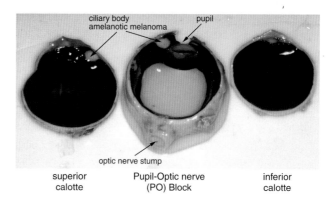

Figure 1.25

Figure 1.24 The primary cuts in a globe are important if all the features are to be displayed in a paraffin section. Upper left: a second cut in a globe is made with a large dermatome blade. The first cut reveals a small tumour adjacent to the optic nerve (right). The paraffin section passes through the centre of the nerve, the centre of the tumour, and the centre of the anterior segment. The clinical diagnosis was a retinoblastoma but pathologically the tumour was a small benign glial tumour (astrocytic hamartoma, see Chapter 11).

Figure 1.25 Oblique cuts are made in this globe to pass through a superonasal tumour in the ciliary body. The central pupil-optic nerve block is subsequently processed for paraffin histology and the calottes are retained for specialised investigation.

Table 1.1 A summary of the special stains used in routine diagnostic histopathology.

Type of stain	Reactions (colours)	Diagnostic use	Figure
Alcian blue	Mucopolysaccharides (blue)	Macular dystrophy Thyroid eye disease (muscle)	1.26
Alizarin red	Chelates calcium (red)	Calcification in tissues, e.g. band keratopathy	1.27
Bodian	Axons (black)	Optic atrophy	1.28
Colloidal iron	Mucopolysaccharide (blue)	Macular dystrophy Thyroid eye disease (muscle)	1.26
Gram	Bacteria: differing cell wall staining characteristics Gram positive (dark blue) Gram negative (red)	Identification and classification of bacteria	1.29
Loyez	Myelin (black)	Demyelinating diseases (e.g. multiple sclerosis) Optic atrophy	1.30
Masson trichrome	Epithelium (red) Connective tissue (green)	Cornea: damage to Bowman's layer Lens: fibrous metaplasia	1.21, 1.31
Periodic acid-Schiff (PAS)	Basement membranes (bright pink)	Cornea: epithelial basement membrane, Descemet's membrane Lens: capsule Retina: inner limiting membrane Others: fungal elements	1.32
Prussian blue (Perls')	Ferrous (Fe^{2+}) and ferric (Fe^{3+}) iron (dark blue)	Iron-containing salts and blood products, e.g. metallic foreign body and haemorrhage	1.33
van Gieson (combined with elastin stain = elastin van Gieson)	Muscle (yellow) Connective tissue (red) Often combined stain for elastin (black)	Giant cell arteritis to demonstrate fragmentation of internal elastic lamina	1.34
von Kossa	Phosphates in calcified tissue (black – precipitated as a silver salt)	Calcification in tissues, e.g. band keratopathy	1.35
Ziehl–Neelsen	Acid-fast bacilli *Mycobacterium* sp. *Nocardia* sp. (pink staining rods)	Identify acid-fast pathogens in inflammatory tissue	1.36

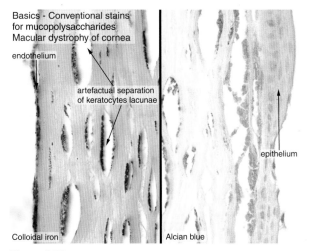

Basics - Conventional stains for mucopolysaccharides
Macular dystrophy of cornea

endothelium

artefactual separation of keratocytes lacunae

epithelium

Colloidal iron   Alcian blue

Figure 1.26

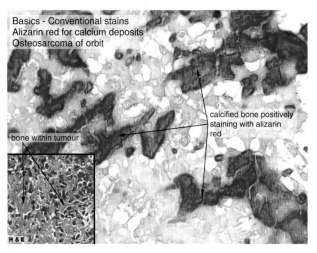

Basics - Conventional stains
Alizarin red for calcium deposits
Osteosarcoma of orbit

bone within tumour

calcified bone positively staining with alizarin red

H&E

Figure 1.27

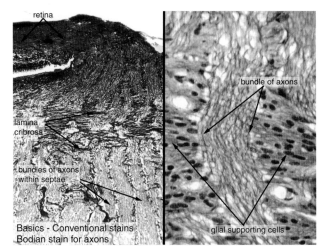

retina

lamina cribrosa

bundles of axons within septae

bundle of axons

glial supporting cells

Basics - Conventional stains
Bodian stain for axons

Figure 1.28

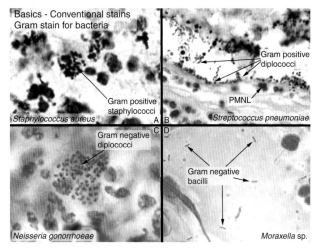

Basics - Conventional stains
Gram stain for bacteria

Gram positive staphylococci

Gram positive diplococci

PMNL

Staphylococcus aureus   A B   Streptococcus pneumoniae

Gram negative diplococci   C D

Gram negative bacilli

Neisseria gonorrhoeae   Moraxella sp.

Figure 1.29

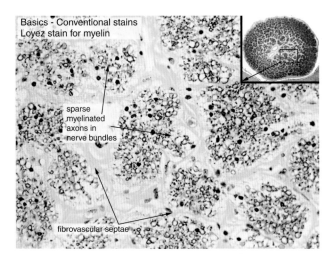

Basics - Conventional stains
Loyez stain for myelin

sparse myelinated axons in nerve bundles

fibrovascular septae

Figure 1.30

Figure 1.26 In macular dystrophy of the cornea, mucopolysaccharides accumulate in the endothelium, in the keratocytes, and in clumps beneath the epithelium. The best way to demonstrate the presence of mucopolysaccharides is to use the colloidal iron (left) or the Alcian blue (right) stains. NB: Mucopolysaccharides do not stain with H&E.

Figure 1.27 Alizarin red stain is used to identify calcium salts. This example shows calcified bone spicules within an osteosarcoma which arose in the orbit of a child who was previously treated by irradiation for a retinoblastoma. The inset shows the appearance of the tumour in an H&E section.

Figure 1.28 In an H&E section (see Figure 1.13) it is not possible to identify individual axons. The Bodian stain is one of the stains used for this purpose. Normal axons are so fine that they are not easily identified at low magnification (left). At high magnification, only segments of the sinuous axons are seen (right).

Figure 1.29 Examples of common pathogenic bacteria as seen in a Gram stain. (A) Gram positive staphylococci are dark blue in colour and occur in clumps. (B) Gram positive diplococci (Streptococcus pneumoniae) are smaller than staphylocci and possess a capsule. Both A and B can be the cause of postoperative endophthalmitis. (C) Gram negative diplococci (Neisseria gonorrhoeae) can be found in conjunctival swabs in adults with unresolving conjunctivitis and in neonates infected during birth (ophthalmia neonatorum). (D) Gram negative bacilli (Moraxella sp.) may be identified in a corneal scrape from a chronic ulcer.

Figure 1.30 Myelin sheaths are demonstrated by the Loyez stain. The inset is a transverse section through the optic nerve of a patient suffering from tobacco-alcohol amblyopia: the centre of the nerve is pale (axial demyelination). The high power view shows the transition from bundles containing sparse myelin sheaths on the left to more densely packed myelin sheaths on the right.

Basics - Conventional stains
Masson trichrome stain for collagen

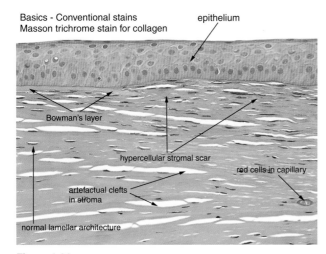

Figure 1.31

Basics - Conventional stains
Periodic acid Schiff (PAS)
for basement membranes

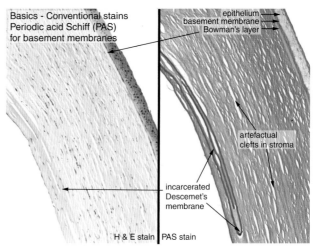

Figure 1.32

Basics - Conventional stains
Prussian blue stain for iron salts

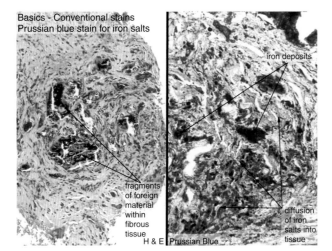

Figure 1.33

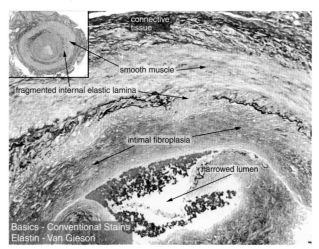

Figure 1.34

Basics - Conventional stains
Von Kossa for phosphate salts

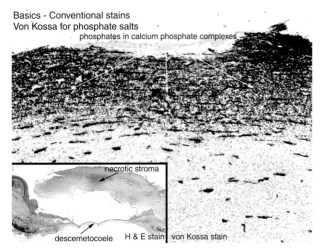

Figure 1.35

Figure 1.31 Masson trichrome stain is frequently used in corneal pathology. In this example, previous trauma has disrupted the Bowman's layer and the adjacent stroma is replaced by an irregular fibrous scar tissue. The epithelium stains pink (and red cells are red!).

Figure 1.32 By comparison with an H&E stain (left), a PAS stain (right) is used to demonstrate basement membranes. In this example, there is a post-traumatic detachment of Descemet's membrane which is incarcerated in the posterior corneal stroma. The stain also demonstrates a thickened epithelial basement membrane secondary to corneal oedema. Clefts in the stroma are artefactual and do not represent corneal oedema.

Figure 1.33 In a standard H&E section, the presence of iron in metallic foreign material in fibrous tissue cannot be determined. The Prussian blue stain demonstrates iron salts within the metallic particles and the widespread diffusion into the surrounding tissue.

Figure 1.34 The van Gieson stain is also a trichrome stain and is used to differentiate between muscle (yellow) and connective tissue (red). When combined with a stain for elastic tissue (black), fragmentation of the internal elastic lamina can be demonstrated in degenerative disease of the temporal artery.

Figure 1.35 The von Kossa stain reacts with phosphates to form a black precipitate. It is used to identify calcium phosphate complexes in tissues. In this example, the patient suffered from alkali burns which were intensively treated with phosphate buffered solutions. The extent of calcium phosphate deposition is not apparent in the H&E stained section (inset).

Other techniques

Immunohistochemistry

This technology has brought about a revolution in diagnostic and research pathology and has superseded electron microscopy. Precise identification of cells by type is achieved by applying a specific antibody to an antigenic epitope within the cell. The antibody is subsequently labelled with a chromogen which can be visualised by light or fluorescence microscopy. The number of specific antibodies which are commercially available is ever increasing (Table 1.2). For example, there are at least 25 antibodies to specifically identify T- and B-cell subsets and macrophages in benign and malignant states (Figure 1.37). Similarly, a battery of immunohistochemical reagents is applied to poorly differentiated tumours when the H&E appearance is inconclusive (for example in metastatic disease). In ophthalmic pathology, the standard brown chromogen (peroxidase-antiperoxidase: PAP) is of limited value in the study of pigmented tissues; as an alternative, red chromogens (alkaline phosphatase) are more helpful (Figure 1.37).

Electron microscopy/immunoelectron microscopy

The transmission electron microscope (TEM) focuses electrons to resolve cell structures at a high magnification (for example up to ×100 000). This was a valuable tool prior to immunohistochemistry and was mainly used to identify cell organelles (for example melanosomes) and viral particles. The principles applied in immunohistochemistry can also be applied at the ultrastructural level. Antibodies are labelled with very small gold particles that appear as black dots in micrographs. The technique can localise epitopes within cellular organelles and membranes – this is essentially a research tool.

The scanning electron microscope (SEM) focuses a raster of electrons on tissue surfaces. It is particularly useful for the study of the corneal endothelium.

Polymerase chain reaction (PCR)

Specific DNA or RNA sequences can characterise pathogenic organisms or cellular constituents. Only very small samples of tissue are required (for example aqueous or vitreous tap). This technique breaks down nuclear chromatin into sequences and a particular sequence (for example unique constituents of viruses or bacteria) under investigation is amplified to a level that allows rapid detection using gel electrophoresis.

In situ hybridization

This technique also relies on the ability to cut segments of nuclear proteins with specific enzymes. The fragments are identified by immunohistochemical techniques in routine light microscopy. The advantage is that the precise location of the protein fragments can be visualised within the tissue.

Flow cytometry

This research tool is used to identify cells types within a population (for example lymphoid proliferations). A suspension of cells is labelled with fluorescent antibodies specific for antigen determinants on the surfaces of the different cell types. The flow cytometer differentiates and quantifies the different cell types (for example B and T cells).

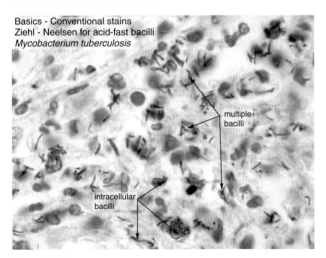

Figure 1.36

Figure 1.36 An immunosuppressed patient who succumbed to tuberculosis. Acid-fast organisms stained with Ziehl–Neelsen were plentiful in a choroidal microabscess.

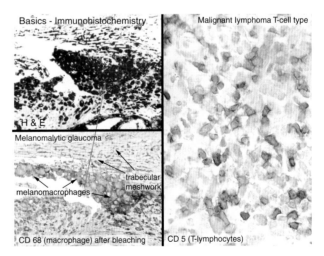

Figure 1.37

Figure 1.37 Immunohistochemistry is helpful in the diagnosis of benign and malignant conditions. In heavily pigmented tissues, it is necessary to bleach the melanin prior to application of a specific antibody labelled with a red chromogen. In this case, the angle in the trabecular meshwork is blocked by macrophages (CD68 positive) laden with melanin pigment derived from a necrotic melanoma of the ciliary body (melanomalytic glaucoma – left upper and lower). In the case of a malignant T-cell lymphoma, a brown chromogen (peroxidase-antiperoxidase: PAP) is used to label the anti-T-cell antibody (CD5, right). Note that not all the malignant cells express the epitope.

Table 1.2 A summary of the antibodies used in immunohistochemistry.

Antibody	Antigen	Diagnostic use
Anti-actin/myoglobin	Contractile filaments in smooth and striated muscle	Tumours derived from muscle, e.g. rhabdomyosarcoma (Figure 1.38)
Desmin	Intermediate filaments in smooth and striated muscle	Tumours derived from muscle, e.g. rhabdomyosarcoma (Figure 1.38)
Carcinoembryonic antigen (CEA)	High MW glycoprotein normally present in gastrointestinal epithelial cells	Metastatic adenocarcinomas to ocular tissues, adnexal skin tumours, sebaceous carcinoma
CD1–79+	Components of T and B cells, and macrophages	Many uses to identify cells in inflammatory infiltrates and in lymphomas (Figure 1.37)
Cytokeratin/CAM 5.2/AE1/AE3	Intermediate filaments in epithelial cells	Carcinomas derived from epidermis (Figure 1.39)
Epithelial membrane antigen (EMA)	Initially used for epithelial cells and carcinomas	Sebaceous carcinoma
Factor VIII-related antigen	Endothelial cell constituents	Neovascularisation and vascular tumours (Figure 1.40)
Glial fibrillar acidic protein (GFAP)	Glial cell constituents	Normal: glial cells and astrocytes (Müller cells) in retina Disease: preretinal membranes and astrocytic tumours (gliomas) of the optic nerve
HMB45/melan-A	Intracytoplasmic antigen in melanocytes	Identifies cells of melanocytic origin (active naevi and malignant melanomas – Figure 1.41)
S-100	Constituents of cells of neural crest lineage	Peripheral nerve tumours and melanocytic tumours
Vimentin	Intermediate filaments Cells of mesenchymal origin	Differentiation of spindle cell tumours, e.g. leiomyoma

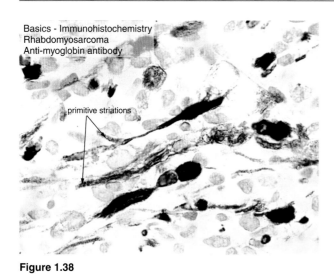

Figure 1.38

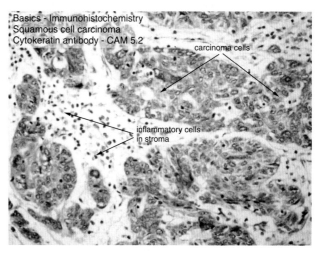

Figure 1.39

Figure 1.38 In poorly differentiated spindle cell tumours, an H&E section will not provide a specific diagnosis. In this example, an antibody against myoglobin demonstrates the protein within the cytoplasm of some of the tumour cells to confirm a diagnosis of embryonal rhabdomyosarcoma. Note that not all the tumour cells express the epitope.

Figure 1.39 In metastatic tumours, the primary site may not be evident on first presentation so that immunohistochemistry can be helpful in suggesting the origin. In this example of an orbital biopsy, CAM 5.2 labelled with peroxidase-antiperoxidase (PAP) demonstrates the characteristics of squamous epithelium. A primary bronchial carcinoma was the source. This specimen was negative for carcinoembryonic antigen which excluded a primary gastrointestinal carcinoma.

Table 1.3 A summary of routine media used in bacteriology.

Name of media	Appearance	Common pathogens cultured
Nutrient agar	Transparent pale yellow	Routine screening
Blood agar	Opaque blood red	Gram positive cocci and rods Fungi
Chocolate agar	Opaque brown	Gram negative cocci
MacConkey's agar	Transparent pink	Gram negative rods
Meat broth	Small bottle containing fragments of meat	Anaerobic rods
E. coli on non-nutrient agar	Pale yellow with a surface layer	Acanthamoeba previously a common cause of keratitis secondary to contact lens wear
Lowenstein–Jensen media	Opaque green media on a slope	Mycobacteria

Microbiology

The microbiology is here presented in context with the pathology commonly encountered in ophthalmic practice. It is important for ophthalmologists to be aware of *basic* microbiological techniques and the selection of media for an accurate diagnosis of infective conditions (Table 1.3). This text is not intended to be comprehensive, and for more specialised accounts the reader should consult the appropriate reference works.

Media

Organisms have specific growth requirements which are provided by the standard media (Table 1.3; Figures 1.42, 1.43). The majority of organisms will grow in normal atmosphere but some proliferate in a low oxygen environment (anaerobes).

Stains
Gram stains
The initial diagnosis of a bacterial or fungal infection can be made rapidly using a Gram stain on a smear taken from an infected site (Table 1.4; Figure 1.36).

Common organisms associated with chronic ophthalmic disease
1 Mycobacteria (Gram positive, acid alcohol fast bacilli – Figure 1.36):
  * *M. tuberculosis:* conjunctivitis and uveitis. Culture in Lowenstein–Jensen media.
  * *M. leprae:* eyelid paralysis, corneal ulceration, and uveitis. Culture in armadillos.

Table 1.4 Common organisms associated with acute conjunctivitis, keratitis, and endophthalmitis.

	Gram positive	Gram negative
Cocci	*Staphylococcus* sp. *Streptococcus* sp.	*Neisseria* sp.
Rods	*Corynebacteria* sp. *Listeria* sp. *Clostridium* sp. *Proprionibacterium* sp.: a facultative anaerobe and a common cause of late stage endophthalmitis following cataract surgery	*Escherichia* sp. *Klebsiella* sp. *Pseudomonas* sp. *Haemophilus* sp. *Moraxella* sp.

2 Atypical mycobacteria: "swimming pool" conjunctivitis.
3 *Actinomyces:* dacryocystitis. Gram positive felt-like network of branching filaments.

Common fungal pathogens
These grow on Sabauraud's media.
1 *Candida* sp.: common cause of corneal ulceration. Non-branching septate hyphae with budding yeasts.
2 *Aspergillus* sp.: keratitis, endophthalmitis, and orbital cellulitis. Branching septate hyphae.
3 *Mucor* sp.: rare cause of orbital cellulitis in association with diabetic ketoacidosis. Large branching septate hyphae.

Examination techniques

Postgraduate examinations will rely either on microscopic glass slides and the microscope or photomicrographs to test the knowledge of the candidates. In the former case, familiarity with a microscope is advantageous!

Microscopic glass slides

Viewing the slide with the naked eye can be invaluable in locating the essential pathology (for example intraocular or extraocular tumour) and the opportunity to measure dimensions. If the abnormality is not readily evident, a useful procedure is to examine a section of an eye from front to back, i.e. cornea, angles, iris, lens, vitreous, retina, optic nerve, and retroocular tissues.

Advice on the detection of specific pathological features is provided at the start of each chapter.

Micrographs

The use of photographic material is increasingly common. The illustrations will be of specific diagnostic pathological entities which will be similar to those presented in this text.

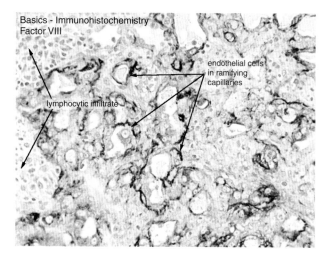

Figure 1.40

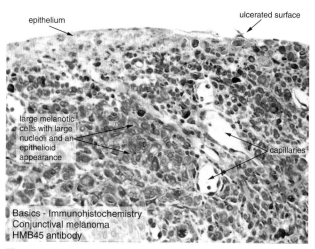

Figure 1.41

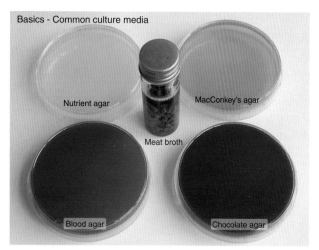

Figure 1.42

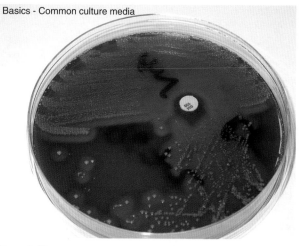

Figure 1.43

Figure 1.40 Factor VIII antibody is used to identify blood vessels in reactionary and neoplastic proliferations. This example is taken from an inflammatory mass in which there is striking angiogenesis in a dense inflammatory cell infiltrate (bacillary angiomatosis).

Figure 1.41 HMB45 is used for identification of melanocytic proliferations (benign and malignant). The extensive infiltration and nuclear pleomorphism indicate malignancy in this conjunctival amelanotic melanoma. Inflammatory cells within the tumour are the result of surface ulceration. The brown PAP label can be used in amelanotic melanomas but pigmented tumours require bleaching.

Figure 1.42 The standard agar plates used for isolation of pathogenic bacteria.

Figure 1.43 A positive culture on blood agar. The β-haemolytic streptococcus has haemolysed the red cells around each colony. A sample of the colony will be smeared onto a glass slide for Gram stain identification. The weak sensitivity to gentamicin is exhibited by the absence of colonies surrounding the antibiotic disc. This antibiotic is ineffective in the treatment of Gram positive cocci.

Chapter 2
Eyelid and lacrimal sac

Eyelid

Diseases originating in the eyelid are commonly encountered by the clinician and thus a common source of material submitted to the pathologist. The role of the pathologist is to provide a definitive diagnosis, to ascertain the clearance of a malignant tumour so that the clinician can plan for additional treatment if necessary, and to predict recurrence. Pathology in the eyelid can vary from the most benign cysts to invasive carcinomas and the specimens can range in size from tiny fragments to exenteration specimens.

An appreciation of the normal anatomy is important in understanding the different pathological processes that can occur in the eyelid.

Normal eyelid

Anatomy

The anatomy of an eyelid can be simplified into four layers (Figure 2.1):
1 Skin, which is formed by the epidermis and dermis.
2 Striated muscle, formed by the orbicularis oculi.
3 Tarsal plate containing the Meibomian glands.
4 Conjunctival mucosa.

The anatomical grey line is located between the eyelashes and the Meibomian orifices and marks the anterior border of the tarsal plate. The mucocutaneous junction where the epithelium changes from epidermal to conjunctival type is present just behind the opening of the tarsal glands. The dermis contains blood vessels, lymphatics, and nerves, all of which can be a source of benign or malignant tumours.

In the upper lid, the levator palpebrae superioris inserts into the upper border of the tarsal plate by an aponeurosis which also contains the smooth fibres of Müller's muscle (Figure 2.2).

How to examine an eyelid specimen

Macroscopic
A tumour will be excised close to the edge if the surgeon considers it benign. In the case of a suspected malignant tumour, the surgeon will remove surrounding normal tissue for clearance (up to 5 mm if possible). The specimens will be ellipsoid, rectangular, or pentagonal, and may extend to the full thickness of the lid. In the latter, it should be possible to identify the grey line and lashes (Figures 2.3, 2.23), and the tarsal plate in the cut surface (Figures 2.44, 2.54).

Microscopic
The specimen will be lined on one surface by epidermis which is covered with bright red (eosinophilic) keratin. The basal layer of the epidermis is undulating due to the presence of rete pegs. Small pilosebaceous follicles are present in the superficial dermis and these structures are often referred to as adnexal glands. These are the features of skin and they can only be found on the outer surface of the eyelid:

- *Epidermis* (Figure 2.4): the basal layer is cuboidal. The squamous cell layer consists of polygonal cells. The superficial cells are flattened and contain keratin granules. The horny or keratin layer is very thin in the lid. A thin space containing fine cytoplasmic processes (prickles) identifies the cells in the squamous layer. This is important as an identification feature for tumours derived from the squamous cell layer (refer to squamous carcinoma).
- *Melanocytes:* the cells with clear cytoplasm in the basal layer are melanocytes.
- *Dermis:* the fibrofatty tissue in the dermis contains elastic fibres. The arterioles, venules, lymphatics, and nerves are present throughout.
- *Muscle:* the striated muscle fibres of the orbicularis oculi possess nuclei which are located at the edge of the cell membrane. Smooth muscle nuclei are located centrally.
- *Tarsal plate:* dense collagenous tissue surrounds the elements of the Meibomian gland.
- *Adnexal structures:* the glands of Zeis are of sebaceous type and are located at the lid margin. The glands of Moll are of sudoriferous type (Figure 2.1). Accessory lacrimal glands are present at the upper edge of the tarsal plate (Wolfring) and in the fornix (Krause).
- *Tarsal conjunctiva:* see Chapter 3.

Infections

Bacterial

Bacterial infection occurs in the adnexal glandular structures of the eyelid producing a purulent reaction – hordeolum or stye. Organisms leading to granulomatous reactions (for example *Mycobacterium leprae*) are exceedingly rare.

Necrotising fasciitis
A synergistic infection of *Streptococcus pyogenes* (group A) and *Staphylococcus aureus* results in massive destruction of the eyelid and adjacent orbital tissue. Treatment requires extensive surgical clearance and high dose antibiotics. The histological appearance is that of a purulent exudate between necrotic tissue planes: clumps of bacteria are easily recognised.

Viral

Wart/verruca vulgaris
A wart appears as a solitary, slow growing, well circumscribed nodule lined on the surface by crumbly or spiky keratin. Treatment is usually by surgical excision or cryotherapy. Infection by the human papilloma virus (HPV) has been demonstrated using viral culture and immunohistochemistry.

Macroscopic examination reveals a hyperkeratotic nodule with surrounding skin. Histologically there is hyperplasia and folding of the epidermis due to viral stimulation. The major part of the tumour is formed by keratin. The diagnostic feature is the presence of cells with clear cytoplasm in the superficial layers (Figure 2.5).

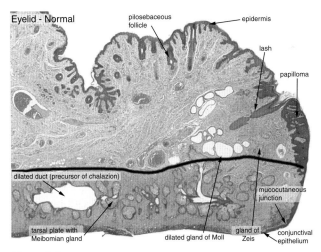

Eyelid - Normal

Figure 2.1

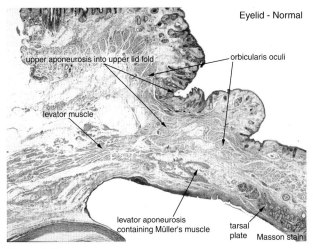

Eyelid - Normal

Figure 2.2

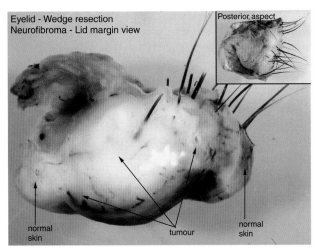

Eyelid - Wedge resection
Neurofibroma - Lid margin view

Posterior aspect

Figure 2.3

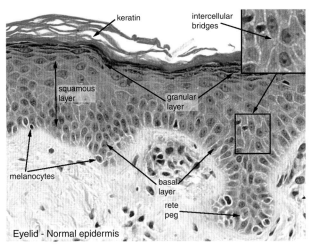

Eyelid - Normal epidermis

Figure 2.4

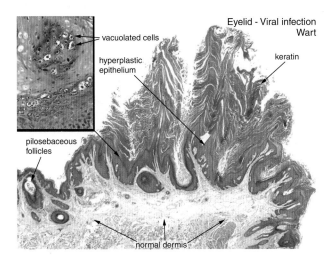

Eyelid - Viral infection
Wart

Figure 2.5

Figure 2.1 This example shows the normal anatomical constituents of the eyelid. However, a small papilloma located at the eyelid margin has obstructed the ducts of the gland of Moll with secondary dilatation. The papilloma is also obscuring the anatomical grey line, which is located between the eyelashes and the ducts of the Meibomian gland; the grey line demarcates the beginning of the anterior border of the tarsal plate (superimposed black line).

Figure 2.2 In the Masson stain, muscle fibres are red and the fibrous tissue is green. The stain illustrates the location of the striated muscle fibres of the orbicularis oculi and levator palpebrae superioris. The smooth muscle bundles of Müller's muscle are present within the aponeurosis. The lid fold is formed by an extension of the levator fibres into the skin – a feature of the Caucasian eyelid.

Figure 2.3 A wedge resection of a potentially malignant tumour which, on histology, was proven to be a neurofibroma. Note the clearance margin of normal tissue around the tumour. The inset shows the posterior aspect of the specimen.

Figure 2.4 Micrograph to show the layers of the normal epidermis. The inset shows the intercellular bridges in the squamous layer.

Figure 2.5 A wart is characterised by massive keratinisation (hyperkeratosis). The infected cells are vacuolated and contain clumps of viral particles (inclusion bodies) seen as small dense blue granules (inset). Normal skin is present at the edge of the wart.

Molluscum contagiosum

A common viral skin infection (pox virus) of childhood: it presents as umbilicated nodules that may be either solitary or multiple. The virus is spread by fomites in children or by direct contact in adults. Treatment may be conservative, although a large range of modalities are available: curettage, excision, cryotherapy, and electrodessication.

Specimens may be derived from curettings or excision biopsies (Figure 2.6). The tumour may also have the appearance of a basal cell carcinoma and a wedge resection may be submitted.

The nodule is well circumscribed (Figure 2.6). The central area of the mass is filled with necrotic cells which explain the umbilication. The infected cells in the superficial squamous layer are hyperplastic. The presence of proliferating viral particles causes the cell contents to be replaced by pink granular material. This becomes basophilic when the dead cells are shed (Figure 2.7).

Spillage of viral particles can produce a follicular conjunctivitis.

Inflammation

Chalazion

This lipogranulomatous inflammation within the Meibomian gland is common in clinical practice.

Clinical presentation
The condition in the acute stage appears as a generalised painful swelling, more commonly in the lower lid. A chalazion may resolve spontaneously or progress to the chronic stage at which there is a tense ovoid mass within the tarsal plate. The size of such masses can vary from 1 mm to several times the thickness of the eyelid.

This condition may be recurrent and it is important in the differential diagnosis to consider the possibility of a sebaceous gland carcinoma.

Pathogenesis
Initially the ducts of the Meibomian gland are obstructed by inspissated secretion of fatty material. Retention of lipid material within the gland and spillage into the surrounding tissues induces a lipogranulomatous inflammatory reaction. This process may be recurrent, but histology of multiple recurrences is mandatory to exclude *sebaceous gland carcinoma* (see below).

Possible modes of treatment
Incision and curettage of the persistent cystic mass are usually successful.

Macroscopic
In the early stages the submitted material is friable and pale yellow in colour while in delayed excisions the fibrous residue is white and firm.

Microscopic
Most commonly the lipogranulomatous reaction is restricted to the tarsal plate but may track anteriorly or posteriorly to mimic a malignant tumour (Figure 2.8). The free fat spaces represent the release of lipid from necrotic Meibomian gland cells.

The cellular infiltrate is a classic giant cell granulomatous reaction with lipid globules in the cytoplasm of macrophages and also within multinucleate cells (Figure 2.9). Lymphocytes and plasma cells are abundant and recurrent inflammation proceeds to reactionary fibrosis.

Tumours

Tumour-like masses in the eyelid are commonly encountered in clinical practice and often a clinical diagnosis is unreliable. The spectrum extends from a benign cyst to a highly malignant metastasising tumour. The rate of growth is an important feature in distinguishing benign from malignant variants. The majority of tumours are derived from the epidermis and are UV or viral induced. However, tumours derived from any intrinsic eyelid tissue may be encountered (for example muscle, nerve, melanocytes, adnexal).

Benign

Cysts
Sudoriferous cysts
Sudoriferous cysts, or sweat gland cysts, are derived from the ducts of the glands of Moll which are lined by a cuboidal epithelium surrounded by a smooth muscle layer (myoepithelium). The cysts appear as solitary or multiple subcutaneous translucent swellings at the lid margin. Presumed fibrosis constricts the ducts and continuing secretion of the glands leads to the development of cysts, which are easily excised *in toto*.

The thin walled cysts contain clear or milky fluid with a smooth interior (Figure 2.10). The characteristic histological feature is a double layer of cells on the inner surface. The inner cells are cuboidal and the outer layer is of myoepithelial origin (Figure 2.11).

Epithelial inclusion cysts (epidermoid and dermoid)
Obstruction of the duct of a pilosebaceous follicle creates cysts which are lined by stratified squamous epithelium (epidermoid or retention cysts). A dermoid cyst is a second type of cyst also lined by stratified squamous epithelium and is formed when embryonic ectodermal rests are displaced into the lid or orbit.

The essential difference between the two types is the presence of pilosebaceous follicles in the wall of a dermoid cyst.

Epidermoid cysts These firm pale nodules on the eyelid skin surface often have a punctum and clinically are referred to as "sebaceous cysts". Continued formation of keratin within the lumen is responsible for the foul-smelling granular yellow content. Rupture of an epidermoid cyst with the release of keratin during surgery can induce a giant cell granulomatous reaction. Dividing a fixed specimen demonstrates the yellow greasy and flaky content.

The cysts are lined by stratified squamous epithelium and the lumen contains keratin (Figures 2.12, 2.13).

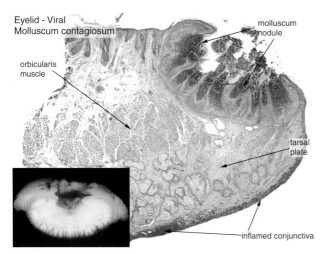

Eyelid - Viral
Molluscum contagiosum

molluscum
nodule

orbicularis
muscle

tarsal
plate

inflamed conjunctiva

Figure 2.6

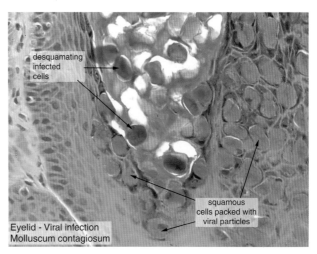

desquamating
infected
cells

squamous
cells packed with
viral particles

Eyelid - Viral infection
Molluscum contagiosum

Figure 2.7

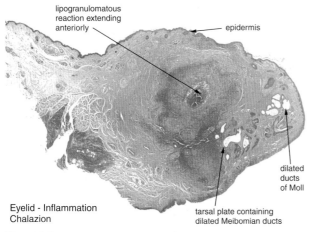

lipogranulomatous
reaction extending
anteriorly

epidermis

dilated
ducts
of Moll

Eyelid - Inflammation
Chalazion

tarsal plate containing
dilated Meibomian ducts

Figure 2.8

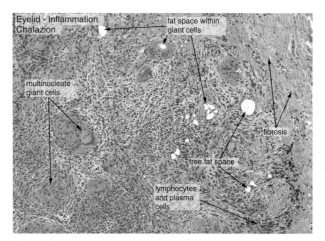

Eyelid - Inflammation
Chalazion

fat space within
giant cells

multinucleate
giant cells

fibrosis

free fat space

lymphocytes
and plasma
cells

Figure 2.9

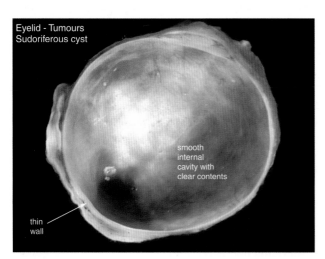

Eyelid - Tumours
Sudoriferous cyst

smooth
internal
cavity with
clear contents

thin
wall

Figure 2.10

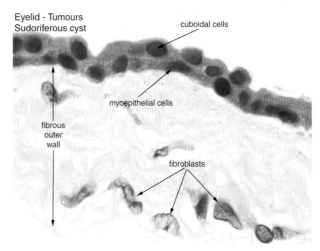

Eyelid - Tumours
Sudoriferous cyst

cuboidal cells

myoepithelial cells

fibrous
outer
wall

fibroblasts

Figure 2.11

Figure 2.6 A wedge excision was performed because the molluscum nodule was thought to be a basal cell carcinoma. The inset shows the cut surface of a different molluscum contagiosum excised with a margin of normal skin. Note the central umbilication. The central crater contains necrotic cells, shown in detail in Figure 2.7.

Figure 2.7 Viral particles proliferating within the cytoplasm of the squamous epithelial cells have a "smudgy" pink appearance. Cell death releases the vital particles from the surface of the crater.

Figure 2.8 Extension of a chalazion into the anterior part of the eyelid led to a clinical suspicion of a sebaceous gland carcinoma and the mass was widely excised.

Figure 2.9 A florid chalazion demonstrates all the features of a lipogranulomatous reaction with prominent fat spaces and multinucleate giant cells. In biopsies of recurrent chalazia, there is often more fibrosis than is shown here.

Figure 2.10 The absence of solid material within the cavity is highly suggestive of a cyst derived from a sweat gland duct (the contents wash out when the cyst is cut open).

Figure 2.11 The fibrous wall is lined internally by an inner cuboidal cell layer and an outer flat myoepithelial layer, thus retaining the features of a normal sweat gland duct.

Dermoid cysts These cysts occur in children and are usually solitary and present as slowly growing painless masses in the upper lid.

The pathogenesis is of interest. In embryonic life, the face is formed by processes (frontal, nasal, maxillary) which extend forwards and fuse. Incarceration of ectoderm between the frontal and maxillary processes results in the formation of cysts. The incarcerated ectoderm also forms pilosebaceous follicles so that a dermoid cyst contains hairs. Rupture (spontaneous or traumatic) releases highly irritant lipid and keratin into the surrounding tissues resulting in a chronic granulomatous reaction.

Treatment is by surgical excision although care must be taken to avoid rupture and spillage of contents.

An excised specimen appears as a smooth intact ovoid mass with a thin wall containing pultaceous yellow white material and obvious hairs (Figure 2.14).

Microscopy shows the lumen to contain keratin and hair. The walls are similar in appearance to an epidermoid cyst but include hair follicles and sebaceous follicles (pilosebaceous follicles – Figure 2.15).

Xanthelasmas

Xanthelasmas are common superficial skin nodules that increase in frequency in the middle-aged and the elderly. Associated hyperlipidaemia should be suspected although more than 50% of patients are normolipaemic. The nodules are bilateral and have a pale yellow appearance (Figure 2.16). Treatment is usually conservative as the nodules often recur but for cosmesis, surgical excision, laser ablation, or topical treatments may be requested.

Microscopic examination reveals large clusters of ovoid cells with eccentric nuclei in the dermis (Figure 2.17). The cytoplasm of the cells is almost translucent and appears as pale granular material ("foamy cytoplasm") which stains positively for fat in a frozen section.

Naevi

The term naevus is most commonly applied to a tumour formed by melanocytic proliferation. This abnormality is present at birth, but with the onset of puberty, these tumours can grow in size and pigmentation. There are three main types:

1 Junctional.
2 Intradermal.
3 Compound.

This classification is based on the anatomical location of the melanocytic proliferation. In embryonic life melanocytes migrate from the neural crest to reach the basal layer of the epidermis, i.e. at the junction between the epidermis and the dermis, hence the term *junctional naevus*. Arrested migration of melanocytes explains the proliferation of these cells in the dermis, i.e. *intradermal naevus*. Most commonly, however, the two types coexist to form a *compound naevus*. In all forms of naevi, the immunohistochemical reactions are positive with melan-A, HMB45, and S100.

Junctional naevus

Junctional naevi appear as flat areas of increased pigmentation (black or brown) which may vary in size. The melanocytic proliferation is confined to the epidermis.

Clinically, an increase in size of a flat pigmented patch with nodule formation is strongly suggestive of malignant transformation to a melanoma.

Histologically, in a junctional naevus, the melanocytic proliferation is confined to the lower layers of the epidermis and usually takes the form of small clusters of cells. It is important to appreciate that melanocytes are clear cells and pigmentation is the result of transfer of pre-melanosomes from the parent melanocytes to the adjacent epidermal cells (Figure 2.18).

Intradermal naevus

Clusters of heavily pigmented spindle cells are present in the dermis. The potential for malignant transformation is far less than for junctional naevi.

Compound naevus

The melanocytes are present in clusters within the epidermis and in the dermis, where the cells in the deeper clusters become smaller and more mature (Figure 2.19).

Benign tumours of the epidermis

The distinction between basal cell and squamous cell tumours is based on the degree of cellular differentiation and maturation. Basal cell papillomas contain cells which resemble the cells of the basal layer of the epidermis throughout the tumour. In squamous cell papillomas there is differentiation from basal cells to prickle cells, granular cells, and keratin.

Basal cell papilloma (BCP)/seborrhoeic keratosis

This common slowly growing tumour presents as a well circumscribed nodule with cauliflower-like appearance. It may be pigmented. The aetiology of this tumour is unknown. The treatment may be conservative, although the tumour is usually excised for cosmetic reasons or if there is a suspicion of malignancy.

The tumour will have the appearance of a closely excised nodular mass which projects from the skin surface (Figure 2.20). The surface is sometimes lined by flaky keratin (which is why the obsolete term "seborrhoeic keratosis" was used).

The majority of cells are uniform and basophilic (Figures 2.21, 2.22). The abnormal tumour cell surface predisposes to infection and secondary inflammation is seen as a lymphocytic infiltrate in the base of the tumour. The key histological feature is the lack of maturation from basal to squamous cell type (see Figure 2.4).

Squamous cell papilloma (SCP)

Hyperkeratotic tumours projecting from the surface of the lid are relatively common. The tumour may be of a viral aetiology or may be a benign proliferation of epidermal cells. The clinical presentation is in the form of a slowly growing, well circumscribed warty lesion. The treatment outlined in BCPs applies to SCPs.

The appearance in an excised specimen is similar to a basal cell papilloma except that the surface is heavily keratinised (Figure 2.23). Keratinisation may take the form of finger-like processes (filiform).

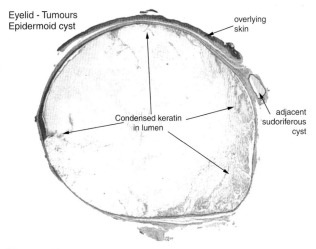

Eyelid - Tumours
Epidermoid cyst

overlying skin

Condensed keratin in lumen

adjacent sudoriferous cyst

Figure 2.12

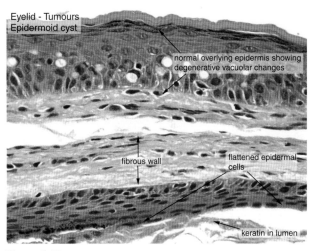

Eyelid - Tumours
Epidermoid cyst

normal overlying epidermis showing degenerative vacuolar changes

fibrous wall

flattened epidermal cells

keratin in lumen

Figure 2.13

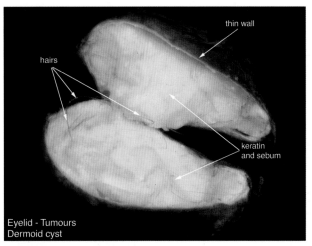

thin wall

hairs

keratin and sebum

Eyelid - Tumours
Dermoid cyst

Figure 2.14

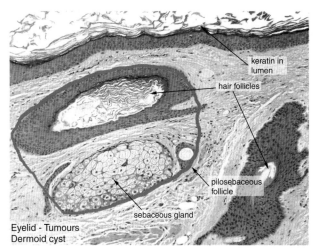

keratin in lumen

hair follicles

pilosebaceous follicle

sebaceous gland

Eyelid - Tumours
Dermoid cyst

Figure 2.15

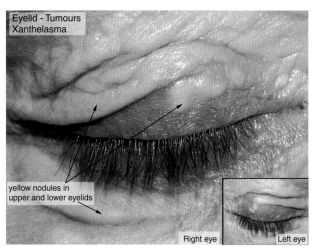

Eyelid - Tumours
Xanthelasma

yellow nodules in upper and lower eyelids

Right eye   Left eye

Figure 2.16

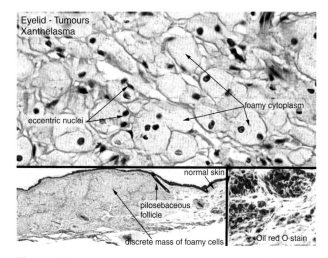

Eyelid - Tumours
Xanthelasma

foamy cytoplasm

eccentric nuclei

normal skin

pilosebaceous follicle

discrete mass of foamy cells   Oil red O stain

Figure 2.17

Figure 2.12 Low power view of a complete epidermoid cyst excised with overlying skin. The cyst contains keratin. Distortion of the adjacent duct of a sweat gland has given rise to a concurrent sudoriferous cyst.

Figure 2.13 In an epidermoid cyst, the epidermis lining the wall becomes compressed by the compacted keratin. Compare the thickness with that of the overlying epidermis which shows secondary degenerative vacuolar changes.

Figure 2.14 The diagnosis of a dermoid cyst is made when the lumen contains hair in addition to keratin and sebum (fatty materials secreted by sebaceous follicles).

Figure 2.15 The hallmark histological feature of a dermoid cyst is the presence of pilosebaceous follicles (outlined in red) in the wall, which is lined by stratified squamous epithelium.

Figure 2.16 In this patient, the upper and lower eyelids on both sides contain yellow plaques (xanthelasmas).

Figure 2.17 The plaque in xanthelasma is formed by well circumscribed masses of foamy cells (lower left). The cells have well defined cytoplasmic membranes and faintly staining granular material in the cytoplasm: this displaces the small nuclei (upper). The lipid within the cells stains positively with Oil red O (lower right).

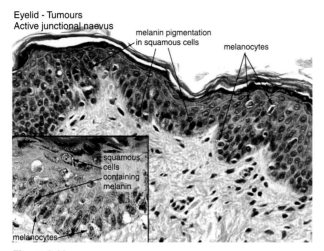

Eyelid - Tumours
Active junctional naevus

melanin pigmentation
in squamous cells

melanocytes

squamous
cells
containing
melanin

melanocytes

Figure 2.18

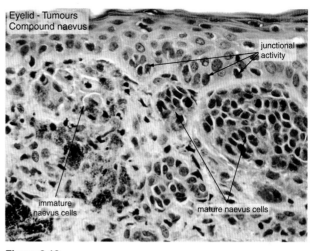

Eyelid - Tumours
Compound naevus

junctional
activity

immature
naevus cells

mature naevus cells

Figure 2.19

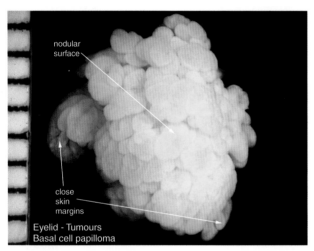

nodular
surface

close
skin
margins

Eyelid - Tumours
Basal cell papilloma

Figure 2.20

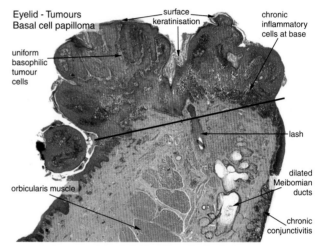

Eyelid - Tumours
Basal cell papilloma

surface
keratinisation

chronic
inflammatory
cells at base

uniform
basophilic
tumour
cells

lash

orbicularis muscle

dilated
Meibomian
ducts

chronic
conjunctivitis

Figure 2.21

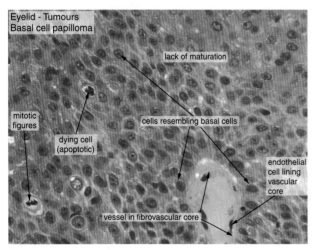

Eyelid - Tumours
Basal cell papilloma

lack of maturation

mitotic
figures

cells resembling basal cells

dying cell
(apoptotic)

endothelial
cell lining
vascular
core

vessel in fibrovascular core

Figure 2.22

Figure 2.18 In an active junctional naevus, the melanocytes (clear cells) transfer melanin into the squamous cells and the melanin-containing cells are carried to the surface. The difference between melanocytes with clear cytoplasm and squamous cells containing melanosomes is shown in the inset.

Figure 2.19 A compound naevus is characterised by proliferating melanocytes in the basal epidermis and clumps of "naevus cells" in the dermis. The clusters of naevus cells show varying degrees of maturation and melanin content.

Figure 2.20 A basal cell papilloma is easily identified both clinically and pathologically. The appearance is that of a cauliflower at low magnification.

Figure 2.21 This basal cell papilloma was excised with the underlying eyelid because there was a suspicion of malignancy. The tumour is growing away from the underlying dermis and is therefore more likely to be benign ("away from the patient"). The superimposed black line indicates the margins of the tumour. The basophilic appearance of the tumour is due to the presence of cells which retain the staining characteristics of the epidermal basal layer.

Figure 2.22 A basal cell papilloma is formed by cells of uniform size and shape. Intercellular spaces or bridges are not prominent.

The tumour cells show marked differentiation from basal to squamous with the formation of a granular layer and a thick keratin layer (Figure 2.24). Intercellular spaces are prominent and contain cytoplasmic bridges. Keratin formation can occur within the proliferating cells (dyskeratosis) (Figure 2.25). Inflammatory changes in the adjacent dermis can occur and are due to bacterial proliferation in the keratin.

Keratoacanthoma

This is an uncommon skin tumour with a characteristic presentation of rapid growth and hyperkeratosis. Rapid growth within 3 months produces an ovoid tumour mass with a central keratin core. It can mimic a squamous cell carcinoma both clinically and pathologically. The tumour can reach a large size and occupy most of the anterior surface of an eyelid. Spontaneous resolution can occur but surgical excision is effective.

The excision is usually wide and the specimen contains a well defined umbilicated nodule with a central keratinised core and a smooth rounded peripheral surface (Figure 2.26).

If on histology the tumour is well demarcated, of squamous type, with a flat base, and hyperkeratosis in the central part, the diagnosis is keratoacanthoma (Figure 2.27). The cellular component is relatively small and confined to a layer at the base of the tumour. Here, there are islands of well differentiated squamous cells (Figure 2.28). Normal epidermis at the edge of the tumour favours the diagnosis of keratoacanthoma because in squamous carcinomas the adjacent epidermis shows the changes of premalignancy (see below).

Premalignant changes

Actinic/solar/senile keratosis

Overexposure to sunlight is followed by precancerous changes in the epidermis. Solar keratosis is more common in Caucasians, especially those with an outdoor lifestyle. This condition can progress to squamous cell carcinoma.

Clinically, solar keratosis appears as a flat, scaly plaque of variable size (15–20 mm) and irregular periphery.

The pathogenesis is well understood – UV light to the epidermis damages the DNA control of cell proliferation.

The neoplastic proliferation is confined to sectors of the epidermis, and here there are areas where the basal cells possess the features of malignant cells (Figures 2.29, 2.30). A secondary effect of rapid cell division is that nuclei are carried through to the keratin layer (parakeratosis).

UV radiation to the dermis is associated with changes in the elastin which becomes clumped (solar elastosis).

Treatment is usually in the form of cryotherapy – excision is unusual.

Malignant – common

Derived from epidermis

Malignant epidermal carcinomas can be divided into basal cell carcinoma and squamous cell carcinoma. In terms of incidence, basal cell carcinoma is by far the commonest malignant skin tumour encountered in clinical practice.

Immunohistochemical markers (CAM 5.2, AE1, and AE3) which label cytokeratins, or the intermediate filaments, react positively with cells of epidermal origin.

Basal cell carcinoma (BCC)

The commonest skin tumour involving the eyelids, especially the lower. It is more common in Caucasians with a history of extensive sunlight exposure.

Clinical presentation

An elderly patient will typically present with a well circumscribed firm nodular or cystic lesion that is slow growing with development of a rolled edge and a central ulcer (Figure 2.31). This type of BCC is usually solitary and is easily eradicated. The rarer variant, sclerosing (scirrhous) type, which presents as a firm plaque with poorly defined margins is difficult to treat due to its imprecise boundaries (see below).

Pathogenesis

UV damage to the epidermis, especially in Caucasians who lack pigment protection and are exposed to strong sunlight as part of their profession or pastime, for example fishermen.

Possible modes of treatment

Local excision would be most common, but for nodular types other modalities have been preferred including laser ablation, cryotherapy, radiation, photodynamic, chemotherapy, and electrodessication treatment. A biopsy may be performed to confirm the diagnosis and would be helpful in planning the definitive procedure.

Macroscopic

Most commonly, the specimen takes the form of an ellipsoidal or pentagonal excision bearing a central nodular tumour that may or may not be ulcerated. The sclerosing variant requires wide excision (Figure 2.32). Extensive spread may require radical exenteration (Figure 2.33) and adjuvant therapy.

The recognition of tumour extension by multiple samples of the edge of the specimen is standard procedure in many centres (see Chapter 1). Evidence of tumour at the surgical excision line of the specimen is an indication for further treatment.

For practical purposes, basal cell carcinomas do not metastasise but scirrhous basal cell carcinomas are known to locally invade the medial part of the orbit (Figure 2.33).

Microscopic

The morphological appearances can be subdivided into two basic types:

1 *Nodular*. Synonymous term: solid, including cystic variants (see below).
2 *Sclerosing*. Synonymous terms: morphoeic, cicatrising, scirrhous.

Both types can exist within a single tumour. The diagnosis in each type relies on the identification of *palisading basal cells* at the periphery of the tumour cell nests.

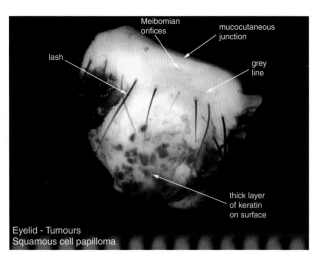

Eyelid - Tumours
Squamous cell papilloma

Figure 2.23

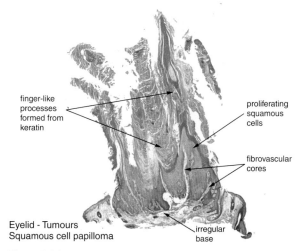

Eyelid - Tumours
Squamous cell papilloma

Figure 2.24

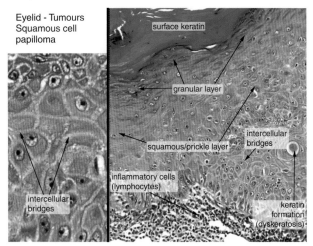

Figure 2.25

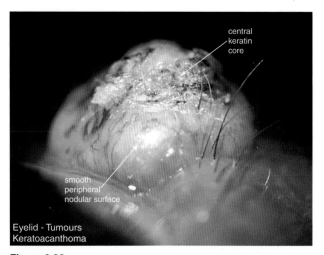

Eyelid - Tumours
Keratoacanthoma

Figure 2.26

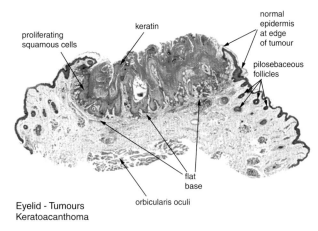

Eyelid - Tumours
Keratoacanthoma

Figure 2.27

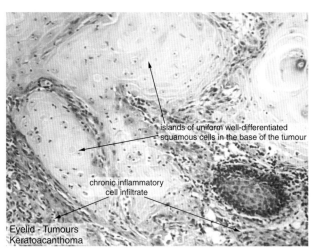

Eyelid - Tumours
Keratoacanthoma

Figure 2.28

Figure 2.23 A "wedge" excision of the lower lid bearing a heavily keratinised squamous cell papilloma. Note the normal surface anatomy.

Figure 2.24 The bulk of squamous papilloma consists of finger-like processes of keratin. The presence of proliferating squamous cells is revealed by the pinker cytoplasm (compared with a basal cell papilloma). The base is uneven (compare with a keratoacanthoma – see below).

Figure 2.25 Proliferating squamous cells are more eosinophilic than those in a basal cell papilloma, and the spaces between them contain intercellular bridges (left). Abnormal keratin granules are present within individual cell cytoplasm – this is referred to as dyskeratosis.

Figure 2.26 The clinical and macroscopic appearances of a keratoacanthoma are typical in that the tumour is umbilicated with a central keratin core. A history of rapid growth (within 12 weeks) is a helpful clinical indicator.

Figure 2.27 A block excision of the eyelid was performed after a clinical misdiagnosis of squamous cell carcinoma. Note that the rounded edge is formed by normal epidermis. The keratoacanthoma has a flat base and is widely cleared.

Figure 2.28 While the major part of the tumour consists of keratin, islands of proliferating squamous cells are present at the base. Note the inflammatory cell infiltration.

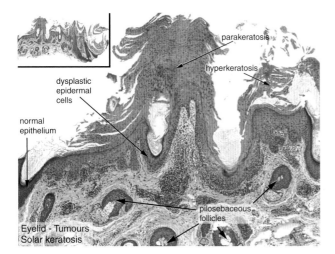

Figure 2.29

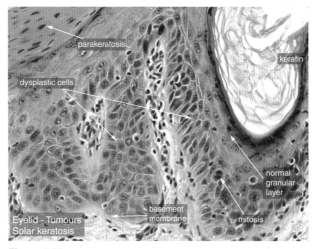

Figure 2.30

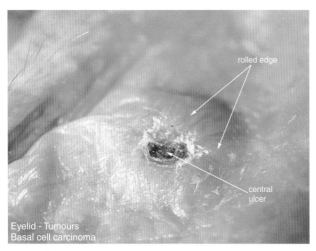

Figure 2.31

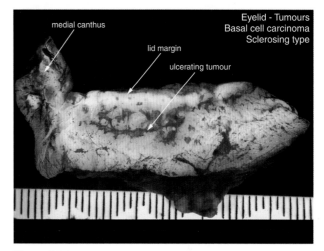

Figure 2.32

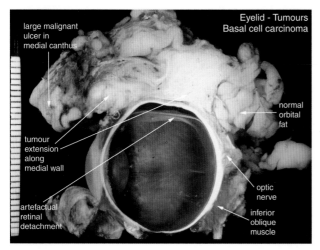

Figure 2.33

Figure 2.29 Precancerous field change (inset) occurs in regions of the epidermis and these take the form of alternating sectors of hyperkeratosis and parakeratosis (migration of nuclear fragments into the keratin layer) with marked dysplasia of the basal epidermal cells (see Figure 2.30). The adjacent epidermis (to the left) is of normal appearance.

Figure 2.30 Dysplastic cells vary in size, shape, and polarity within the basal layers of the epidermis. The basement membrane is intact. Penetration of this membrane is an indicator of invasion and the presence of a squamous cell carcinoma.

Figure 2.31 The typical clinical appearance of a basal cell carcinoma of the lower eyelid. The centre of the tumour is ulcerated and the edges are rolled.

Figure 2.32 Basal cell carcinomas of sclerosing type must be widely excised and frozen sections may be used to confirm clearance intraoperatively. This specimen is taken from the left lower lid and, unlike the more common nodular counterpart, the sclerosing variant has a poorly defined edge.

Figure 2.33 When recognition and treatment are delayed, a sclerosing basal cell carcinoma may infiltrate widely throughout the orbital tissue. This exenteration specimen has been divided in the horizontal plane to demonstrate the extent of tumour spread.

Nodular/solid In this subtype of BCC, nests of tumour cells of varying size invade the dermis to reach the underlying muscle (Figure 2.34). Necrosis within large tumour nodules leads to the formation of cysts which can increase in size and mimic an epidermoid cyst (Figure 2.35). Loss of surface integrity predisposes to ulceration which is usually in the centre – the largest part of the tumour (Figure 2.36). Surrounding inflammation is a common feature.

The tumour cells possess scanty cytoplasm, hence the basophilic (blue) colour of the tumour (Figure 2.37). Within each cell nest or nodule, the cells at the periphery are arranged in a palisade fashion (Figure 2.38).

Pari passu proliferation of melanocytes sometimes gives a pigmented appearance to a basal cell carcinoma.

Sclerosing The characteristic feature of this subtype is the presence of small tumour cell nests within dense fibrous tissue which differs from the large discrete nodular masses seen in the solid subtype. The predominance of fibrous tissue explains the clinical and low-power histological appearance of this type of basal cell carcinoma. At the periphery of the tumour the islands are often small and inconspicuous so that it may be difficult to assess clearance. See Figure 2.32 for the macroscopic appearance of this tumour.

The presence of larger elements resembling a solid basal cell carcinoma can facilitate the diagnosis (Figure 2.39). Within the dense fibrous tissue, the islands of tumour cells are small and inconspicuous (Figures 2.39, 2.40), so that histological determination of clearance requires care. Nonetheless, the detailed architecture of the cells resembles those of the solid type (Figure 2.41). The fibrous tissue contains a mixed inflammatory cell infiltrate – lymphocytes, mast cells, and macrophages (Figure 2.41).

Adenoid variant

This is a rare subset of a solid basal cell carcinoma which has an atypical architecture. The cells are arranged in cords and acini resembling glandular tissue. The matrix surrounding the cords contains mucopolysaccharides (Figure 2.42).

Squamous cell carcinoma

This tumour is much rarer than basal cell carcinoma and it may arise *de novo* or from existing solar keratosis.

Clinical presentation

A heavily keratinised nodular tumour that may be ulcerated is present on the eyelid. The margins are less distinct compared with a nodular basal cell carcinoma. Lymphoid metastases to preauricular or submandibular lymph nodes and perineural infiltration are late events.

Aetiology and pathogenesis

The aetiology is thought to be multifactorial including: UV exposure, ionising radiation, chronic irritation, and the human papilloma virus.

Possible modes of treatment

Surgical excision is preferred. Other modalities include cryotherapy and irradiation.

Macroscopic

The most commonly submitted specimen would be a wide excision biopsy. The tumour appears as a heavily keratinised or ulcerated mass with irregular edges. Tumours excised from the central part or lateral part of the lid are usually adequately cleared (Figures 2.43, 2.44). Adequate excision from tumours in the medial canthus is more difficult due to close association of neighbouring structures and a predilection for orbital invasion.

Intraorbital spread requires exenteration (Figures 2.45, 2.46) or irradiation.

Microscopic

The tumours can be graded as stages I–IV according to the level of dedifferentiation, which in the most extreme example may be of spindle cell type. Completely undifferentiated tumours often require immunohistochemical identification for cytokeratins (CAM 5.2, AE1, and AE3).

The tumour at low power may arise in a pre-existing solar/actinic keratosis (Figure 2.47) or, at a later stage, be ulcerated (Figure 2.48). Ulceration occurs because the malignant cells are unable to maintain normal surface protection which leads to secondary infection and leucocytic infiltration (Figure 2.49). The underlying tissue response to ulceration is lymphocytic infiltration. In addition, the malignant cells have the capacity to induce fibrosis (desmoplastic reaction).

In a well differentiated tumour, the cells show the stages of normal differentiation with the formation of prickle cells and keratin. There is considerable variation in the size and shape of the tumour cells and mitotic figures are plentiful (Figures 2.50, 2.51).

In poorly differentiated squamous cell carcinomas, the nest-like squamous differentiation is lost, but intercellular bridges are still identified (Figure 2.52).

Derived from adnexal glands: sebaceous gland carcinoma (SGC)

Benign and malignant tumours can arise from pilosebaceous follicles and from sebaceous glands (Meibomian and Zeiss). The benign tumours are clinically similar to other nodular tumours described above but are rare and of more interest to pathologists than ophthalmologists! Sebaceous gland carcinoma is of importance to ophthalmologists because it mimics common inflammatory conditions (chalazion and blepharoconjunctivitis) of the eyelid and has a more aggressive behaviour than either basal cell carcinoma or squamous cell carcinoma. Sebaceous carcinomas are usually nodular in form and are unilateral, but an ability to spread within the epidermis simulates a chronic blepharoconjunctivitis (masquerade syndrome).

Eyelid - Tumours
Basal cell carcinoma

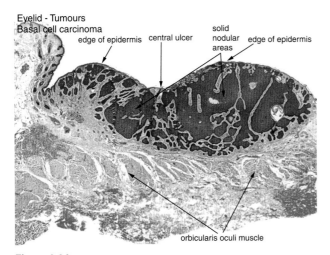

Figure 2.34

Eyelid - Tumours
Basal cell carcinoma

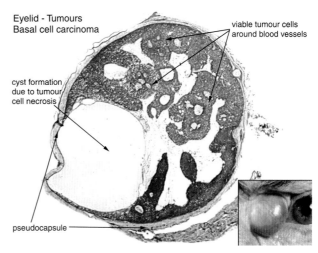

Figure 2.35

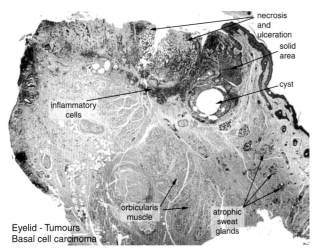

Eyelid - Tumours
Basal cell carcinoma

Figure 2.36

Eyelid - Tumours
Basal cell carcinoma

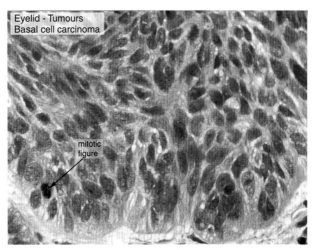

Figure 2.37

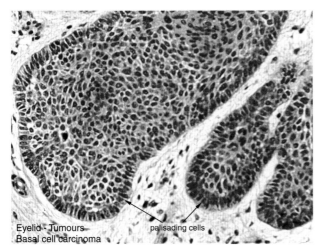

Eyelid - Tumours
Basal cell carcinoma

Figure 2.38

Figure 2.34 The basophilic (*"if it's blue, it's bad"*) appearance of the tumour cells is characteristic of the commonest form of basal cell carcinoma (nodular). Cells form large solid areas and smaller nests and the base of the tumour extends to the orbicularis muscle, i.e. the tumour is growing *into* the patient. The epidermis covers the periphery of the tumour but is absent in the central part where it is ulcerated.

Figure 2.35 A patient presented with a rapidly growing cystic tumour at the medial canthus (inset). The clinical diagnosis was of an infected epidermoid cyst and the mass was excised without overlying skin. On histology, there are extensive areas of necrosis leading to cyst formation but viable tumour is present around the blood vessels. The basal cell carcinoma is surrounded by a pseudocapsule.

Figure 2.36 In this wedge resection of a clinical basal cell carcinoma, the tumour has outgrown its blood supply leading to large areas of infarction and necrosis (rodent ulcer). Destruction of the surface epidermis leads to secondary infection.

Figure 2.37 Detailed examination of a basal cell carcinoma reveals tumour cells which vary in shape but are relatively uniform in size. There is no evidence of maturation to prickle or squamous cells and mitotic figures are identified in every high power field.

Figure 2.38 The most important diagnostic feature in basal cell carcinoma is the "palisading" arrangement of the cells at the periphery of the nests.

Eyelid - Tumours
Basal cell carcinoma - Sclerosing type

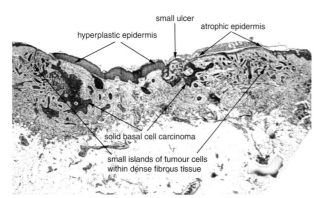

hyperplastic epidermis
small ulcer
atrophic epidermis
solid basal cell carcinoma
small islands of tumour cells within dense fibrous tissue

Figure 2.39

Eyelid - Tumours
Basal cell carcinoma - Sclerosing type
solid tumour mass
small islands of tumour cells inducing formation of dense fibrous tissue
inflammatory cell infiltrate (lymphocytes)

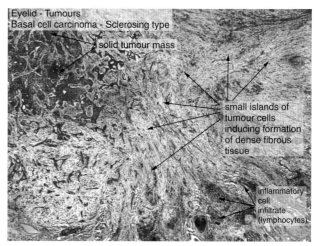

Figure 2.40

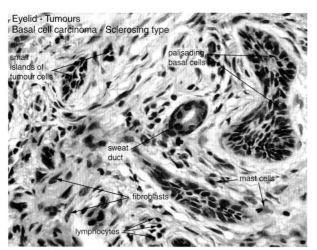

Eyelid - Tumours
Basal cell carcinoma - Sclerosing type
small islands of tumour cells
palisading basal cells
sweat duct
mast cells
fibroblasts
lymphocytes

Figure 2.41

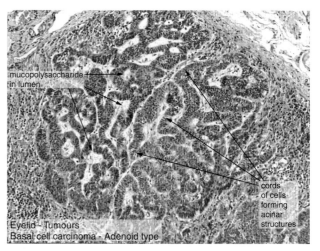

mucopolysaccharide in lumen
cords of cells forming acinar structures
Eyelid - Tumours
Basal cell carcinoma - Adenoid type

Figure 2.42

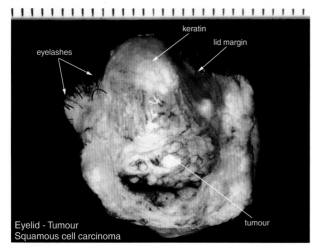

eyelashes
keratin
lid margin
tumour
Eyelid - Tumour
Squamous cell carcinoma

Figure 2.43

Figure 2.39 In a sclerosing basal cell carcinoma, the infiltrating cells are often inconspicuous within dense fibrous tissue. Fibrous contraction (cicatrisation) leads to distortion of the surface of the lid. The overlying epidermis varies in thickness between hyperplasia and atrophy.

Figure 2.40 The clinical and pathological difficulty in determining surgical limits of a sclerosing basal cell carcinoma can be demonstrated by histology of the edge. The fibrous tissue proliferation partially obscures the small islands of infiltrating malignant cells.

Figure 2.41 Small islands of tumour cells within dense fibrous tissue are characteristic of a sclerosing basal cell carcinoma. Note that pallisading is not evident in the smallest tumour cell nests. Inflammatory cells (mast cells and lymphocytes) are present within the fibrous tissue.

Figure 2.42 Since all forms of basal cell carcinomas are derived from pluripotent ectoderm stem cell lines, it is reasonable to assume that there is a potential for differentiation into adnexal type tissues. The adenoid variant more closely resembles a tumour of sweat glands. The Alcian blue–PAS stain reveals mucopolysaccharides in the spaces enclosed by the cords of the tumour cells.

Figure 2.43 An elderly patient presented with a slowly growing hard mass in the lower eyelid. A pentagonal excision was performed to remove a large squamous cell carcinoma.

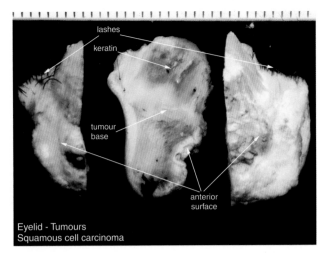

lashes

keratin

tumour base

anterior surface

Eyelid - Tumours
Squamous cell carcinoma

Figure 2.44

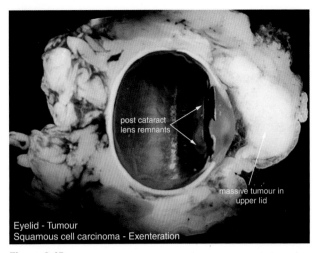

post cataract lens remnants

massive tumour in upper lid

Eyelid - Tumour
Squamous cell carcinoma - Exenteration

Figure 2.45

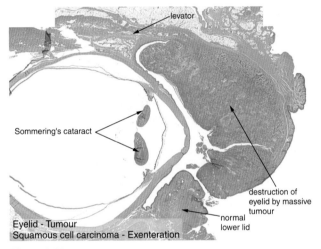

levator

Sommering's cataract

destruction of eyelid by massive tumour

normal lower lid

Eyelid - Tumour
Squamous cell carcinoma - Exenteration

Figure 2.46

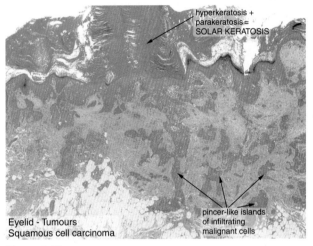

hyperkeratosis + parakeratosis = SOLAR KERATOSIS

pincer-like islands of infiltrating malignant cells

Eyelid - Tumours
Squamous cell carcinoma

Figure 2.47

Eyelid - Tumour
Squamous cell carcinoma

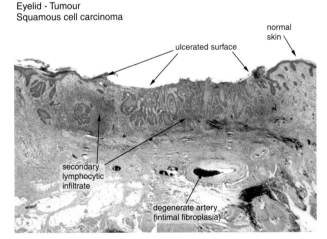

normal skin

ulcerated surface

secondary lymphocytic infiltrate

degenerate artery (intimal fibroplasia)

Figure 2.48

Figure 2.44 The specimen in Figure 2.43 has been cut vertically to remove a central block (see "Macroscopic examination or specimen 'grossing' " in Chapter 1), which is positioned to show the cut surface. This reveals the deep invasion of a squamous cell carcinoma into the substance of the lid. In practice, clearance blocks would be taken from the lateral and medial borders.

Figure 2.45 Macroscopic appearance of an exenteration specimen for squamous cell carcinoma with extensive invasion of the upper lid. Prior to the exenteration, the patient had cataract surgery which was only partially successful, leaving behind a Sommering's cataract.

Figure 2.46 Low power microscopic appearance of an exenteration specimen for squamous cell carcinoma with extensive invasion of the upper lid. (Same case as that shown in Figure 2.45.)

Figure 2.47 Squamous carcinomas often arise in sectors of solar/actinic keratosis. The surface still maintains integrity and there is little secondary inflammation. The malignant cells are inducing a fibroblastic reaction.

Figure 2.48 Ulceration is a common occurrence in squamous carcinomas and this leads to extensive lymphocytic infiltration and fibrosis. The inflammatory process also damages the walls of underlying blood vessels.

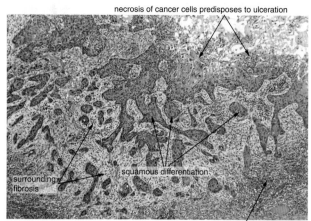

necrosis of cancer cells predisposes to ulceration

squamous differentiation

surrounding fibrosis

Eyelid - Tumour / Squamous cell carcinoma   lymphocytic infiltrate

Figure 2.49

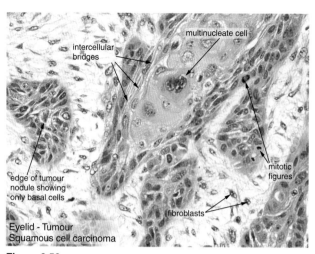

multinucleate cell

intercellular bridges

mitotic figures

edge of tumour nodule showing only basal cells

fibroblasts

Eyelid - Tumour
Squamous cell carcinoma

Figure 2.50

Eyelid - Tumour
Squamous cell carcinoma

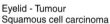

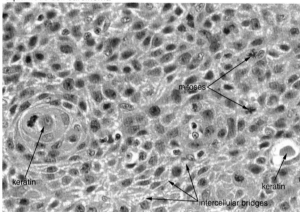

mitoses

keratin

keratin

intercellular bridges

Figure 2.51

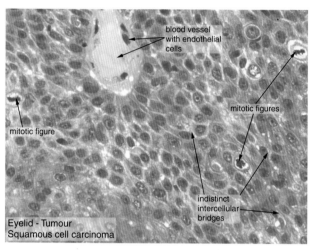

blood vessel with endothelial cells

mitotic figures

mitotic figure

indistinct intercellular bridges

Eyelid - Tumour
Squamous cell carcinoma

Figure 2.52

Figure 2.49 Even at moderate magnification, it is possible to see that within the islands of malignant cells there is differentiation to form squamous cells. The surface cells of the tumour disintegrate and provide a substrate for bacterial infection with secondary leucocytic inflammatory infiltration. The underlying dermal tissue responds to the inflammatory process in the form of lymphocytic infiltration.

Figure 2.50 In three dimensions, the finger-like extensions of a squamous cell carcinoma are cut in different planes so that some islands contain basal cells.

A section which passes through the central part of an island reveals differentiation into squamous cells and shows intercellular bridges and the formation of bizarre cells such as malignant multinucleated cells. Fibroblasts are prominent in the stroma.

Figure 2.51 In a moderately differentiated squamous cell carcinoma, it is still possible to identify intercellular bridges and keratin formation.

Figure 2.52 A poorly differentiated squamous cell carcinoma will still retain intercellular bridges albeit indistinct ones.

Clinical presentation

- Yellow nodule that may or may not be ulcerated.
- Plaque-like lesion.
- Chronic blepharoconjunctivitis especially with loss of lashes (Figure 2.53).
- Recurrent eyelid inflammation similar to a chalazion.
- Metastasis to lymph nodes and viscera if correct diagnosis is delayed. It is more common in the elderly, females, and in the upper lid.

Pathogenesis

Unknown.

Possible modes of treatment

Wide surgical excision or exenteration is preferred. Adjunctive radiotherapy for advanced cases (but the tumour has a tendency to be radioresistant).

Macroscopic

If a sebaceous carcinoma is suspected, the pathologist should be informed and fresh (unfixed) tissue should be submitted immediately for frozen section for fat stains (normal tissue processing removes fat).

Specimens submitted may present as:

- a lid wedge excision including a pale yellow nodular tumour (Figure 2.54)
- fragments resembling the granular material seen in a chalazion
- an exenteration (Figure 2.55).

Microscopic

Nodular tumours Revision of the normal histology provides a better understanding of the variable appearance of sebaceous gland carcinoma (Figure 2.56). The basic element of a sebaceous gland is the lobule which is outlined by a single cuboidal basal layer. These cells mature in an orderly fashion into large cells with lipid-laden foamy cytoplasm and a small nucleus. In the neck of the follicle, the cells fragment to release lipid into the ducts (holocrine secretion).

In a well differentiated sebaceous gland carcinoma, the morphology is lobular and the centre of the lobule contains foamy cells. The basal cells may fail to differentiate into foamy cells and the lobules are filled with small basophilic cells (Figure 2.57).

In less well differentiated tumours, the basal cells predominate and the cytoplasm contains small circular spaces which represent the lipid globules which were removed during paraffin processing (Figure 2.58). The lipid is preserved in frozen sections and stains positively with appropriate stains (Figure 2.59).

In completely dedifferentiated tumours, lipid spaces are rare and are seen only in thin sections at high magnification (Figure 2.60). In such advanced cases, the tumour infiltrates the eyelids extensively (Figure 2.61).

Diffuse intraepithelial spread Intraepithelial spread can be extensive (Figure 2.62) and requires high magnification for identification of the limits (Figures 2.63, 2.64). The malignant cells within the normal epithelial cells possess foamy cytoplasm and show nuclear atypia. Fat stains (Figure 2.64) and immunohistochemistry can be helpful in determining the boundaries of spread.

Immunohistochemistry

The central foamy cells are identified with human milk fat globule-1 (HMFG1 – Figure 2.64) and epithelial membrane antigen (EMA). The smaller peripheral basal cells stain with cytokeratin markers (PKK1 MNF116).

Malignant – rare

The following are extremely rare in clinical practice but must be considered in the differential diagnosis in the scenario of rapidly growing tumours.

Metastasis

Suspicion of metastasis should be aroused in the presentation of a rapidly growing tumour of the eyelid. The location of the primary tumours is similar to those described for intraocular metastasis.

Cutaneous melanoma

Malignant melanoma arising from the epidermis of the eyelid is extremely rare and is easily recognised by heavy pigmentation of a rapidly spreading flat area (lentigo maligna) or a nodular tumour. The histological appearances are similar to those described for intraocular melanoma.

Kaposi's sarcoma

Previously extremely rare, the incidence of this tumour has increased along with the increased incidence of the acquired immune deficiency syndrome (AIDS). Rapidly growing erythematous swelling of the eyelid in an immunocompromised patient should lead to a suspicion of this tumour. The histological feature is the presence of malignant spindle cells surrounding vessels with thin walls.

Merkel cell tumour

A smooth elongated ovoid mass projecting from the surface of the upper lid is the characteristic appearance of this tumour. The cells forming the tumour are of neuroendocrine type and are arranged in nests.

Lymphoma

The histological appearances of malignant lymphoid tumours of the eyelid are similar in appearance to conjunctival lymphomas.

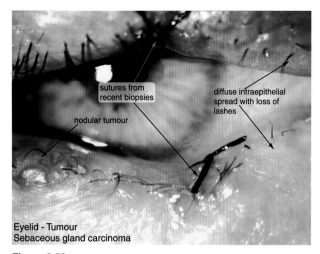

Figure 2.53

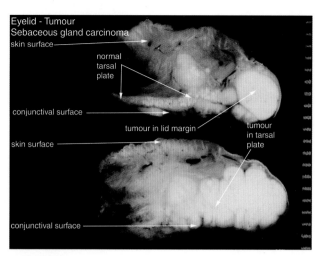

Figure 2.54

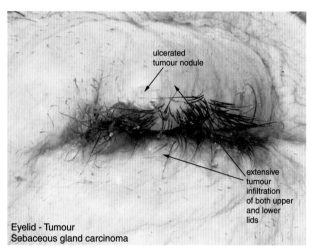

Figure 2.55

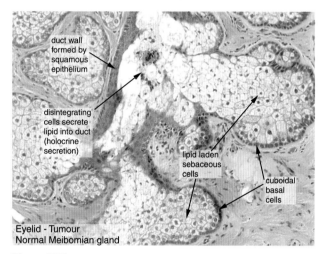

Figure 2.56

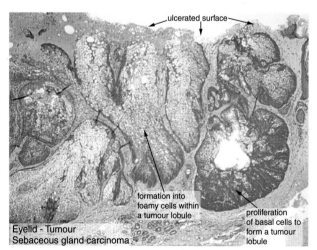

Figure 2.57

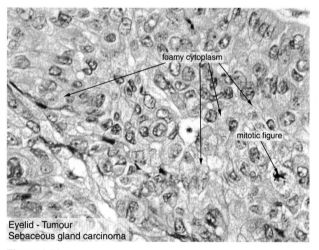

Figure 2.58

Figure 2.53 Slit lamp photograph of a patient presenting with severe unilateral blepharoconjunctivitis. Biopsies of the upper and lower lids were performed and these revealed diffuse intraepithelial spread of a sebaceous gland carcinoma involving both skin and conjunctiva. Note the loss of lashes.

Figure 2.54 Two levels of a wedge excision of an eyelid containing a solid sebaceous gland carcinoma. In the centre of the specimen, the tumour fills the tarsal plate.

Figure 2.55 An exenteration specimen in which there was extensive unilateral tumour infiltration in both lids. The diagnosis was delayed until a lymph node metastasis was identified. The patient ultimately died of lung metastases. See Figure 2.61.

Figure 2.56 To appreciate the morphology of sebaceous gland carcinoma, it is important to revise the normal tissue histology of Meibomian gland lobules and ducts.

Figure 2.57 A well differentiated sebaceous gland carcinoma recapitulates the normal gland by the formation of foamy cells within the centres of the tumour lobules. As the tumour dedifferentiates, cells retain the features of basal cells and form nests and cords within the tumour lobules.

Figure 2.58 In a poorly differentiated sebaceous gland carcinoma, the diagnostic feature is the presence of small clear fat spaces.

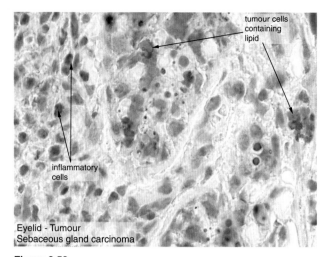

Figure 2.59

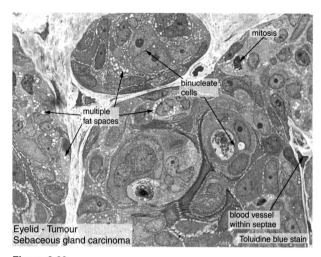

Figure 2.60

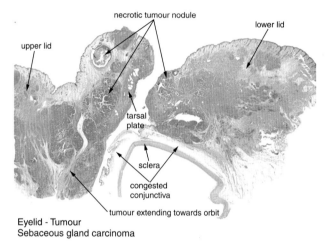

Figure 2.61

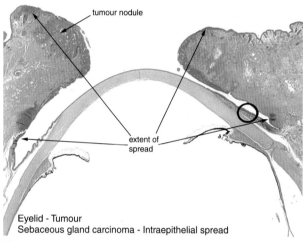

Figure 2.62

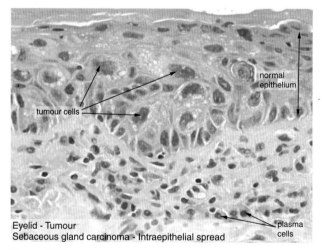

Figure 2.63

Figure 2.59 Lipid within the cytoplasm in a sebaceous gland carcinoma is best demonstrated by the Oil red O stain in fresh frozen sections.

Figure 2.60 In a thin plastic section stained with toluidine blue, the tiny lipid spaces in a sebaceous gland carcinoma can be identified at high magnification. Within the lobules the cells show marked variation in size and shape in this poorly differentiated tumour.

Figure 2.61 Blocks from the specimen shown in Figure 2.55 were taken from the upper and lower lid and recombined to show the extent of infiltration by a sebaceous gland carcinoma in both lids.

Figure 2.62 In a case similar to that shown in Figure 2.53, the intraepithelial spread of a sebaceous gland carcinoma covers the tarsal and bulbar conjunctiva and the adjacent lid margin. A small nodular tumour represents the original focus. The circled area over the limbus indicates the histology shown in Figure 2.63.

Figure 2.63 Histology from the limbus marked with a circle in Figure 2.62. The malignant cells possess foamy cytoplasm which permits the distinction from normal cells that have lost their orderly arrangement due to tumour cell infiltration. The underlying stroma contains lymphocytes and plasma cells.

Soft tissue tumours

Benign

Hamartomas and choristomas

A hamartoma is a benign tumour arising from tissue elements normally present at that site. The most common tissue sources are blood vessels and nerves.

Hamartomas differ from choristomas, which are benign tumours arising from tissues that are *not normally* present at that site.

Vascular

Capillary/cavernous haemangioma Benign tumours composed of either capillaries or larger vessels occur in early childhood. Their clinical appearances are quite distinct and biopsy is rarely indicated. They have a tendency to regress although surgical intervention may be required if there is visual obscuration. See Chapter 5 in haemangiomas of the orbit for a histological description.

Lymphangioma This tumour is formed by dilated lymphatics which contain pink staining lymph. Inspissation leads to compression of the thin-walled lymphatic channels which rupture and induce bleeding and inflammation. This explains the slow enlargement of these hamartomas.

Neural: neurofibroma

Neural tumours are described in Chapter 5.

Malignant

Malignant soft tissue tumours of the eyelid are rare (for example rhabdomyosarcoma) and are identical to those described in Chapter 5.

Lacrimal drainage system

Infections

Dacryocystitis

Inflammation of the lacrimal sac may be acute or chronic.

The patient presents with a painful swelling in the medial canthus. Depending on the patency of the canaliculi, the swelling may be reducible with purulent discharge through the puncti. The aetiology is most commonly secondary to a nasolacrimal duct obstruction with stasis of drainage. In extreme forms, this condition may progress to an orbital cellulitis. Treatment is initially medical with antibiotics to contain the infection, although recurrent or chronic cases may require surgery (dacryocystorhinostomy) during which part of the wall of the lacrimal sac should be sent for histological examination. Numerous Gram positive and Gram negative bacterial pathogens have been isolated from extruded material, with the most common being *Staphylococcus aureus*.

Macroscopic examination of a part of or the whole of an inflamed lacrimal sac reveals a thickened wall and purulent or mucoid material in the lumen (Figure 2.65). On histological examination thickening of the wall is due to lymphocytic infiltration with follicle formation in the submucosa. Purulent exudate in the lumen is responsible for necrosis of the epithelium (Figure 2.66), which also undergoes squamous metaplasia due to chronic irritation (Figure 2.67).

Mucocoele

If chronic inflammation is controlled, a lacrimal sac enlarges due to mucous secretion by the goblet cells in the epithelium.

Dacryolith

Hard stone-like structures may form within the lumen of an inflamed lacrimal sac or canaliculus – so called "dacryolith". These structures are usually formed by inspissated mucous and clumps of bacteria (Figure 2.68, left), but occasionally a foreign body such as a lash may be identified (Figure 2.68, right).

Canaliculitis

Inflammation of the canalicular system is less common than dacryocystitis. Epiphora with surrounding mucopurulent conjunctivitis are the usual clinical features. The canalicular area is inflamed and the associated punctum may be pouting or shut.

Actinomyces israelii is the most commonly identified pathogen. Firm gritty concretions are often evident which present as small yellow "sulphur granules" (Figure 2.69). Histology reveals clumps of fine branching fungal filaments within inflammatory tissue and mucous (Figures 2.69, 2.70).

Numerous other pathogens have been described, including bacterial (for example *Proprionibacterium proprionicum*), fungal (for example *Candida* sp., *Aspergillus* sp.), and viral (HSV/HZV). Canaliculitis may also result from spread of infection from a pre-existing dacryocystitis.

Tumours

Carcinomas of the lacrimal sac are extremely rare, and in some reported series papillomas were not identified. A pre-existing chronic dacryocystitis may complicate the diagnosis. Carcinomas present clinically with a hard mass in the medial canthus with epiphora in the late stage. The tears may be blood stained. Advanced cases may involve the nasopharynx.

The tumours can be papillary (Figure 2.71) or solid. Squamous cell carcinomas can occur and the histology is identical to that described in the eyelid. Transitional carcinomas have an epithelial component consisting of columnar cells which resemble the normal epithelium of the sac (Figures 2.72, 2.73).

Lymphomas of the lacrimal sac have also been described.

Eyelid - Tumour
Sebaceous gland carcinoma - Intraepithelial spread

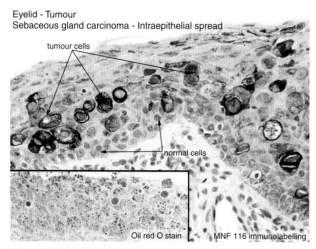

Figure 2.64

Lacrimal drainage system - Chronic dacryocystitis

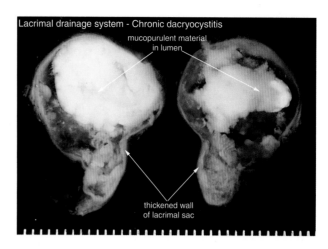

Figure 2.65

Lacrimal drainage system - Chronic dacryocystitis

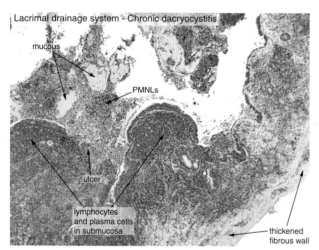

Figure 2.66

Lacrimal drainage system - Dacryocystitis

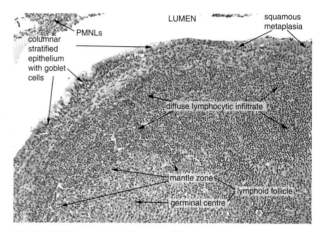

Figure 2.67

Lacrimal drainage system - Chronic dacryocystitis / Dacryolith

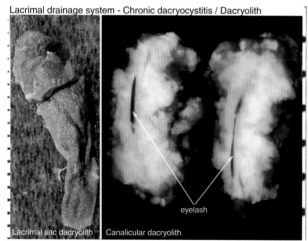

Figure 2.68

Figure 2.64 An immunohistochemical marker for the cytokeratins (MNF116) present in the epidermis and adnexal structures stains malignant sebaceous gland cells infiltrating the conjunctival epithelium. In another case, tissue from the conjunctiva in intraepithelial spread was frozen and stained for lipid (inset). This technique clearly identifies the lipid within tumour cells (Oil red O stain).

Figure 2.65 A patient with chronic dacryocystitis complained of a persistent large swelling of the medial canthus and epiphora. A dacryocystorhinostomy was performed in which intraoperatively an enlarged thickened sac was removed. When the specimen was divided, the lumen contained mucous and purulent material and the sac wall was thickened.

Figure 2.66 Low power illustration of chronic dacryocystitis reveals pus and mucous in the lumen and a dense chronic inflammatory infiltrate in the submucosa. Focal ulceration is a common feature. PMNLs = polymorphonuclear leucocytes.

Figure 2.67 In some specimens, the chronic lymphocytic reaction in the submucosa may develop lymphoid follicles with germinal centres and mantle zones. This example demonstrates metaplasia from the columnar ciliated epithelium (transitional) to squamous epithelium due to chronic irritation.

Figure 2.68 A female patient complained of epiphora but did not refrain from using mascara, hence the brown appearance of the dacryolith which was removed during dacryocystorhinostomy (left). As can be seen, a perfect cast of the lacrimal sac and part of the nasolacrimal duct was obtained! The dacryoliths extracted from the canaliculi (right) are much smaller (compare scales). In this example, a lash behaved as a nidus for inspissation of mucus.

Lacrimal drainage system -
Chronic canaliculitis /
Actinomyces

sulphur granules

cut
surface

clumps of
organisms

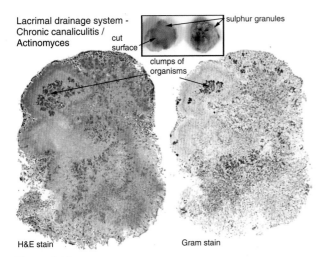

H&E stain

Gram stain

Figure 2.69

Lacrimal drainage system -
Chronic canaliculitis /
Actinomyces

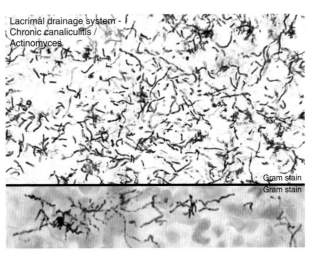

Gram stain

Gram stain

Figure 2.70

Lacrimal drainage system - Lacrimal sac
Transitional cell carcinoma

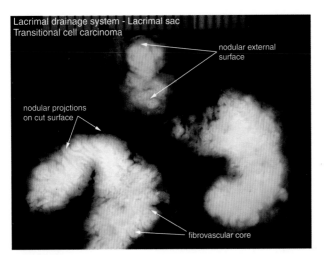

nodular external
surface

nodular projctions
on cut surface

fibrovascular core

Figure 2.71

Lacrimal drainage system - Lacrimal sac
Transitional cell carcinoma

cilia

columnar epithelium

Normal

Transitional papillary carcinoma

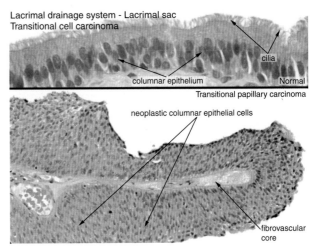

neoplastic columnar epithelial cells

fibrovascular
core

Figure 2.72

Lacrimal drainage system - Lacrimal sac
Transitional cell carcinoma

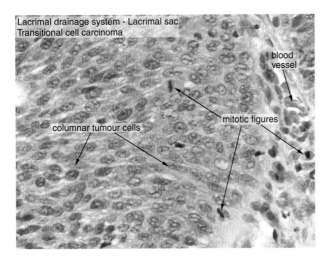

blood
vessel

columnar tumour cells

mitotic figures

Figure 2.73

Figure 2.69 Sulphur granules (inset) extruded from the canaliculus in a case of actinomyces infection have a granular surface. Even at low power, it is possible in an H&E stain and a Gram stain to identify clumps of actinomyces within inspissated mucous (see Figure 2.70).

Figure 2.70 Actinomyces appear as fine branching Gram positive filaments (upper). The morphology of the filaments is improved by a red counterstain (lower).

Figure 2.71 The papillary pattern of growth in a lacrimal sac tumour characterises a transitional cell carcinoma. The cut surface has a nodular appearance and each papillary projection has a central fibrovascular core.

Figure 2.72 In this papillary transitional cell carcinoma (lower), the tumour cells are elongated and have some resemblance to the overlapping nuclei seen in the columnar ciliated epithelium of the normal lacrimal sac (upper).

Figure 2.73 The cells in a poorly differentiated transitional cell carcinoma are elongated and, in this regard, resemble normal columnar epithelium, although there is marked variation in nuclear chromatin. In such tumours, the mitotic rate is high.

Chapter 3
Conjunctiva

Normal

The conjunctiva is a specialised mucous membrane that covers the surface of the globe and the lids. It facilitates movements of the globe and lids while protecting the orbital contents from the external environment. The conjunctiva also contributes to the stability of the tear film by the mucous secretion of the goblet cells.

Sophisticated antigen recognition mechanisms within the conjunctiva form part of a complex immune defence system that also controls antibody production in tears.

Anatomy

The mucous membrane begins at the mucocutaneous junction of the eyelid edge (see Figure 2.1), lines the inner surface of the eyelids (palpebral), and is reflected in the fornices onto the globe (bulbar) as far as the limbus. At the medial canthus there is a conjunctival fold (plica semilunaris). A pink oval structure, the caruncle (medial to the plica semilunaris), contains pilosebaceous follicles.

Histologically, the conjunctival epithelium consists of three layers – basal, wing, and superficial cuboidal (Figure 3.1). The surface cuboidal cells possess microvilli which serve as an attachment mechanism for the mucoid component of the tear film. Other cell types within the epithelium include goblet cells, Langerhans cells, and melanocytes. Melanin pigmentation in the basal layer is a feature of darkly pigmented races.

The stroma contains nerves, blood vessels, and lymphatics: lymphoid follicles are located in the fornices. Lymphocytes and mast cells are scattered throughout. Accessory lacrimal glands are present in the upper border of the tarsal plate (Wolfring) and in the fornices (Krause).

Conjunctival specimens

The opportunity to study conjunctival pathology occurs in the following situations:
- *Conjunctival complete/partial biopsy* of an inflammatory, degenerative, or neoplastic process. Biopsy specimens vary in size (2–10 mm) and will probably consist of irregular pale-white rolled tissue surrounding a mass. If a biopsy is required, it is important to handle the specimen with great care to minimise traumatic artefact. Spreading the specimen onto a piece of filter paper is not recommended (as it may damage the epithelium), but if in doubt the clinician should consult the pathologist for correct tissue handling.
- *Conjunctival scraping*, for example in the diagnosis of adult trachoma inclusion conjunctivitis (TRIC).
- *Impression cytology:* a strip of acetate paper is applied to the surface of the conjunctiva so that the surface cells can be removed. The paper is then stained with appropriate stains, for example Giemsa for malignant cells or PAS for goblet cell density.
- *Exenteration* specimens are submitted in treatment of advanced malignant neoplastic processes.

The various histopathological disorders identified in these specimens will be described in the subsequent sections. A notorious pitfall in histology occurs when the conjunctival epithelium undergoes metaplasia to squamous type (as in keratoconjunctivitis sicca, see below). If the underlying stroma is fibrotic, it is easy to mistake the altered conjunctiva for skin (Figure 3.2). If the stratified epithelium is flat, does not possess rete pegs (characteristic of epidermis), and is not associated with pilosebaceous follicles, it can be assumed that the origin is conjunctival.

Non-specific chronic conjunctivitis

Diffuse inflammatory thickening of the conjunctiva occurs in two forms, papillary and follicular.

Papillary conjunctivitis

Papilla formation in the conjunctiva is a non-specific reaction. The clinical appearances are those of an erythematous conjunctiva with numerous small flat-topped nodules with central vessels. Common causes include:
- bacterial infection
- chronic blepharitis
- allergic conjunctivitis
- contact lens/foreign body irritation.

Microscopic
Papillae are formed by a chronic inflammatory cell infiltrate consisting of lymphocytes, plasma cells, macrophages, and eosinophils (Figures 3.3, 3.18). The shape of the papilla is formed by fibrous septae which tether the swollen stroma by drawing in folds of epithelium.

Diagnosis is made by a conjunctival scrape in which eosinophils are prominent in a Giemsa stained preparation (Figure 3.4).

Follicular conjunctivitis

In some inflammatory processes the reaction takes the form of lymphoid aggregates which appear histologically as small lymphoid follicles. Clinically the follicles resemble small "rice grains" and each is surrounded by blood vessels which is a diagnostic distinction from papillary conjunctivitis. Again the reaction is not specific to one disease. The causes include:
- viral infection (*Molluscum* sp., adenovirus, primary herpes simplex)
- chlamydial infection (see below)
- hypersensitivity to topical medication (see below).

Microscopic
The conjunctival stroma contains small discrete lymphoid follicles which possess a central germinal centre surrounded by mature lymphocytes (Figures 3.5, 3.6).

Conjunctiva - Normal histology

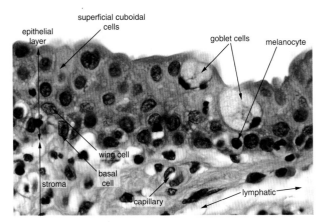

Figure 3.1

Conjunctiva - Epithelial metaplasia
Keratoconjunctivitis sicca

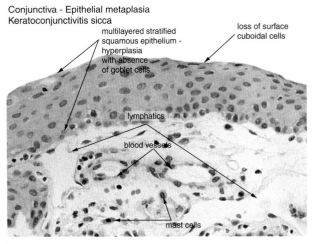

Figure 3.2

Conjunctiva - Papillary conjunctivitis

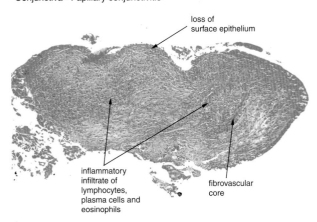

Figure 3.3

Conjunctiva - Papillary conjunctivitis
Scrape

Giemsa stain

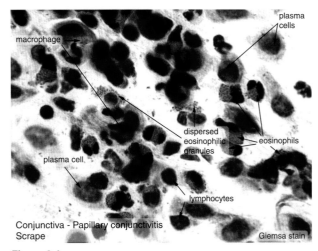

Figure 3.4

Conjunctiva -
Follicular conjunctivitis

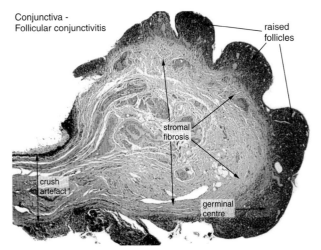

Figure 3.5

Figure 3.1 The conjunctival epithelium is highly specialised and is relatively thin (five to seven layers of cells). The basal layer matures into wing cells, and these differentiate to cuboidal surface cells. The goblet cells are larger than the epithelial cells and possess an eccentric nucleus and clear cytoplasm due to accumulation of mucin. Melanocytes are present in the basal layer. Dendritic cells are also present but are not demonstrated in routine stains. The underlying stroma contains lymphatics and scattered inflammatory cells.

Figure 3.2 In severe keratoconjunctivitis sicca, the epithelium is hyperplastic and the differentiation into cuboidal surface cells is lost. Goblet cells are absent. Without prior knowledge of the tissue origin, it would easy to assume that this is a skin biopsy.

Figure 3.3 It is rarely necessary to perform a biopsy in papillary conjunctivitis. In this archival example, there is surface ulceration and unresolving chronic blepharitis which raises the possibility of more serious disease. The undulation of the surface is due to tethering of the epithelium by fibrous septae which cannot be demonstrated.

Figure 3.4 The diagnosis of papillary conjunctivitis is usually made in a conjunctival scrape in which there is a mixed inflammatory cell infiltrate. Giemsa staining enhances the appearances of eosinophils, which are bilobed and contain bright red granules: when the cells are disrupted, these granules are dispersed. Lymphocytes are the smallest cell with scanty cytoplasm. Plasma cells have irregular nuclear chromatin and more cytoplasm than lymphocytes. Macrophages possess kidney-shaped nuclei and are larger than plasma cells.

Figure 3.5 When this conjunctival biopsy was performed, a clamp was placed across the base of the fold resulting in crush artefact (to the annoyance of the pathologist). At the apex of the fold, the superficial stroma contains collections of lymphocytes (follicles). In one follicle, the section passes through a germinal centre. The underlying stroma is fibrous which indicates a chronic inflammatory process.

Specific inflammatory conditions

Allergic eye disease

Vernal conjunctivitis (spring catarrh)

As the name suggests, this allergic papillary conjunctivitis occurs in the spring in sensitised atopic individuals exposed to airborne antigens such as pollen. The diagnosis is based on the history and clinical appearance, and can be supported by a conjunctival scrape if necessary. The histological features are those of papillary conjunctivitis as described above.

Eye drops/toxic follicular conjunctivitis

Almost every type of topical ophthalmic medication has been linked to follicular conjunctivitis (see above for histology):
- antibiotics: neomycin, gentamicin
- antiviral agents: idoxuridine, triflurothymidine
- miotics: dipivefrine, pilocarpine
- ocular antihypertensive medications: apraclonidine, eserine
- mydriatics: atropine, adrenaline (epinephrine)
- solution preservatives: thiomersol, benzalkonium chloride.

Autoimmune

Keratoconjunctivitis sicca (KCS) – dry eye

Adequate lubrication of the ocular surface depends on the normal aqueous tear production by the main lacrimal gland and accessory lacrimal glands (Krause and Wolfring). The outermost lipid (secreted by Meibomian glands) and innermost mucous layers (secreted by goblet cells of the conjunctiva) function to provide tear film stability.

There are many causes of "dry eye", but the two most pathologically important are age-related lacrimal gland atrophy (non-Sjögren's syndrome KCS) and chronic autoimmune inflammation (Sjögren's syndrome).

Clinical presentation
The patient complains of ocular irritation and redness. Some will observe a lack of tears. There may be an increased incidence of blepharitis.

Sjögren's syndrome sufferers may have associated generalised dry mucous membrane symptoms (oral and urogenital tracts). The incidence of systemic lymphoma is increased and appropriate investigations should be carried out.

Pathogenesis
Age-related atrophy is poorly understood but the incidence is greater in elderly women. Chronic infection may pass upwards through the ducts of the lacrimal gland to initiate periductal fibrosis and secondary atrophy of the glandular tissue.

Sjögren's syndrome is an autoimmune systemic disease that can be primary or secondary in association with collagen disorders.

Genetics
High HLA association exists for both primary and secondary Sjögren's syndrome (for example HLA B8).

Possible modes of treatment
Principles of treatment involve:
1 Investigation and diagnosis of KCS.
2 Treatment of the cause.
3 Artificial tear supplementation.
4 Surgical procedures designed to increase tear retention by decreased draining and evaporation.

The reader is best advised to refer to a clinical textbook for further details.

Microscopic: lacrimal gland histology
In age related atrophy, the lobules decrease in size due to fibrous replacement and fatty infiltration (Figure 3.7). Often the process is selective and many lobules retain normal architecture (Figure 3.8).

In Sjögren's syndrome, destruction is widespread and there is fibrous tissue replacement and dense lymphocytic infiltration (Figure 3.9).

Irrespective of the cause of a defective tear film, the conjunctival epithelium responds by metaplasia to a stratified squamous type. The loss of goblet cells with a reduction in mucous secretion compounds the epithelial abnormality by destabilising the tear film (Figures 3.2, 3.10).

Ocular cicatricial pemphigoid (OCP)

Ocular cicatricial pemphigoid (OCP) is a rare chronic disorder that is characterised by recurrent conjunctival surface bullae and blistering with eventual scarring.

Other names include: benign mucosal pemphigoid, cicatricial pemphigoid, benign mucous membrane pemphigoid, ocular pemphigoid.

Clinical presentation
OCP is a bilateral disease and is more common in elderly women.

The disease may initially present as a burning and foreign body sensation with mucous discharge. Acute blistering may not be evident but there is progressive subepithelial scarring characterised by shallowing of the fornices and formation of fibrous bands leading to symblepharon. Trichiasis may occur when there is extensive lid scarring. Eventually there is surface keratinisation of both the cornea and conjunctiva.

Dry eye is a common symptom due to the obliteration of the ducts of the lacrimal gland by the scarring process. In addition, loss of goblet cells and absence of mucous production exacerbates epithelial metaplasia.

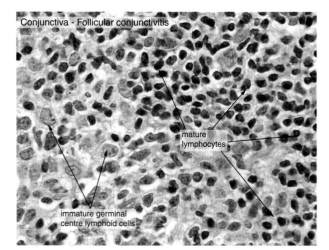

Conjunctiva - Follicular conjunctivitis

mature lymphocytes

immature germinal centre lymphoid cells

Figure 3.6

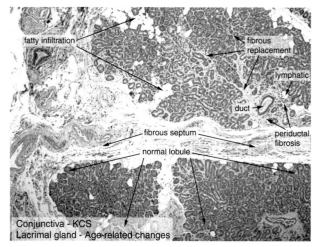

fatty infiltration

fibrous replacement

lymphatic

duct

fibrous septum

periductal fibrosis

normal lobule

Conjunctiva - KCS
Lacrimal gland - Age-related changes

Figure 3.7

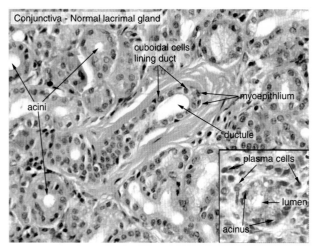

Conjunctiva - Normal lacrimal gland

cuboidal cells lining duct

myoepithlium

acini

ductule

plasma cells

lumen

acinus

Figure 3.8

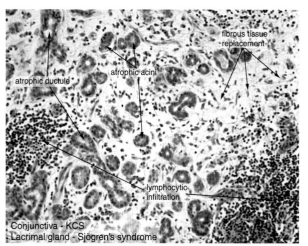

atrophic ductule

atrophic acini

fibrous tissue replacement

lymphocytic infiltration

Conjunctiva - KCS
Lacrimal gland - Sjögren's syndrome

Figure 3.9

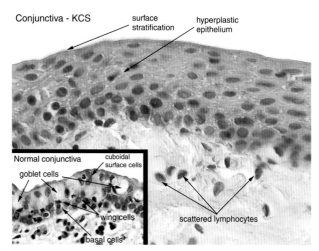

Conjunctiva - KCS

surface stratification

hyperplastic epithelium

Normal conjunctiva

cuboidal surface cells

goblet cells

wing cells

basal cells

scattered lymphocytes

Figure 3.10

Figure 3.6 Each nodular raised area in follicular conjunctivitis has the appearance of a follicle in a lymph node. The germinal centre contains immature lymphoid cells of varying size and shape. The cells gradually mature into small lymphocytes as they progress towards the periphery.

Figure 3.7 The normal lacrimal gland contains acini and ducts forming lobules separated by fibrous septae. The changes that occur in normal ageing are shown in the upper lobule in which there is fibrosis extending from the duct into the lobule. Fatty infiltration is present at the periphery of the lobule.

Figure 3.8 In the centre of a lobule, bilayered ductules are present. Cuboidal cells line the inner surface and are surrounded by contractile myoepithelium which promotes the flow of tear fluid (this is relevant to the histogenesis of lacrimal gland tumours which possess cells derived from both constituents of the ductules – see Chapter 5). The adjacent acini secrete water solutes, salts, and antibacterial agents (for example lysozyme). Plasma cells are present in the stroma around the acini (inset): the plasma cells secrete immunoglobulins which are transported across the cuboidal cell cytoplasm into the lumen.

Figure 3.9 In Sjögren's syndrome, there is extensive destruction of the lacrimal gland lobules with fibrous replacement; lymphocytic infiltration is prominent.

Figure 3.10 The conjunctival epithelium responds to an inadequate tear film by metaplasia to a stratified squamous architecture with hyperplasia. Goblet cells are absent. The inset shows normal epithelium containing plentiful goblet cells for comparison.

Pathogenesis

OCP is a type II autoimmune disorder (humoral) characterised by complement binding IgG and IgA deposits within the epithelial basement membrane.

Possible modes of treatment

Treatment is difficult and the reader should refer to standard texts.

Principles will include lubrication, lid surgery for trichiasis, as well as mucous membrane grafts for deficient conjunctiva. Immunosuppressants have been used to suppress the disease progression.

Due to the altered surface environment, cataract surgery is best done using a clear corneal incision.

Macroscopic and microscopic

Tissue available for study is usually in the form of a conjunctival biopsy – the specimen should be partitioned for immunofluorescence and immunohistochemistry before fixation for routine histology.

Consultation with the pathologist is essential.

Histopathology

The changes are not regarded as specific for this disease. Widening of the intercellular spaces and separation of the epithelium from the stroma (bulla) are the common findings (Figure 3.11). The stroma contains a dense mixed inflammatory cell infiltrate.

Immunohistochemistry

Immunolabelling for immunoglobulins, especially IgG, reveals localisation in the basement membrane of the epithelium (Figure 3.12). The inflammatory cell infiltrate contains T and B cells.

In many cases it may not be possible to identify IgG deposits, especially if the biopsy is taken at a later stage of the disease.

Stevens–Johnson syndrome (SJS)

In comparison with OCP, Stevens–Johnson syndrome (SJS) affects younger patients (10–30 years) and is a systemic inflammation of the skin and mucous membranes of acute onset. There is a male predominance.

Other names include: erythema multiforme major; toxic epidermal necrolysis is an extreme variant.

Clinical presentation

Generalised systemic signs of malaise and fever with cutaneous and mucosal eruptions.

In the acute phase which lasts for 2–3 weeks, ocular signs include bilateral swollen inflamed eyelids with crusting, a mucopurulent conjunctivitis with chemosis, bullae, and eventual ulceration.

When the acute phase subsides, conjunctival scarring and symblepharon may result. Ocular surface abrasion and

infection are secondary to trichiasis. Dry eyes can occur with a mechanism similar to OCP.

Pathogenesis and genetics

Many cases are thought to be either drug related (for example antibiotics like sulphonamides and anticonvulsants) or postinfectious (for example herpes simplex virus and mycoplasma). There have been numerous HLA associations including B12 and Bw44.

This disease is characterised by an immune complex vasculitis. The stroma contains T-helper cells.

Possible modes of treatment

The patient requires acute admission for systemic support. Ocular treatment is mainly restrictive to artificial tears and topical antibiotics, although some clinicians use topical and systemic steroids. Other ophthalmic treatment would deal with the chronic complications which are similar to OCP.

Macroscopic and microscopic

Most diagnostic pathological investigations would be in the form of skin biopsies. Conjunctival biopsies are rarely necessary.

The histological pattern is non-specific but features to be sought include vasculitis, epithelial oedema, and separation. The stroma is oedematous and infiltrated by lymphocytes and plasma cells (Figure 3.13).

Immunohistochemistry

Immune complex deposition (IgA, IgG, and complement) is demonstrated in the walls of blood vessels (type III immune reaction).

Granulomatous conjunctivitis

The common forms of granulomatous conjunctivitis are mycobacterium related and sarcoidosis. The features of a mycobacterial infection are similar to that described in Chapter 8.

Sarcoidosis

Currently the measurement of serum angiotensin converting enzyme (ACE) levels in the blood and chest X-rays are helpful in providing the diagnosis of this condition. In an overt case, small pale nodules in the conjunctiva may be evident and can be readily biopsied.

Microscopic

The main pathological feature is the presence of non-caseating giant cell granulomatous reactions in the superficial stroma (Figures 3.14, 3.15). The central pale cells are classified as epithelioid histiocytes, which are modified macrophages.

Conjunctiva - Ocular cicatricial pemphigoid

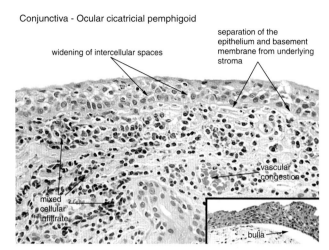

Figure 3.11

Conjunctiva - Ocular cicatricial pemphigoid
Immunohistochemistry

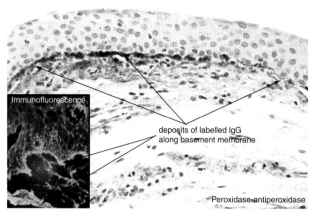

Figure 3.12

Conjunctiva - Stevens-Johnson syndrome

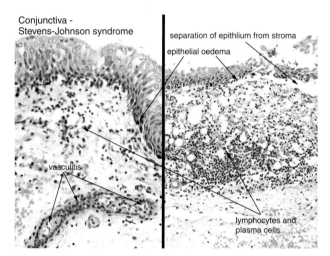

Figure 3.13

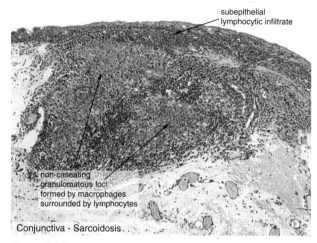

Conjunctiva - Sarcoidosis

Figure 3.14

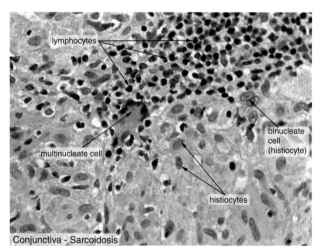

Conjunctiva - Sarcoidosis

Figure 3.15

Figure 3.11 A conjunctival biopsy in ocular cicatricial pemphigoid reveals a loss of goblet cells in a hypoplastic epithelium. The intercellular spaces are widened due to oedema. There is tendency for the epithelium to separate from the stroma to form a bulla as shown in the inset.

Figure 3.12 Immunohistochemical labelling to identify IgG reveals a dense deposit in the basement layer of the conjunctival epithelium (peroxidase-antiperoxidase reaction) in the early stage of the disease. The inset shows the immunofluorescent equivalent performed on a frozen section. The cell nuclei stain orange and the fluorescein labelled IgG appears apple-green.

Figure 3.13 The pathological changes in Stevens–Johnson syndrome are based on an autoimmune vasculitis with stromal infiltration of lymphocytes and plasma cells (left). The inflammatory round cells localise beneath the oedematous epithelium which separates from the oedematous stroma, thus creating a bulla (right).

Figure 3.14 Compact non-caseating granulomas are characteristic of sarcoidosis in a conjunctival biopsy. The central part of a granuloma contains histiocytes which have kidney-shaped nuclei and pink cytoplasm. The clumps of histiocytes are surrounded by a layer of lymphocytes.

Figure 3.15 Details of a non-caseating granuloma in sarcoidosis. Occasionally two cells fuse to form binucleate cells. Multinucleate giant cells with nuclei condensed around the periphery are found occasionally.

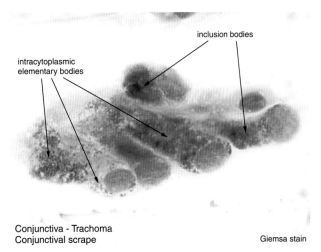

Conjunctiva - Trachoma
Conjunctival scrape   Giemsa stain

Figure 3.16

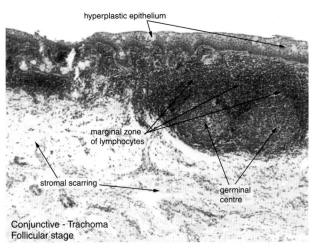

Conjunctive - Trachoma
Follicular stage

Figure 3.17

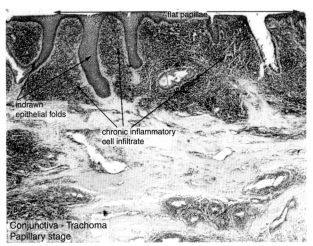

Conjunctiva - Trachoma
Papillary stage

Figure 3.18

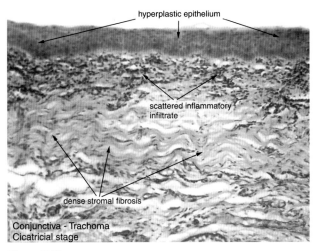

Conjunctiva - Trachoma
Cicatricial stage

Figure 3.19

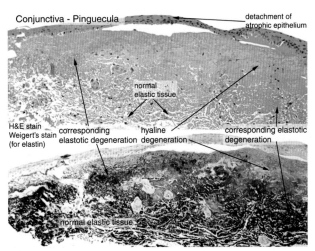

Figure 3.20

Figure 3.16 A conjunctival scrape can be used for identification of chlamydial infection. In the early stages of infection by *Chlamydia trachomatis*, the organisms are identified in the cytoplasm as elementary bodies. As the organisms proliferate they condense to form inclusion bodies (Giemsa stain).

Figure 3.17 Follicular conjunctivitis is a feature of the early stage of chlamydial infection. The blood vessels are surrounded by lymphocytes which migrate to form follicles beneath the hyperplastic epithelium.

Figure 3.18 At a further stage the disease progresses to a papillary conjunctivitis in which flattened papillae are formed by masses of inflammatory cells beneath the hyperplastic epithelium. Foci within the epithelium are tethered by fibrous strands so that processes of epithelium appear to extend into the superficial stroma.

Figure 3.19 At the late stage there is complete fibrous replacement of the conjunctival stroma. The epithelium is metaplastic to stratified squamous type and goblet cells are absent.

Figure 3.20 In an H&E section of a pinguecula (upper), the identification of degenerate elastin fibres is difficult. The fibres resemble coiled red strands. Pingueculae also contain areas of hyaline degeneration and, sometimes, keratinoid deposits (not shown). The overlying epithelium is detached in sectors. A stain for elastin (lower) demonstrates the strand-like appearance of the degenerate elastin in the tissue shown above. The hyaline material is homogeneous and hypocellular. Note that the elastotic degeneration stains in a similar manner to the abundant underlying normal elastic tissue.

Infective (bacterial)

Trachoma

Conjunctival infection by *Chlamydia trachomatis* is the commonest cause of global blindness. Various immunotypes are present in the Chlamydiaceae (A–K). A, B, Ba, and C immunotypes cause endemic trachoma. The pathogen is an obligate intracellular organism as it does not possess intrinsic glycolytic systems to convert glucose to glucose-6-phosphate. Transmission by flies, poverty, and poor sanitation are the factors which maintain reinfection. Infection by *Chlamydia trachomatis* is rare in temperate climates.

The disease is easily diagnosed clinically and is classified into five stages. Confirmation of the early stage can be made by a conjunctival scrape showing organisms within epithelial cells in a Giemsa stained preparation (Figure 3.16).

The disease progresses to a follicular conjunctivitis (Figure 3.17) and is followed by a papillary stage (Figure 3.18).

Repeated or continuing infection leads to stromal fibrosis and contractual scarring (Figure 3.19) on the inner surface of the eyelid causing entropion. The resultant trichiasis abrades the corneal surface resulting in ulceration, scarring and, ultimately, blindness.

The diagnosis was made in the past by the identification of inclusion bodies and elementary bodies in a conjunctival scrape. Currently the diagnosis is made using mainly immunofluorescence, although ELISA and PCR techniques can be utilised.

Adult inclusion conjunctivitis/ophthalmia neonatorum

The subtypes D–K of the Chlamydiaceae cause a follicular conjunctivitis in adults. Unlike trachoma, transmission is venereal or by hand to eye and is associated with genitourinary infection.

Chlamydial infection is the most common cause of ophthalmia neonatorum. Infection occurs in the birth canal and results in a papillary conjunctivitis.

Identical laboratory techniques are applied in all forms of chlamydial infection (see section on "Trachoma" above).

Degenerative conditions

Degeneration of the stroma leads to fibrosis and deposition of abnormal elastic tissue (elastotic degeneration). Fibrous tissue may also degenerate to form an amorphous acellular mass (hyaline degeneration).

Pinguecula/pterygium

Elastotic degeneration occurring in the conjunctival stroma can give rise to two clinical variants which are separately classified according to location:

1 *Pinguecula (pl. pingueculae):* a nodular grey-white nodule of the conjunctiva located often in the nasal or temporal bulbar conjunctiva but not involving the cornea.
2 *Pterygium (pl. pterygia):* a wing-shaped grey-white thickening located either in the nasal or temporal limbus with an apex extending towards the cornea. Superficial blood vessels feature prominently and point towards the apex of the mass.

The geographic distribution of individuals with pterygia and pingueculae is more frequent in sunny climates. The location of the degenerative processes confined by the palpebral fissure also implicates UV exposure. Wind and dust are factors that may exacerbate the conditions.

The treatment is often conservative using topical lubricants to minimise surface irritation and inflammation. Surgical excision may be for cosmesis, chronic inflammation, or when pterygia distort the cornea and cause a visual disturbance.

Pathology

The specimen may be submitted as a triangular or oval grey-white flat mass. Superficial blood vessels may be apparent.

The histological appearances of pingueculae and pterygia are basically identical (Figures 3.20, 3.21). The epithelium varies between atrophy, hyperplasia, metaplasia, and dysplasia (see section on "Conjunctival intraepithelial neoplasia" below). The stroma contains hypocellular areas of degenerate hyalinised collagen. Intermingled in these areas are large clumps of red staining strands which stain positively for elastin (elastotic degeneration). It is important to appreciate that in these areas of actinic damage, the epithelium can undergo precancerous and cancerous change (squamous cell carcinoma).

Weigert's elastica and elastica van Gieson are special stains to demonstrate elastotic degeneration.

Pseudopterygium

A pseudopterygium extends from the bulbar conjunctiva onto the cornea, and in this regard it resembles a pterygium. The process is secondary to corneal damage (trauma or peripheral ulceration) and, unlike a pterygium, can occur anywhere along the 360 degrees of the corneal periphery. Clinically, the ability to pass a probe beneath the apex is a useful diagnostic feature. Histologically, a pseudopterygium consists of fibrovascular tissue which *does not* contain foci of elastotic degeneration (Figure 3.22). The epithelium often extends around the fibrovascular mass.

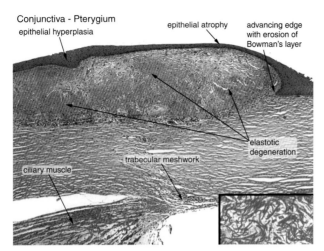

Conjunctiva - Pterygium

epithelial hyperplasia

epithelial atrophy

advancing edge with erosion of Bowman's layer

elastotic degeneration

ciliary muscle

trabecular meshwork

Figure 3.21

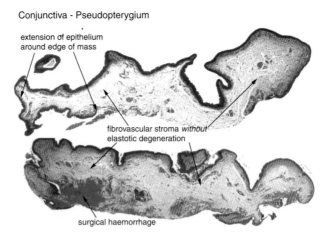

Conjunctiva - Pseudopterygium

extension of epithelium around edge of mass

fibrovascular stroma *without* elastotic degeneration

surgical haemorrhage

Figure 3.22

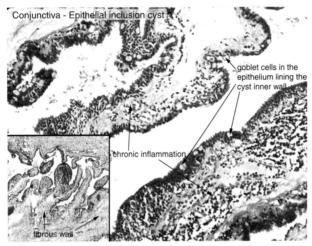

Conjunctiva - Epithelial inclusion cyst

goblet cells in the epithelium lining the cyst inner wall

chronic inflammation

fibrous wall

Figure 3.23

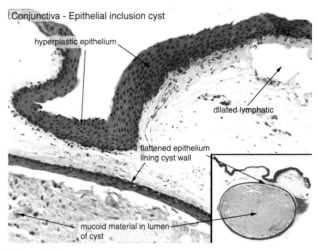

Conjunctiva - Epithelial inclusion cyst

hyperplastic epithelium

dilated lymphatic

flattened epithelium lining cyst wall

mucoid material in lumen of cyst

Figure 3.24

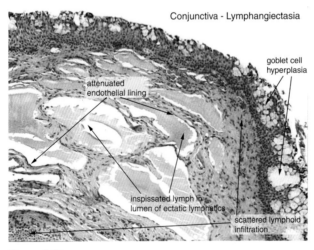

Conjunctiva - Lymphangiectasia

goblet cell hyperplasia

attenuated endothelial lining

inspissated lymph in lumen of ectatic lymphatics

scattered lymphoid infiltration

Figure 3.25

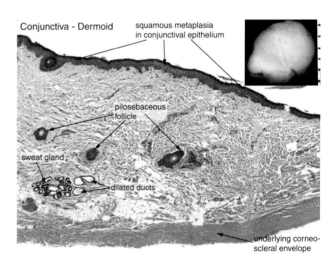

Conjunctiva - Dermoid

squamous metaplasia in conjunctival epithelium

pilosebaceous follicle

sweat gland

dilated ducts

underlying corneo-scleral envelope

Figure 3.26

Tumours

Benign tumours

Epithelial inclusion cysts

Most frequently, cysts are due to previous trauma with incarceration of conjunctival epithelial nests in the stroma.

These cysts can be of variable size and appear as discrete round or oval masses in the stroma. Transillumination will demonstrate that the fluid content is opaque. Microscopy will reveal lining cells resembling conjunctival epithelium on the inner surface of the wall (Figure 3.23). The milky content of the cyst is the result of secretion of mucin by goblet cells and desquamation of epithelial cells. The epithelium in the cyst may undergo metaplasia to a squamous cell type (Figure 3.24).

Hamartomas and choristomas

Tumourous malformations are of two types: those which are formed from tissues normally present at that site are *hamartomas* and those which contain tissues which are *not* normally present at that site are *choristomas*.

Lymphatic cyst/lymphagiectasias

Hamartomatous malformations of lymphatics leads to the formation of multiple small cysts or larger swollen cystic structures lined by an attenuated endothelium (Figure 3.25). Lymph can become inspissated and this leads to rupture of dilated lymphatics and a secondary inflammation in the conjunctival stroma. Lymphatic cysts occur when ectatic lymphatics coalesce. These hamartomatous malformations may include a vascular component.

Angiomas

Angiomas of the conjunctiva can occur and are of the capillary type (see Chapter 5).

Dermoid

A dermoid of the conjunctiva appears at birth and is an example of a choristoma because the tumour contains elements derived from skin. It is assumed that a fragment of dermal ectoderm is misplaced into the conjunctival precursors during embryogenesis.

Most commonly a dermoid forms a solid ovoid white mass (occasionally hair-bearing) at the limbus. However, a tumour formed by fat and fibrous tissue (dermolipoma) may be present as a soft tissue swelling located in the fornix.

Histologically, a solid dermoid contains adnexal structures within fibrofatty tissue (Figure 3.26).

Naevi

Conjunctival naevi are thought to be present at birth but only manifest in adult life with increased pigmentation or size. They are classified in the same manner as eyelid naevi (see Chapter 2). A small flat pigmented area is due to proliferation of melanocytes within the epithelium and is called a *junctional naevus*. A nodular tumour is formed when stroma contains proliferating melanocytes and the term *intrastromal naevus* is applied. If naevus cells are present in both the epithelium and stroma, the term *compound naevus* is applied: this tumour is also nodular.

Clinical presentation

The tumour presents commonly as a static nodule with variable pigmentation. A rapid increase in size or pigmentation should lead to a suspicion of malignant transformation to a melanoma. Malignant transformation is very rare. However, at least 20% of melanomas arise from pre-existing naevi.

Figure 3.21 In a pterygium, the degenerative process extends onto the cornea as a plaque and there appears to be collagenolysis extending into the peripheral stroma. The plaque contains foci of elastotic degeneration shown at high magnification in the insert. The abundant hyalinisation of the ciliary muscle (detached by artefact) indicates that this patient is elderly.

Figure 3.22 The illustration shows two levels through a pseudopterygium. Compared with a pterygium, the stroma of a pseudopterygium does not contain areas of elastotic degeneration and it may be possible to identify extension of the epithelium around the edges of the fibrovascular stroma.

Figure 3.23 A large epithelial inclusion cyst was ruptured during excision. As a result the cyst collapsed and the mucosal lining formed folds (inset). The epithelium lining the inner surface of the cyst is of conjunctival type.

Figure 3.24 Secretion of mucin and the release of cell debris causes expansion of a conjunctival cyst and the epithelial lining becomes flattened with a loss of goblet cells. The overlying normal conjunctival epithelium is metaplastic and hyperplastic due to mechanical irritation.

Figure 3.25 Large dilated lymphatics within the stroma of the conjunctiva are the characteristic diagnostic feature of lymphangiectasia. This example was included because it also shows goblet cell hyperplasia which sometimes occurs in areas of irritation.

Figure 3.26 A solid white mass was present at the limbus at birth. The mass was excised with a strip of normal cornea and sclera (inset). Histology reveals a fibrofatty mass containing skin adnexal structures (pilosebaceous follicles and sweat glands). The epithelium has undergone metaplasia to a stratified squamous type with keratinisation. Note that without the visible underlying sclera, it would be easy to regard this as a skin biopsy.

Possible modes of treatment
Usually conservative. Surgical excision for cosmesis or enlargement.

Macroscopic
An ellipse of conjunctiva may contain a flat black area (junctional naevus) or a small nodule of variable pigmentation and dimensions of up to 8 mm (intrastromal or compound naevi).

Microscopic
In a compound naevus, the cells are small and of uniform size (Figure 3.27). Pigmentation may not be a prominent feature. The cells form clusters within the epithelium and within the stroma. The cellular proliferation is accompanied by incarceration of epithelium to form cysts and enlargement of such cysts can lead to tumour enlargement and give rise to suspicion of malignant transformation.

Special investigations/stains
The Masson–Fontana stains melanin which appears as black granules.

Immunohistochemistry
Naevus cells stain positively for melan-A, S-100, and HMB-45 (same reactivity with melanomas).

Amyloid

An amyloid nodule deposited within the conjunctiva appears as a well demarcated pale subconjunctival mass. This condition may occur as part of a systemic amyloidosis or be secondary to chronic inflammatory disorders such as trachoma and chronic keratitis. Amyloid deposition can also be found in the vitreous and retinal vessels, but most commonly involves the orbit and lacrimal gland (see Chapter 5).

Papillomas

Papillomas are common in the conjunctiva and may be present in two forms:
1 *Papillary/pedunculated:* vascular, cauliflower-like tumours.
2 *Placoid/sessile:* ovoid pink swellings.
   The pathogenesis is related to infection by the human papilloma virus – type 16/18 is implicated in the papillary form.
   Treatment is usually by total excision including a frill of normal conjunctiva.

Macroscopic
1 *Papillary/pedunculated tumours:* when the ovoid mass is bisected, a fibrovascular core is evident (Figure 3.28).
2 *Placoid/sessile:* an ovoid mass containing prominent blood vessels.

Complications/secondary effects
Excessive growth can lead to infection and infarction. Metaplasia to a squamous epithelium can result secondary to mechanical irritation and UV exposure. Malignant transformation to a squamous cell carcinoma has been known to occur in both papillary and placoid types but is rare.

Microscopic
1 *Papillary/pedunculated:* the conjunctival origin (as opposed to skin) is easily identified by the presence of goblet cells within the epithelium (Figures 3.29, 3.30).
2 *Placoid/sessile:* the surface of the mass of proliferating metaplastic (squamous) cells is smooth. Fibrovascular cores project into the thick layer of epithelial cells (Figure 3.31).

Premalignant and malignant tumours

Epithelial-based neoplasia

Conjunctival intraepithelial neoplasia (CIN)
In the preceding text, reference has been made to squamous metaplasia in the conjunctival epithelium. In certain circumstances (for example pingueculae and pterygia), this change exposes the epithelium to the risk of neoplastic transformation.

The term conjunctival intraepithelial neoplasia (CIN) is used to describe a spectrum of patterns of cellular proliferation which range from dysplasia to frank carcinoma-in-situ. The essential feature of CIN is that the *neoplastic cells have not penetrated the underlying basement membrane.* The clinical appearances are often similar and definitive diagnosis and management often relies on the biopsy and histopathological examination. NB: The acronym CIN in general pathology refers to cervical intraepithelial neoplasia.

Clinical presentation
Usually unilateral, located in the interpalpebral fissure, and close to the limbus. The tumour is usually flat with a gelatinous texture and may have a pale white surface (leukoplakia) due to an oedematous keratin layer.

Pathogenesis
This condition is more common in the elderly, particularly those with a long history of ultraviolet light exposure. The human papilloma virus has also been implicated. Other factors may include smoking and carcinogen exposure.

Possible modes of treatment
Complete or partial excision biopsy is important for classification. Adjuvant cryotherapy is commonly applied. Topical mitomycin therapy has been described but is controversial.

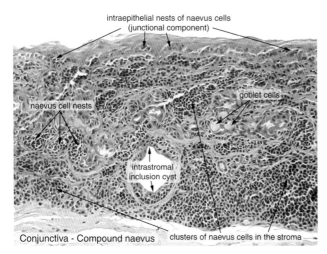

intraepithelial nests of naevus cells
(junctional component)

naevus cell nests

goblet cells

intrastromal
inclusion cyst

Conjunctiva - Compound naevus

clusters of naevus cells in the stroma

Figure 3.27

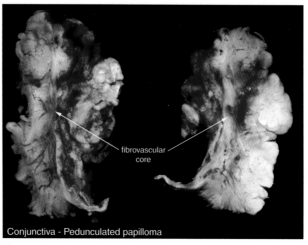

fibrovascular
core

Conjunctiva - Pedunculated papilloma

Figure 3.28

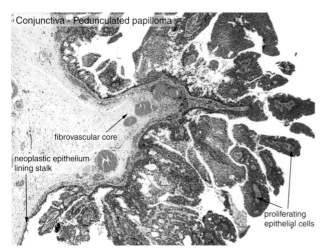

Conjunctiva - Pedunculated papilloma

fibrovascular core

neoplastic epithelium
lining stalk

proliferating
epithelial cells

Figure 3.29

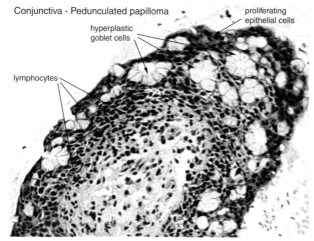

Conjunctiva - Pedunculated papilloma

proliferating
epithelial cells

hyperplastic
goblet cells

lymphocytes

Figure 3.30

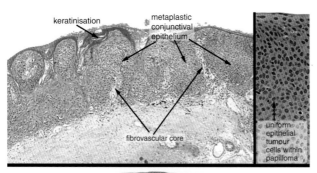

keratinisation

metaplastic
conjunctival
epithelium

uniform
epithelial
tumour
cells within
papilloma

fibrovascular core

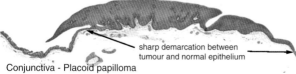

sharp demarcation between
tumour and normal epithelium

Conjunctiva - Placoid papilloma

Figure 3.31

Figure 3.27 In a compound naevus of the conjunctiva, the epithelium contains nests of naevus cells. Within the stroma there is a dense infiltrate of naevus cells which also tend to form nests in the base of the tumour. A feature of a compound naevus is the presence of small epithelial cysts among the naevus cell clusters. The cysts enlarge due to goblet cell secretion and give an impression that the tumour is increasing in size.

Figure 3.28 This conjunctival papilloma has been bisected to demonstrate the fibrovascular core which supports the proliferating epithelial cells (see Figures 3.29, 3.30).

Figure 3.29 A low power micrograph of part of a typical conjunctival papilloma to show finger-like processes of fibrovascular tissue lined by epithelial cells of the conjunctival type.

Figure 3.30 Mechanical irritation of conjunctival papilloma leads to secondary inflammation seen as inflammatory cell infiltration within the fibrovascular core. Proliferating epithelial cells on the surface encompass clusters of goblet cells, which are easily recognised by their clear cytoplasm and eccentric nuclei.

Figure 3.31 Upper left: placoid/sessile conjunctival papillomas differ from the pedunculated variant in that the proliferating cells tend to be of the squamous type and the goblet cells are absent. Keratinisation may be a feature. At high magnification, the tumour cells are relatively uniform in size (upper right). The lower figure shows the sharp demarcation between a placoid papilloma and normal epithelium.

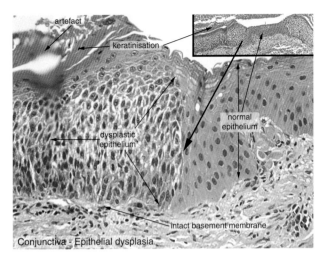

Figure 3.32

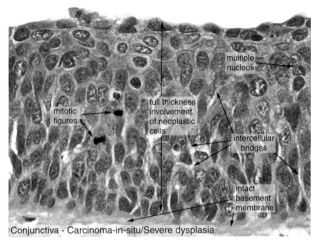

Figure 3.33

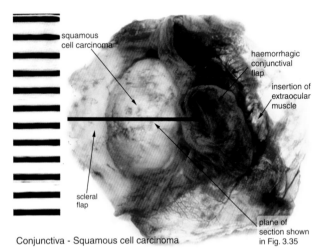

Figure 3.34

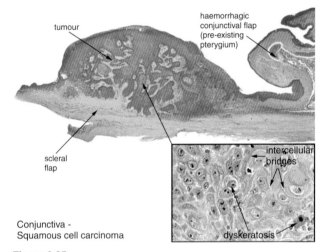

Figure 3.35

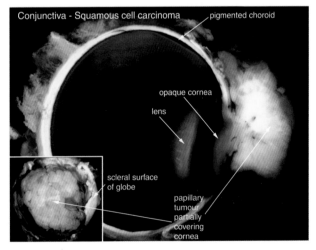

Figure 3.36

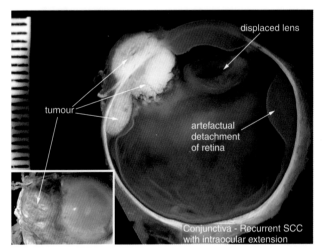

Figure 3.37

Conjunctival dysplasia

This represents the benign end of the CIN spectrum.

Microscopically, sharply demarcated areas/sectors of the epithelium will be thickened by proliferating squamous cells with varying degrees of differentiation (Figure 3.32). Cytokeratin markers (for example CAM 5.2) confirm an epithelial origin.

Carcinoma-in-situ (CIS): severe dysplasia

This represents the more malignant variant of CIN. The change may be extensive within the conjunctiva in an exenteration for invasive squamous cell carcinoma specimens.

Microscopically, the proliferating cells occupy the full thickness of the epithelium and possess all the characteristic cytological features of a squamous cell carcinoma but *the basement membrane remains intact* (Figure 3.33).

These tumours stain positively with cytokeratin markers which are useful in excluding invasion of the basement membrane.

Squamous cell carcinoma (SCC)

A rare conjunctival tumour that has an increased incidence in sun-drenched countries. It may arise *de novo*, from a pre-existing pterygium, or an area of CIN.

Clinical presentation

A non-pigmented mass that has a gelatinous texture located within the interpalpebral fissure. The surface may be keratinised and friable. The tumour often extends onto the cornea but is not strongly adherent.

Pathogenesis

Presumed UV damage.

Possible modes of treatment

Complete excision with cryotherapy to the edges. Partial sclerectomy may be required. Topical mitomycin C has been used and is effective.

If tumour involvement was so extensive that preservation of the globe is not possible by a local excision, enucleation or exenteration will be required for extensive ocular or orbital involvement.

Pathology

The specimen may be in the form of a conjunctival excision biopsy and usually includes a scleral flap (Figure 3.34). Histologically, squamous carcinomas which arise in the conjunctival and corneal epithelium are commonly well differentiated (Figure 3.35).

An enucleation specimen is submitted when the tumour proliferation is extensive (Figure 3.36).

Previous intervention with scleral resection and inadequate clearance may lead to penetration of the globe (Figure 3.37).

Melanocytic neoplasia

Primary acquired melanosis (PAM)

Clinical presentation

This umbrella term to classify diffuse pigmented tumours of the conjunctiva describes a spectrum that extends from benign acquired melanosis (primary acquired melanosis (PAM) without atypia) to PAM with mild, moderate, or severe atypia.

The condition occurs in middle age or in later life as an expanding diffuse flat pigmentation in the conjunctiva and is usually unilateral. Previously, pigmentation was not present at that site and this excludes a junctional naevus. A histopathological diagnosis is important because one form of acquired melanosis may be the source of a malignant melanoma.

Figure 3.32 In conjunctival dysplasia, the dysplastic sectors are separated by sectors of normal epithelium. The dysplastic spindle-shaped cells show variations in size and shape of nuclei, and occasional mitotic figures can be identified. The basement membrane is intact. Although intercellular bridges are not prominent, the presence of a space between the cells indicates the squamous epithelial nature of the tumour.

Figure 3.33 By comparison with mild dysplasia, the cells in carcinoma-in-situ possess more of the features of a frank carcinoma (prominent nucleoli within irregularly shaped nuclei) with plentiful mitotic figures. The basement membrane remains intact so this is "preinvasive" carcinoma. In some areas, intercellular bridges can still be demonstrated.

Figure 3.34 An excision specimen for a conjunctival squamous cell carcinoma usually includes a scleral flap for clearance. Clinically, the tumour has a gelatinous appearance with numerous surface blood vessels. In a fixed specimen, the tumour is more opaque. The brown appearance of the conjunctival flap is due to intraoperative bleeding. A section through the specimen is shown in Figure 3.35.

Figure 3.35 The histological section of the specimen in Figure 3.34 shows that the tumour is widely cleared. The inset shows the features characteristic of a well differentiated squamous cell carcinoma with prominent intercellular bridges and intracytoplasmic keratinisation (dyskeratosis).

Figure 3.36 In the developing world, treatment may be delayed as in this enucleation specimen in a black African. Initial examination of the specimen suggests that the cornea is completely covered by a large papillary tumour (inset). A cut across the eye and the tumour reveals a conjunctival and partial corneal location without penetration of the corneoscleral envelope. Subsequent histology confirms the clinical diagnosis of squamous cell carcinoma.

Figure 3.37 In this case, a conjunctival squamous cell carcinoma was initially treated by local resection and sclerectomy. Histopathological examination of the specimen revealed inadequate clearance. A year later, the patient presented with a mass at the limbus (inset) with visual disturbance due to lens displacement. Intraocular spread was identified and enucleation was carried out. Examination of the interior of the globe reveals tumour penetration of the sclera with intraocular spread. The retina is detached artefactually and the cloudy appearance is due to formalin fixation.

Clinically it is impossible to make a reliable distinction between the benign and premalignant forms of acquired melanosis.

It is important to appreciate that intraepithelial melanocytic proliferation represents a field change and pigmentation can occur spontaneously in any area of the conjunctiva. In the premalignant form multiple biopsies are necessary.

Possible modes of treatment
1 Observation.
2 Excision biopsy to identify the subtype of acquired melanosis or if malignancy is suspected.
3 Cryotherapy to larger areas.
4 Topical antimetabolites (mitomycin C) are also used.

Macroscopic
A typical specimen in PAM will be an ellipse of pigmented tissue often bearing a nodular brown mass (Figure 3.38). PAM will also be seen in exenteration specimens when there is multifocal development of a malignant melanoma (Figure 3.39).

Microscopic
There are two histopathological subgroups differing in malignant potential:
1 *Benign acquired melanosis (BAM) or primary acquire melanosis without atypia:* melanocytic proliferation is confined to the basal layer and the melanosomes are transferred into the normal superficial epithelial cells (Figure 3.40).
2 *Primary acquired melanosis with atypia:* this may be classified as mild, moderate, or severe (see below). PAM with severe atypia is a serious condition due to the possibility of transformation to a malignant melanoma.

The specimens will either be a biopsy of conjunctiva bearing pigmented areas or an exenteration for malignant transformation (Figures 3.39, 3.40).

Classification is based on the appearance of the infiltrating malignant melanocytes and the extent of infiltration to the superficial layers. In mild atypia, the infiltration is confined to the basal and wing cell layers (Figure 3.41 left). In moderate atypia, the basal and wing cell layers are affected more extensively and the superficial layers are still spared (Figure 3.42). In severe atypia, the full thickness of the epithelium is infiltrated by malignant melanocytes which show marked variation in nuclear size and shape (Figure 3.41 right). As in the CIN counterpart, the basement membrane remains intact.

Complications/secondary effects
There is a risk of transformation to a malignant melanoma.

Repeated cryotherapy causes stromal fibrosis and distortion of the lids with entropion and corneal trauma. Eradication is difficult if the limbus and cornea are affected. Mitomycin destroys melanocytes but induces changes in the epithelium which modify the normal histological appearance.

Special investigations/stains
Masson–Fontana stain is useful to determine the extent of melanin deposition (Figure 3.40 inset).

Immunohistochemistry
Melan-A, HMB45, and S-100 are useful to confirm the diagnosis in amelanotic cases.

Melanoma
Conjunctival melanomas are unilateral and are rare (2% of ocular malignancies). Metastatic spread is to the regional lymph nodes.

Clinical presentation
The patient is typically Caucasian and middle aged or elderly.

Melanomas are usually unilateral and present as pigmented or non-pigmented masses in the conjunctiva. Seventy five per cent of cases arise from pre-existing PAM (Figure 3.39). The remainder arise *de novo* or in a pre-existing naevus. Increased overlying vascularity may be evident in malignant transformation.

Examination of the regional lymph nodes for metastatic spread is mandatory. This is particularly important in the case of PAM when the melanoma often arises in the fornix: in this location, the melanoma is identified later than a tumour arising in the bulbar conjunctiva and the prognosis is worse.

Possible modes of treatment
Although rare, the management of conjunctival melanomas may be difficult. Once diagnosis is confirmed by biopsy, complete surgical excision with cryotherapy to the edges is commonly performed. There is an increasing tendency to use topical cytotoxics (for example mitomycin-C).

If PAM is present, treatment is as described above.

Exenteration is required if the tumour is too large for local excision or is invading the orbit. An early exenteration does not improve the overall survival rate.

Macroscopic
Melanomas of the conjunctiva are not necessarily pigmented and the external and cut surfaces may be white. The specimen will usually be in the form of an excision biopsy (Figure 3.43). Exenteration specimens are rare and diagnosis is obvious on macroscopic examination (Figures 3.39, 3.44)!

In the case of the conjunctival excision biopsy, examination of the frill in different quadrants is important to ascertain surgical clearance and to identify and classify the degree of atypia in PAM.

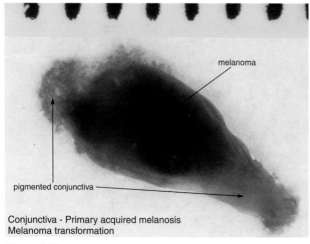

Conjunctiva - Primary acquired melanosis
Melanoma transformation

Figure 3.38

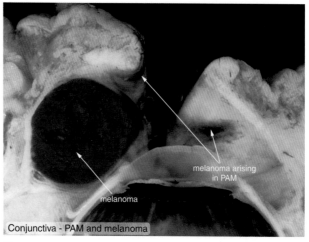

Conjunctiva - PAM and melanoma

Figure 3.39

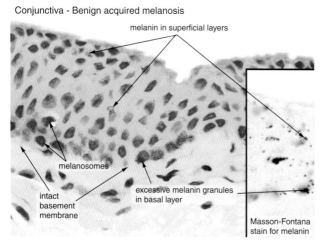

Conjunctiva - Benign acquired melanosis

Figure 3.40

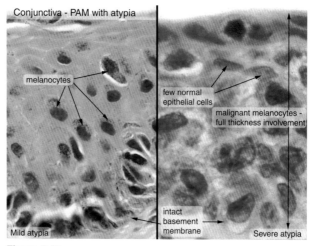

Conjunctiva - PAM with atypia

Figure 3.41

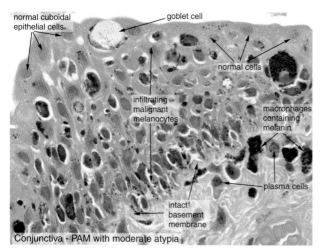

Conjunctiva - PAM with moderate atypia

Figure 3.42

Figure 3.38 A middle-aged female patient with widespread pigmentation of the conjunctiva developed a pigmented tumour nodule in the bulbar conjunctiva. The illustration shows the excision specimen with a pigmented nodule surrounded by a heavily pigmented conjunctiva. Histology confirms a malignant melanoma arising in primary acquired melanosis with severe atypia.

Figure 3.39 An elderly male patient presented with a mass in the lower eyelid. Eversion of the eyelid revealed a large pigmented mass in the tarsal conjunctiva of the lower lid. Elsewhere, the conjunctiva contained smaller nodular pigmented tumours within widespread pigmentation. It was not possible to salvage the globe due to the extensive conjunctival involvement and an exenteration was carried out. The figure illustrates the anterior part of the exenteration specimen to show melanomas arising in primary acquired melanosis with severe atypia.

Figure 3.40 In benign acquired melanosis, the melanocytes are cells with clear cytoplasm within the epithelium and are of uniform size. The melanosomes are transferred to normal epithelial cells and are carried through to the surface. The Masson–Fontana stain for melanin (inset) shows the melanin pigment granules in the more superficial layers of the epithelium.

Figure 3.41 At the extreme ends of the spectrum, it is easy to differentiate mild and severe primary acquired melanosis with atypia. In mild atypia, the nuclei of the melanocytes are of relatively normal size and nucleoli are not easily identified. Melanocytic proliferation does not reach the superficial layers of the epithelium. In severe atypia, there is marked variation of the size and shape of nuclei with full thickness involvement from the basal to the superficial layers. In both examples, the basement membrane remains intact.

Figure 3.42 Differentiation between the grades of malignancy in primary acquired melanosis is subjective. This example shows sparing of the superficial layers by the infiltrating malignant melanocytes (which vary markedly in size and shape); it would be reasonable to regard this as moderate atypia.

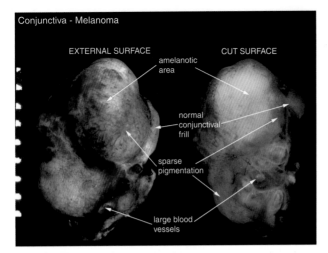

Figure 3.43

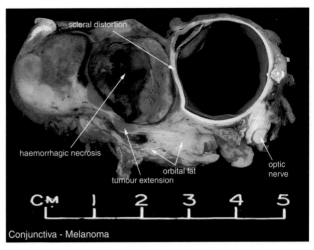

Figure 3.44

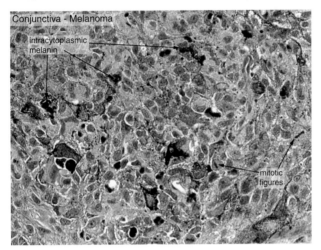

Figure 3.45

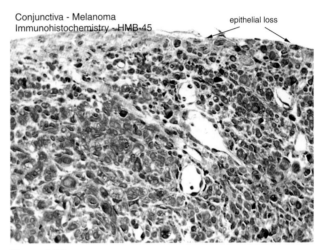

Figure 3.46

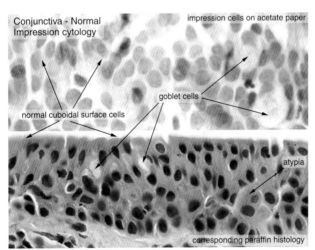

Figure 3.47

Figure 3.43 This is the macroscopic appearance of a relatively large amelanotic conjunctival melanoma (8 × 8 × 6 mm) which was excised with a frill of normal conjunctiva. The tumour is devoid of pigment in one area and is partially pigmented elsewhere.

Figure 3.44 This exenteration specimen contains a partially pigmented malignant melanoma of the conjunctiva. The tumour is almost twice the size of the globe and rapid growth has led to haemorrhagic necrosis. The patient refused surgical treatment for more than a year.

Figure 3.45 The round shape of the cells and prominent intercellular spaces in conjunction with intracytoplasmic melanin classifies the tumour as an epithelioid melanoma.

Figure 3.46 In a suspected case of amelanotic melanoma, the melanocytic origin of the tumour cells is confirmed by the use of immunohistochemical markers – in this example HMB45.

Figure 3.47 Impression cytology provides an opportunity to study the conjunctival surface cells (upper). The epithelial cells on the acetate sheet are of normal size and shape, and goblet cells are present. A paraffin section from the same area shows that there is some atypia in the basal layers but the surface cells are normal (lower).

Microscopic

Conjunctival melanomas can be spindle, epithelioid, or mixed as in uveal melanomas (see Chapter 11). Mitotic figures are often more frequent than in uveal tumours (Figure 3.45). A prominent lymphocytic infiltrate is often present.

Immunohistochemistry

The tumour will react with melan-A, S-100, and HMB45 markers (Figure 3.46).

Impression cytology

The technique for impression cytology is described above. In many publications, this is used to assess surface cells and the presence of goblet cells (Figure 3.47). In the authors' institution, the technique was used to identify malignant melanocytes in the surface layer in cases in which PAM with severe atypia was suspected (Figures 3.48, 3.49).

Lymphoproliferative disease

During life, lymphoid tissue develops in the conjunctival stroma, particularly in the fornices. It has been known for several decades that lymphoproliferative disorders occurring beneath mucosal surfaces (for example gastrointestinal and respiratory systems) have a better prognosis with treatment and such tumours are classified as mucosa-associated lymphoid tumours (MALT). Many primary conjunctival lymphoproliferative tumours are considered to be of MALT type and the spectrum ranges from benign reactionary lymphoid hyperplasia to frank malignant lymphoma. Experience with MALT conjunctival lymphomas has shown that there is often a transformation in recurrences from the more benign variant to the malignant variant (multistep neoplasia).

Because lymphoproliferative disorders are clinically indistinguishable, the classification is entirely the responsibility of the pathologist. The grade of malignancy governs the treatment.

Clinical presentation

Reactive and malignant lymphoid proliferations present in the same way as localised or diffuse conjunctival swellings, which are classically salmon pink in colour. The common sites are the bulbar conjunctiva and the fornix.

The primary tumours may be unilateral or bilateral, or may represent an extension from an orbital lymphoma (see Chapter 5). In addition, conjunctival lymphoid tumours, reactive and malignant, can develop as part of a disseminated disease. It is extremely important that any patient presenting with lymphoid neoplasia in the conjunctiva be referred for general and oncological assessment for systemic involvement.

Possible modes of treatment

Excision biopsy followed by low dose radiotherapy (about 10 Gy) is commonly successful in ablating primary conjunctival lymphomas.

Systemic disease will be treated appropriately by an oncologist.

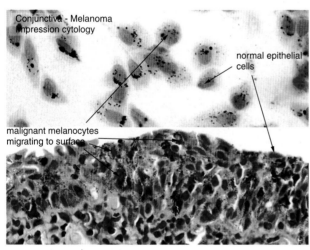

Figure 3.48

Figure 3.48 In primary acquired melanosis with moderate atypia, malignant melanocytes migrate to the surface and are accompanied by normal epithelial cells containing melanosomes. The separation of the two cell types is subjective and requires experience – much depends on the size and nuclear chromatin arrangement. The combined figure shows the impression cytology (upper) with the corresponding histology (lower).

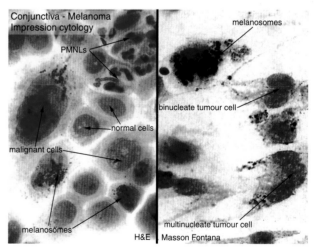

Figure 3.49

Figure 3.49 In frank melanocytic malignancy, the malignant cells on the acetate paper possess nuclei which vary markedly in size (left) and are sometimes binucleate or multinucleate (right). Normal cells are also present. PMNLs = polymorphonuclear leucocytes.

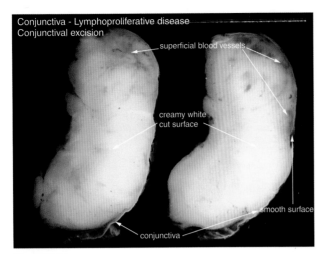

Conjunctiva - Lymphoproliferative disease
Conjunctival excision

superficial blood vessels

creamy white
cut surface

smooth surface

conjunctiva

Figure 3.50

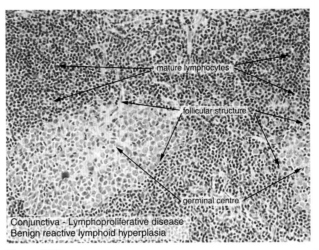

mature lymphocytes

follicular structure

germinal centre

Conjunctiva - Lymphoproliferative disease
Benign reactive lymphoid hyperplasia

Figure 3.51

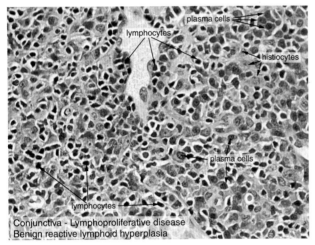

plasma cells

lymphocytes

histiocytes

plasma cells

lymphocytes

Conjunctiva - Lymphoproliferative disease
Benign reactive lymphoid hyperplasia

Figure 3.52

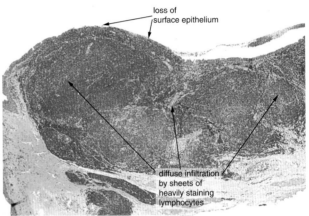

loss of
surface epithelium

diffuse infiltration
by sheets of
heavily staining
lymphocytes

Conjunctiva - Lymphoproliferative disease
Malignant lymphoma

Figure 3.53

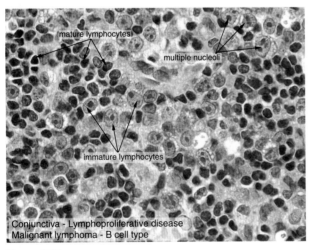

mature lymphocytes

multiple nucleoli

immature lymphocytes

Conjunctiva - Lymphoproliferative disease
Malignant lymphoma - B cell type

Figure 3.54

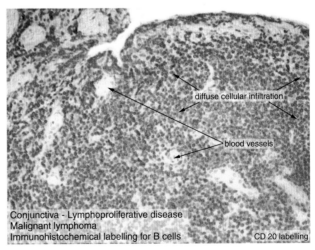

diffuse cellular infiltration

blood vessels

Conjunctiva - Lymphoproliferative disease
Malignant lymphoma
Immunohistochemical labelling for B cells

CD 20 labelling

Figure 3.55

Macroscopic

The specimen will usually be in the form of a conjunctival (excision) biopsy (Figure 3.50). The external surface is smooth and the cut surface has a characteristic homogeneous white appearance.

Histopathology and immunohistochemistry

Immunohistochemistry using markers for B- and T-cell subtypes have refined the diagnosis and classification of conjunctival and orbital lymphomas.

As described above, a wide histological spectrum of lymphoproliferative disease exists ranging from benign to malignant. For the purpose of this text, the two extremes of lymphocytic proliferations are described:

1 *Benign reactive lymphoid hyperplasia:* there may be a follicular pattern resembling that seen in a lymph node (Figure 3.51). The cell population is mixed and includes lymphocytes, plasma cells, and histiocytes (Figure 3.52). Immunohistochemistry will show that the lymphocytes are of two types: B and T cell and this is referred to as polyclonality.

2 *Malignant lymphoma:* at low power, the conjunctival stroma contains sheets of densely blue-staining (basophilic) lymphocytes (Figure 3.53). In a high power view from an H&E section (Figure 3.54) the cell maturation is varied with intermingled primitive and mature lymphocytes. Immunohistochemistry will show that the cells are monoclonal and the B-cell type is by far the most common (Figure 3.55).

Figure 3.50 The diagnosis of conjunctival lymphoproliferative disease can be made on macroscopic examination. The ovoid mass is smooth and the cut surface is creamy white or tan coloured. The salmon-pink clinical appearance is due to superficial vascularity. The classification, however, depends on the histological and immunohistochemical findings.

Figure 3.51 In benign reactive lymphoid hyperplasia of the conjunctiva, the large mass contains lymphocytic proliferations which recapitulate those seen in a normal lymph node. Follicles are present and are formed by pale staining immature cells in the germinal centre surrounded by a mantle of small lymphocytes (see Figures 3.6, 3.17).

Figure 3.52 At high power, it is possible to identify inflammatory cells of different types in a reactionary process (for example lymphocytes, plasma cells, and histiocytes). The clear spaces around the lymphocyte nuclei are due to a shrinkage artefact. Compare with the neoplastic infiltration shown in Figure 3.54.

Figure 3.53 A suspicion of a malignant infiltrate is aroused at low power by the presence of sheets of basophilic cells in the conjunctival stroma ("if it's blue, it's bad!").

Figure 3.54 In a malignant infiltrate, the sheets of lymphoid cells are of the same type (monoclonality) but of varying maturity from lymphoblasts to mature lymphocytes. The nuclear features of primitive lymphocytes include coarse chromatin and multiple nucleoli. Mitotic figures are often found but are not demonstrated in this example.

Figure 3.55 Immunohistochemistry demonstrates that every cell in this tumour is positively labelled with a B-cell marker (CD20 in this case) demonstrating monoclonality. This establishes that the malignant lymphoma is of B-cell type (peroxidase-antiperoxidase label).

Chapter 4
Cornea

Normal

Anatomy

The cornea is a highly specialised structure which possesses the following vital functions: a clear refractive interface, tensile strength, and protection of the intraocular contents from the external environment. It has an elliptical shape with the dimensions 10.6 mm vertically and 11.7 mm horizontally.

Histologically the cornea consists of five layers (Figure 4.1):

1 *Epithelium* (50 μm): consisting of five or six layers (Figure 4.2). These layers are divided into:
   (a) Basal cell layer: cuboidal cells where cell division occurs.
   (b) Wing cells: the second layer is wing shaped to fit over the rounded anterior surface of the basal cells (Figure 4.3).
   (c) Superficial cells: the next three layers become increasingly flattened as they progress towards the surface due to mitotic activity in the basal cell layer. The most superficial cells detach from the surface as a normal process of "wear-and-tear". The cells of the epithelium are attached by desmosomes (Figure 4.3) and the basal layer is attached to Bowman's layer by an anchoring complex (Figure 4.3). Knowledge of the ultrastructure is relevant to appreciate some of the important pathological processes to be described.
2 *Bowman's layer:* a thin homogeneous layer which serves as a base for the epithelial anchoring system. Once destroyed, this layer is never replaced. Its absence indicates previous trauma or ulceration.
3 *Stroma* (500 μm): the keratocytes are spindle cells with long branching interconnecting processes which are never visualised in routine histological sections. These cells lie between lamellae which contain bundles of uniformly spaced collagen fibrils. The interfibrillar spacing is such that any light scattering is cancelled by interference with light rays from adjacent fibrils and is the basis for one of the theories to explain corneal transparency. The orientation of the fibrils varies by 60 degrees between lamellae and this provides structural strength.
4 *Descemet's membrane:* a thin elastic membrane possessing high tensile strength and containing proteoglycans and glycoproteins in addition to collagen (Figure 4.4). The membrane stains intensely pink with the PAS stain. At the ultrastructural level, two zones can be identified – an anterior banded zone which is formed in fetal life and a posterior non-banded zone which increases in thickness throughout adult life (Figure 4.5).
5 *Endothelium:* this monolayer is flattened and cuboidal in section. The endothelial cell population declines with age and this process can be accelerated by certain disease states or surgical intervention. Ultrastructural examination reveals thin interdigitations between cells which increases the surface area available for fluid transport (Figure 4.5). Examination of the posterior surface by scanning electron microscopy reveals that the endothelial cells are arranged in a uniform hexagonal pattern (Figure 4.6).

How to examine a corneal specimen

The increased availability of transplant material due to the establishment of donor tissue eye banks and improved storage systems has led to an escalation in the number of keratoplasty procedures and, consequently, an increase in the number of specimens available for pathological study.

Macroscopic

The specimens submitted are most likely to be in the form of a disc derived from a penetrating or lamellar keratoplasty. The diameter of the disc should be measured (usually 8–10 mm diameter) and both surfaces should be examined for changes such as ulceration, variations in stromal thickness, pigmentation, and the presence of plaques. Retroillumination reveals stromal opacities and neovascularisation.

Figure 4.1 The constituents and relative thicknesses of the layers of a normal cornea.

Figure 4.2 In an H&E section, Bowman's layer is homogeneous and is distinct from the stroma in which there are keratocytes between the collagenous lamellae. The spaces between the lamellae are due to an artefact.

Figure 4.3 At the ultrastructural level, desmosomes form firm attachments between the epithelial cells. The basal layer of the epithelium is attached via hemidesmosomes to Bowman's layer by anchoring filaments which pass through the basement membrane. The filaments merge with anchoring fibrils which are larger and are located in the superficial part of Bowman's layer. The anchoring system is sectioned obliquely and the structures are not clearly seen.

Figure 4.4 By light microscopy (H&E section), Descemet's membrane has two layers – see Figure 4.5 for its ultrastructure. The endothelial cells form a monolayer of flattened cuboidal cells.

Figure 4.5 By transmission electron microscopy, two layers can be identified in Descemet's membrane. The endothelial cells form peripheral interdigitations which increase the cells' surface area to facilitate fluid transport.

Figure 4.6 Scanning electron microscopy of the posterior surface reveals the hexagonal arrangement of the endothelial monolayer. Cytoplasmic processes (microvilli) project from the intercellular borders.

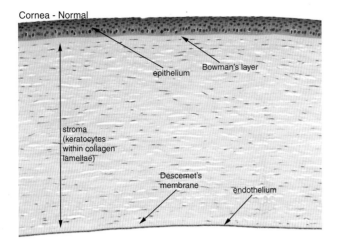

Cornea - Normal

epithelium

Bowman's layer

stroma
(keratocytes
within collagen
lamellae)

Descemet's
membrane

endothelium

Figure 4.1

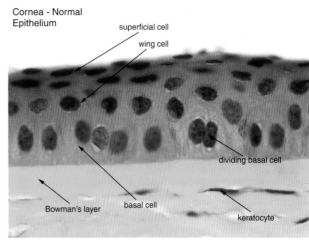

Cornea - Normal
Epithelium

superficial cell

wing cell

dividing basal cell

Bowman's layer

basal cell

keratocyte

Figure 4.2

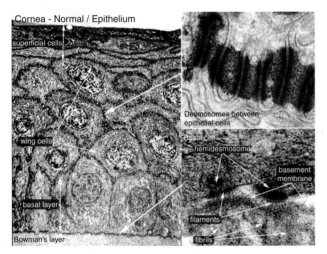

Cornea - Normal / Epithelium

superficial cells

wing cells

basal layer

Bowman's layer

Desmosomes between
epithelial cells

Basal cell
hemidesmosomes

basement
membrane

filaments

fibrils

Figure 4.3

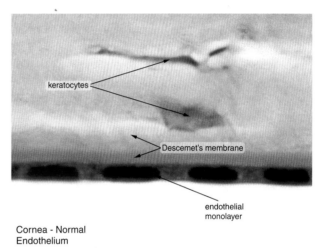

keratocytes

Descemet's membrane

endothelial
monolayer

Cornea - Normal
Endothelium

Figure 4.4

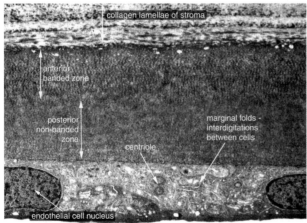

collagen lamellae of stroma

anterior
banded zone

posterior
non-banded
zone

centriole

marginal folds -
interdigitations
between cells

endothelial cell nucleus

Cornea - Normal / Endothelium

Figure 4.5

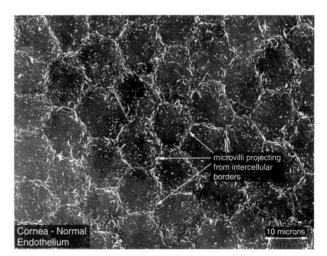

microvilli projecting
from intercellular
borders

Cornea - Normal
Endothelium

10 microns

Figure 4.6

Corneal scrapings

In infective diseases an ulcer will be scraped with a metallic instrument and the material removed is placed in culture and is also smeared onto glass slides for histological examination using special stains. If a fungal or a protozoal infection is suspected, a corneal biopsy may be submitted.

Microscopic

Histological examination should proceed systematically from anterior to posterior:

1 *Epithelium:*
   (a) *Changes in thickness:* hypertrophy (Figure 4.7) or atrophy (Figure 4.8).
   (b) *Oedema:* this is recognised by hyperlucency of basal cell cytoplasm (intracellular oedema – Figure 4.7) and an enlargement of the intercellular spaces (intercellular oedema – Figure 4.7). In advanced oedema, the epithelium separates from Bowman's layer to form a bulla (Figure 4.8).
   (c) *Ulceration:* destruction of the epithelium by microbiological pathogens leads to stromal disintegration and ultimately the rupture of Descemet's membrane. Collagenolysis is promoted by the action of collagenases (metalloproteinases) which are secreted by the intrinsic cells of the tissue (for example epithelial cells and keratocytes), polymorphonuclear leucocytes (PMNLs), and macrophages in addition to the pathogenic organisms. See Chapter 9.

2 *Bowman's layer:*
   (a) *Absence* (Figure 4.7) *or presence* (Figure 4.8): Bowman's layer is lost after traumatic or inflammatory damage.
   (b) *Calcification (band keratopathy):* tiny deposits of calcium salts are deposited in Bowman's layer in chronic

diseases such as sarcoidosis, uveitis, hyperparathyroidism, and usage of certain topical medications (Figures 4.9, 4.10). This abnormality is more commonly treated by mechanical removal and the application of decalcifying agents such as ethylene-diamine tetra-acetate (EDTA).
   (c) *Pannus:* Bowman's layer may be destroyed by fibrovascular inflammatory infiltrate in chronic disease, for example trachoma (Figure 4.11). See also Figure 4.20.
   (d) *Small breaks:* occur in keratoconus (see below).

3 *Stroma:*
   (a) In paraffin sections, mechanical stresses during microtomy separate the lamellae leaving clefts which are a common artefact and should not be mistaken for oedema.
   (b) *Keratocytes:* absence of keratocytes should raise the suspicion of irradiation, chemical injury, or acanthamoeba keratitis (see below).
   (c) *Scar:* replacement of the lamellae by fibroblasts indicates scarring due to previous ulceration or trauma (surgical and non-surgical). Initially the stroma is replaced by areas containing irregularly arranged plump spindle cells (transformed keratocytes) called myofibroblasts and invading capillaries (Figure 4.12). At a later stage, disorganised dense collagenous tissue is formed (Figure 4.13). See the section on the cornea under "Healing and repair in ocular tissues" in Chapter 9.
   (d) *Neovascularisation:* new blood vessels penetrating the stroma can be recognised by the presence of red cells in the lumen of capillaries (Figure 4.12). In many cases the capillaries are surrounded by inflammatory cells.
   (e) *Stromal deposits:* amorphous deposits in the absence of inflammation within the stroma should raise the suspicion of a dystrophy (see below).

Cornea - Non-specific pathology
Epithelial oedema

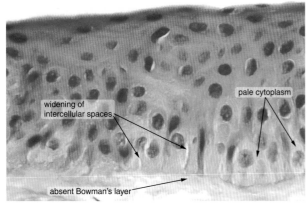

Figure 4.7

Figure 4.7 Corneal oedema can be identified by enlargement of the spaces between the cells and areas of hyperlucent cytoplasm. In this example, the epithelium is greatly increased in thickness to compensate for the loss of Bowman's layer and the surface stroma.

Cornea - Non-specific pathology
Oedema / Bulla formation

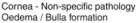
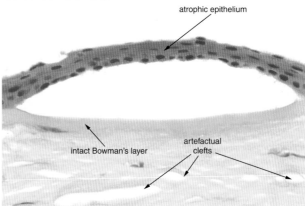

Figure 4.8

Figure 4.8 Excessive fluid movement across the cornea eventually leads to separation of an atrophic epithelium from Bowman's layer with the formation of a bulla. This abnormality is commonly seen in postaphakic corneal decompensation.

Cornea - Non-specific pathology
Band keratopathy

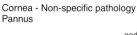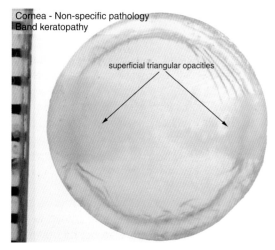

superficial triangular opacities

Figure 4.9

Cornea - Non-specific pathology
Band keratopathy

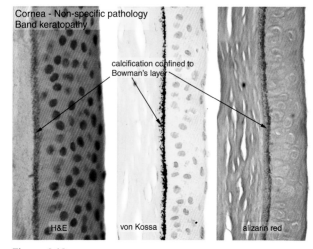

calcification confined to
Bowman's layer

H&E   von Kossa   alizarin red

Figure 4.10

Cornea - Non-specific pathology
Pannus

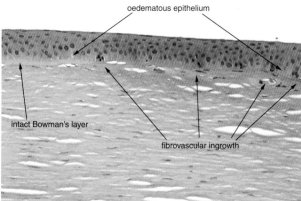

oedematous epithelium

intact Bowman's layer

fibrovascular ingrowth

Figure 4.11

Cornea - Non-specific pathology
Scar / Early stage

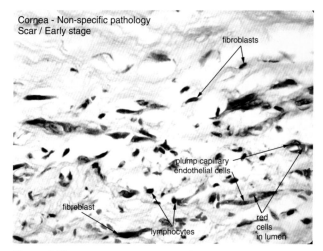

fibroblasts

plump capillary
endothelial cells

fibroblast

lymphocytes

red
cells
in lumen

Figure 4.12

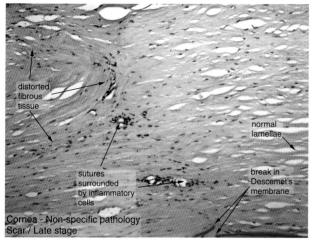

distorted
fibrous
tissue

normal
lamellae

sutures
surrounded
by inflammatory
cells

break in
Descemet's
membrane

Cornea - Non-specific pathology
Scar / Late stage

Figure 4.13

Figure 4.9 A keratoplasty was performed in the treatment of band keratopathy secondary to sarcoidosis but there are many other causes. The calcium deposits are best identified by retroillumination as wing-shaped opacities in the horizontal plane.

Figure 4.10 In an H&E preparation, the calcification appears as fine purple granules restricted to Bowman's layer. The von Kossa stain combines silver salts with calcium phosphate. The alizarin red stains by chelating calcium ions.

Figure 4.11 A common end stage in corneal disease is an ingrowth of fibrovascular tissue (pannus) into the superficial stroma with destruction of Bowman's layer.

Figure 4.12 An early response to any form of damage in the cornea takes the form of invasion by capillaries that contain red cells and transformation of keratocytes into plump spindle cells which have contractile properties, hence the name myofibroblasts. There will also be scattered inflammatory cell infiltrates.

Figure 4.13 An illustration of scar tissue at the site of a clear corneal incision in cataract surgery. A scar is recognised by the disorganised fibrous tissue that is unlike the normal lamella arrangement. The PAS stain reveals a break in Descemet's membrane and the suture material has induced a mild inflammatory response.

4 *Descemet's membrane:*
  (a) *Thickening* may be non-specific. Central nodules or excrescences (guttata) on the posterior surface are pathognomonic of Fuchs' endothelial dystrophy. Peripheral nodules are a non-specific ageing change.
  (b) *Multilayering* behind a Descemet's membrane of normal thickness is indicative of an endothelial dystrophy (for example congenital hereditary endothelial dystrophy (CHED) or iridocorneal endothelial syndrome (ICE)).
  (c) *Breaks in Descemet's membrane* occur after trauma (civil and surgical) and in keratoconus with hydrops (see below).
5 *Endothelium:*
  (a) *Attenuation or absence:* most commonly indicates postaphakic bullous keratopathy.
  (b) *Presence of inflammatory cells:* suggestive of rejection or viral infection.

Ulcerative keratitis

Infectious

Bacterial

Bacterial keratitis
Primary bacterial infection is extremely rare. Factors such as those that disrupt the integrity of surface epithelium expose the stroma and lead to secondary bacterial infection. Such predisposing conditions include bullous keratopathy, connective tissue disorders that affect the corneal periphery and, most importantly, trauma. With the increasing usage of contact lenses, bacterial keratitis has become more common.

Clinical presentation
A painful red eye with a localised abscess in the cornea accompanied by stromal ulceration should arouse clinical suspicion. There may be an acute uveitis with hypopyon.

Advanced untreated cases may result in corneal perforation with hypotonia.

Possible modes of treatment
In view of the overwhelming progression of bacterial keratitis, every effort should be taken to promptly diagnose and treat the infection. A corneal scrape should be performed immediately and sent to a bacteriology laboratory prior to initiation of intensive treatment using topical antibiotics such as cefuroxime and gentamicin. More specific therapy is applied once identification and antibiotic sensitivity of the microorganism is made.

Tectonic surgery is used in cases of impending perforation. The corneal ulcer may be covered by a corneal lamellar graft, conjunctival flap, or an amniotic membrane graft.

A penetrating keratoplasty may be used (see below).

Macroscopic
Three types of specimens may be submitted:
1 Corneal scrape.
2 Keratoplasty (full or partial thickness) specimen. A graft may be performed as an emergency to prevent hypotonia after perforation (Figure 4.14).
3 Enucleation or evisceration specimen from advanced cases. Failure to control pyogenic ulceration and perforation inevitably leads to endophthalmitis (Figure 4.15). Prolonged hypotonia after corneal perforation results in leakage from the choroidal vasculature and exudation into the tissues (Figure 4.16).

Microscopic
A pyogenic ulcer is the response to bacterial infection and is characterised by a dense PMNL infiltrate (Figures 4.17, 4.18).

As the untreated process extends, PMNLs migrate through the iris vessels into the anterior chamber (hypopyon). The anterior uveal tissues are infiltrated by lymphocytes and plasma cells (Figures 4.19, 4.20).

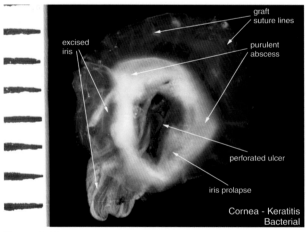

Figure 4.14

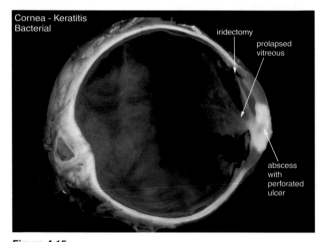

Figure 4.15

Figure 4.14 An ulcer developed within a corneal graft, as is evident from pre-existing suture lines. The patient had an irritated red eye for several days and continued to use his topical steroids. A bacterial keratitis ensued and, at the time of presentation, there was a corneal perforation with iris prolapse. The ulcerated area was excised and replaced by donor tissue. The penetrating keratoplasty specimen contained a large ulcer surrounded by purulent material with iris tissue adherent to the defect.

Figure 4.15 Enucleation was necessary after a corneal ulcer perforated in an aphakic eye (intracapsular cataract extraction). The predisposing cause was a decompensated cornea complicated by bullous keratopathy and secondary infection.

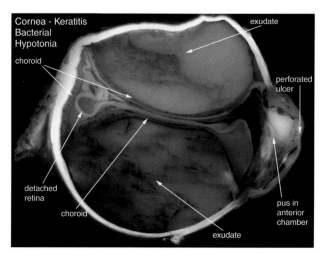

Figure 4.16

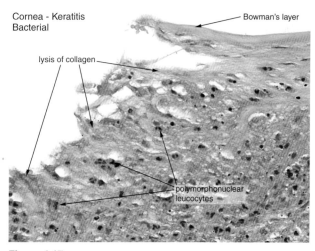

Figure 4.17

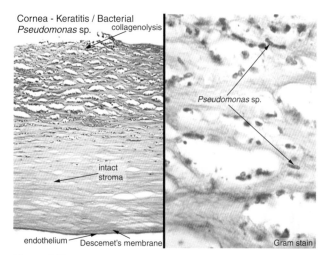

Figure 4.18

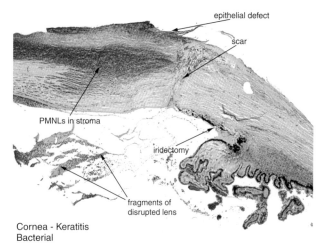

Figure 4.19

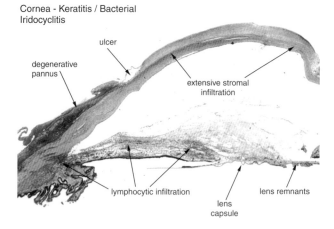

Figure 4.20

Figure 4.16 Intracapsular cataract surgery was complicated by bacterial keratitis. The enucleation specimen shows the effects of prolonged hypotonia after corneal ulceration and perforation. The choroid is detached by exudate which leads to compression of the retina.

Figure 4.17 The stroma at the edge of a pyogenic corneal ulcer contains numerous polymorphonuclear leucocytes (PMNLs) and the epithelium is absent. The lamellar architecture is lost and the frayed collagen is the result of widespread collagenolysis. Bacteria may not be identified if intensive treatment is employed.

Figure 4.18 The superficial half of the cornea has been invaded by *Pseudomonas* sp. (left). Collagenolysis in the infected area is striking in comparison with the stroma of the intact cornea. The organisms appear as short stubby rods and are Gram negative (right).

Figure 4.19 Corneal ulceration complicates secondary glaucoma due to loss of surface integrity in bullous keratopathy. In this archival example, a drainage procedure (Scheie's procedure) failed and the fistula was closed by scar tissue.

Figure 4.20 As ulceration evolves, there is a secondary non-granulomatous iridocyclitis. The peripheral cornea is invaded by fibrovascular tissue and a lymphocytic infiltrate (degenerative pannus). This end stage resulted from bullous keratopathy after complicated cataract surgery.

Sequelae are:

1 *Healing:* scar tissue forms at the site of the previous ulcer (Figure 4.21).
2 *Descemetocoele:* Descemet's membrane is resistant to collagenolysis and repair takes place by growth of the epithelium onto the anterior surface of the membrane (Figures 4.22, 4.23). This condition can remain stable for considerable amounts of time. This condition is more common as a sequel to viral keratitis (see below).
3 *Perforation* (Figures 4.14–4.16).

Special investigations/stains

1 *Gram stain* is used to identify and classify bacteria in tissue (Figure 4.18) and in corneal scrapes (Figures 4.24–4.27). Refer also to Chapter 1. Note that Gram positive bacteria following antibiotic treatment can become Gram negative in appearance.
2 *Brown and Brenn stain* is favoured in the USA. This stain is useful for visualising Gram negative organisms and *Nocardia* sp.
3 *Culture media* are described in Chapter 1. Note the use of antibiotics before scrape or biopsy may render culture media ineffective.

Bacterial crystalline keratopathy

Topical treatment with steroids after surgical interventions of various types (keratoplasty, keratotomy, epikeratoplasty) may be complicated by bacterial proliferation in the stroma. The important feature is that the inflammatory reaction is suppressed. The relative absence of stromal necrosis hints at the importance of metalloproteinase release from the intrinsic cells of the cornea and inflammatory cells (see Chapter 9).

Clinical presentation

White crystalline stromal opacities are evident (Figure 4.28). Cessation of topical steroid therapy rapidly progresses the appearances to that of a typical pyogenic bacterial keratitis. Treatment involves a corneal scrape for culture and sensitivity followed by intensive topical antibiotic.

Pathogenesis

Immunosuppression, usually in the form of steroids, allows unhindered proliferation of bacteria, most commonly *Streptococcus viridans*. It is assumed that the organisms are introduced following minor trauma.

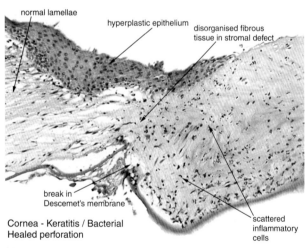

Cornea - Keratitis / Bacterial
Healed perforation

Figure 4.21

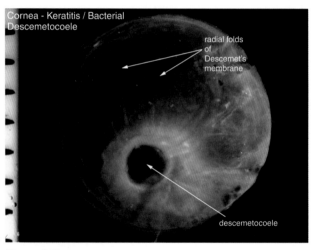

Cornea - Keratitis / Bacterial Descemetocoele

Figure 4.22

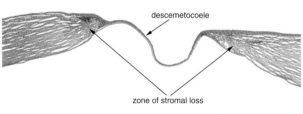

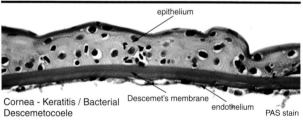

Cornea - Keratitis / Bacterial Descemetocoele

Figure 4.23

Figure 4.21 A small corneal ulcer had destroyed the stroma and had ruptured Descemet's membrane. Bowman's layer is absent. Partial healing has taken the form of disorganised fibrous tissue proliferation. To compensate for corneal thinning, the epithelium is hyperplastic. Inflammatory cell infiltration is sparse due to intensive antibiotic treatment.

Figure 4.22 In a keratoplasty specimen, a descemetocoele appears as a 1–2 mm circular area of extreme thinning. The brown material on the surface is artefactual.

Figure 4.23 A corneal ulcer has destroyed a sector of the stroma (upper) resulting in a descemetocoele. The intact Descemet's membrane (stained red with PAS) is lined by epithelial and endothelial cells (lower).

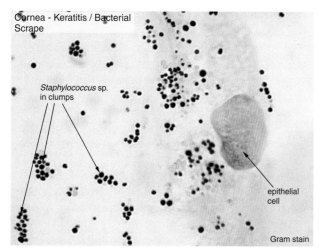

Figure 4.24

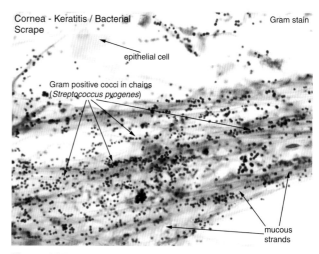

Figure 4.25

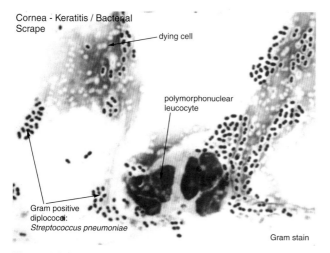

Figure 4.26

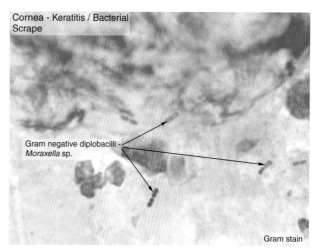

Figure 4.27

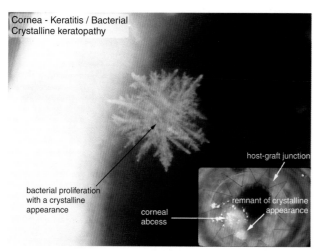

Figure 4.28

Figure 4.24 In a scrape from a corneal ulcer, *Staphylococcus aureus* is Gram positive and forms clumps.

Figure 4.25 *Streptococcus pyogenes* is identified by the chain-like arrangement of the organisms in a Gram stain from a corneal scrape.

Figure 4.26 *Streptococcus pneumoniae* is easily identified as a Gram positive diplococcus surrounded by a capsule. The organisms are intracellular and this excludes the possibility of artefactual contamination.

Figure 4.27 An intractable keratitis was treated by enucleation. Histology of the cornea revealed Gram negative diplobacilli subsequently identified by culture as a *Moraxella* sp.

Figure 4.28 Radiating crystalline opacities are characteristic of bacterial crystalline keratopathy in a patient on topical steroids. Twenty-four hours after the cessation of steroids, the appearance changes to that of a more typical corneal abscess (inset).

Pathology

A corneal scrape or a disc containing opaque white areas will be submitted. There may be evidence of previous surgical intervention or trauma.

On microscopic examination, clumps of bacteria within the stroma are easily identified with a Gram stain. Vascularisation and inflammatory cell infiltration are minimal (Figures 4.29, 4.30).

Fungal

An uncommon infection which tends to affect immunocompromised or debilitated patients. Trauma involving plant material can be a predisposing cause.

Clinical presentation

The slowly progressive corneal opacity is characteristically white with feathery edges and there may be smaller satellite lesions. Suspicion of this condition should arise in predisposed patients, particularly if there is a failure to respond to topical antibiotic treatment.

Possible modes of treatment

Treatment will depend on the correct identification of the fungal organism and includes:
- topical antifungals such as natamycin, myconazole, and amphotericin
- penetrating or lamellar keratoplasty
- enucleation.

Pathology

Specimens may be submitted in the following forms:
1 Corneal biopsy: this would be more common.
2 Keratoplasty (full or partial thickness) specimen.
3 Enucleation specimen.

If a fungal infection is suspected, a tissue sample should be submitted to a mycology laboratory.

Fungi are the largest microbiological pathogens and can be subdivided on the following morphological grounds:
1 *Yeasts:* unicellular organisms that reproduce by budding, but which form hyphae in tissues (Figures 4.31, 4.32).
2 *Filamentous:* multicellular with branching hyphae. These are further subdivided into septate (for example *Aspergillus* sp. – Figure 4.33) or non-septate (for example *Mucor* sp. – see Chapter 5).
3 *Dimorphic fungi:* unicellular organisms which possess a yeast phase in tissues and a mycelial phase in culture (for example *Histoplasma* sp., *Blastomyces* sp., and *Coccidioides* sp.).

Pathogenic fungi invade and destroy the corneal stroma, penetrate Descemet's membrane, and induce a pyogenic inflammatory reaction that can extend into the anterior chamber (Figure 4.34).

Special stains used for identifying fungi
1 *Periodic acid-Schiff (PAS):* stains cell walls, septae (red), and nuclei (blue).
2 *Methenamine-silver* (Grocott–Gomori): stains cell walls (black).
3 *Gram:* stains positive (blue).
4 *Giemsa:* stains organisms (blue).

Protozoal – acanthamoeba

Acanthamoebal keratitis was initially a problem associated with reusable contact lenses cleaned by inappropriate disinfection procedures. These free living protozoa are found in many water sources including tap water and swimming pools. The organisms survive by ingesting bacteria and exist in two forms: a motile trophozoite and a dormant cyst. The latter form is resistant to chemical treatment.

Figure 4.29 In a routine H&E section of bacterial crystalline keratopathy, clumps of bacteria appear as smudgy pink areas. Inflammatory cells are absent from the stroma. The surface is ulcerated and lined by a layer of fibrin.

Figure 4.30 In this example of bacterial crystalline keratopathy, the bacteria are located in the anterior part of the stroma. As is typical, inflammatory cells are absent from the stroma.

Figure 4.31 In this corneal scrape from a corneal ulcer, the budding yeasts of *Candida* sp. are easily demonstrated by a Gram stain. The yeasts are almost as large as the nucleus of an epithelial cell, and therefore much larger than cocci (both stain Gram positive).

Figure 4.32 In a corneal biopsy, the fungal elements of *Candida* proliferate between the lamellae and the keratocytes are destroyed (Gram stain). The inset shows that the yeasts are budding off the hyphae (PAS stain).

Figure 4.33 A silver stain which localises to the cell walls of fungal hyphae is useful for identifying the branching septate hyphae of *Aspergillus* sp. The inset shows a higher magnification of the branching septate hyphae (methenamine silver/Grocott–Gomori stain).

Figure 4.34 Fungal infection is usually most advanced in the posterior corneal stroma and destruction of Descemet's membrane permits access into the anterior chamber. This is a rare type of dimorphic fungus (*Acrimonium* sp.) which possesses branching hyphae and an ability to form yeasts. The patient was struck in the eye by a piece of rotting wood.

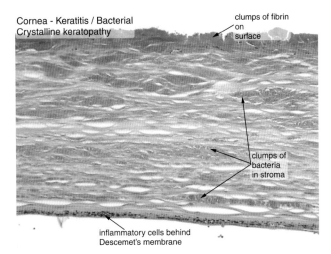

Cornea - Keratitis / Bacterial
Crystalline keratopathy

clumps of fibrin on surface

clumps of bacteria in stroma

inflammatory cells behind Descemet's membrane

Figure 4.29

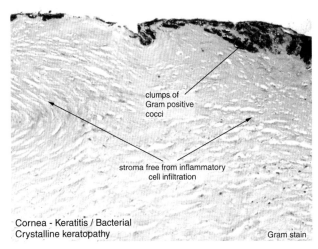

clumps of Gram positive cocci

stroma free from inflammatory cell infiltration

Cornea - Keratitis / Bacterial
Crystalline keratopathy

Gram stain

Figure 4.30

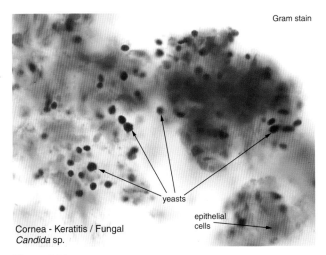

Gram stain

yeasts

epithelial cells

Cornea - Keratitis / Fungal
Candida sp.

Figure 4.31

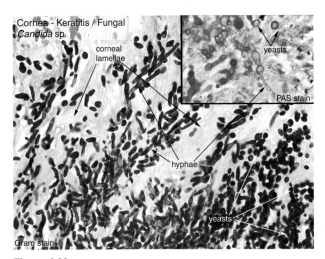

Cornea - Keratitis / Fungal
Candida sp.

corneal lamellae

yeasts

PAS stain

hyphae

yeasts

Gram stain

Figure 4.32

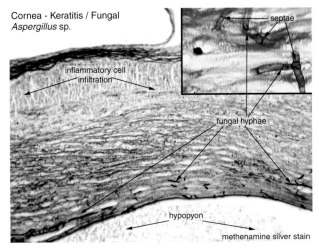

Cornea - Keratitis / Fungal
Aspergillus sp.

septae

inflammatory cell infiltration

fungal hyphae

hypopyon

methenamine silver stain

Figure 4.33

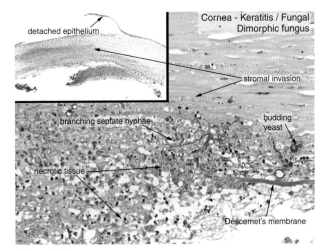

detached epithelium

Cornea - Keratitis / Fungal
Dimorphic fungus

stromal invasion

branching septate hyphae

budding yeast

necrotic tissue

Descemet's membrane

Figure 4.34

Clinical presentation

The patient presents with a painful red eye that in early stages may resemble a bacterial keratitis. Ring infiltrates as well as smaller satellite lesions are common (Figure 4.35). Perineural invasion leads to the appearance of prominent corneal nerves and the patient's discomfort is often out of proportion to the relatively insignificant appearance of the infection. At advanced untreated stages, a hypopyon and scleritis may develop.

Pathogenesis

The most common form of infection occurs when the patient uses soft contact lenses colonised with microorganisms such as bacteria in addition to protozoa. Contaminated contact lens disinfection fluids or washing with tap water are the usual sources of contact lens colonisation.

The protozoon, in sufficient concentration, is capable of invasion of the epithelium. The organism migrates between stromal lamellae and destroys and phagocytoses keratocytes. In many cases, inflammatory cell infiltration is minimal but opportunistic pathogens can induce a pyogenic keratitis.

Diagnosis

The preferred method is to inoculate the material obtained by a corneal scrape onto a confluent layer of *Escherichia coli* grown on non-nutrient agar. Phagocytosis of bacteria is manifest as characteristic streaks in the layer of cultured bacteria. Most microbiology departments require 24 hours' notice in order to prepare the plates.

Examination of wet specimens by phase contrast microscopy allows the identification of trophozoites and cysts.

Confocal microscopy can be used to identify the organisms *in vivo*.

Possible modes of treatment

Topical treatment includes chlorhexidine, polyhexamethylene biguanide (PHMB), propamidine (Brolene), neosporin,

and ketaconazole. The combination of treatment modalities varies among departments. Even though the overall treatment success has improved, the failure rate is based on the fact that none of the medications are cysticidal *in vivo*.

Early surgical intervention by penetrating keratoplasty is preferred to prevent peripheral spread and colonisation.

Paradigm shifts

The use of disposable lenses and the greater awareness of the importance of hygiene have reduced the incidence of infection.

Recent research suggests that other amoebic protozoa (*Vahlkampfia* sp., *Hartmanella* sp.) may be responsible for disease in some individuals.

Macroscopic

1 *Corneal scrape:* by light microscopy, identification of protozoa in corneal scrapes is extremely difficult.
2 *Corneal biopsy:* tiny fragments of tissue are submitted – these are best studied by transmission electron microscopy.
3 *Corneal disc:* retroillumination will show opacification either in the form of haziness or more discrete opacities in secondary infection.
4 *Enucleation:* colonisation of the corneal periphery reduces the success rate of a penetrating keratoplasty due to reinfection of the graft and secondary keratitis resistant to treatment.

Microscopic

At low power, acanthamoebal keratitis should be suspected if the epithelium is absent and the keratocyte content of the stroma is reduced (Figure 4.36).

The organism can be identified in a biopsy or in a keratoplasty specimen using conventional stains (Figure 4.37). In the presence of secondary infection and inflammation, the identification of organisms is much more difficult (Figure 4.38).

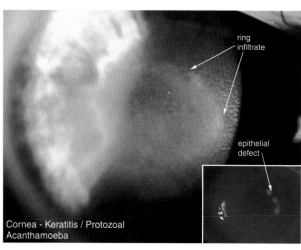

Figure 4.35

Figure 4.35 Slit-lamp photograph to show the ring infiltrate of acanthamoebal keratitis. Fluorescein staining demonstrates the loss of epithelial integrity (inset).

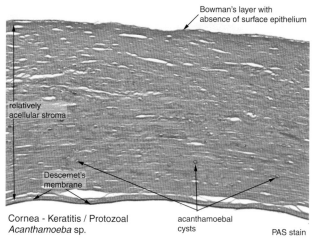

Figure 4.36

Figure 4.36 In a keratoplasty specimen viewed at low power, acanthamoebal keratitis should be suspected if the epithelium is absent, the keratocyte content is reduced, and round or oval structures are scattered throughout the stroma (PAS stain).

Immunohistochemistry

Immunolabelling with an antibody against *Acanthamoeba* provides precise identification (Figure 4.39).

Special investigations/stains

Calcofluor white with fluorescent microscopy is recommended by some authors.

Viral

The DNA viruses, herpes simplex and herpes zoster, are the commonest viral infections of the cornea.

Herpes simplex

Clinical presentation

Primary infection Vesicular eruptions, usually in children, involving the eyelids and lips (cold sores). Corneal involvement is rare. A minor follicular conjunctivitis may occur.

Recurrent infection

1 *Acute stage:* a unilateral painful red eye with superficial ulceration taking the form of club shaped finger-like processes (dendritic/dendritiform). Fluorescein stains the epithelial defect and Rose Bengal identifies dead epithelial cells along the edge of the defect.

2 *Chronic stage:* the disease may progress to ulceration, scarring, or perforation (necrotising form) or to non-necrotising forms – see below.

Pathogenesis

Following primary infection involving the eyelids or the labial mucosa, the herpes simplex virus (HSV) migrates to the trigeminal ganglion and lies dormant. A variety of possible triggers (for example UV light, trauma, menstruation, steroids) reactivate the virus which migrates along the sensory nerves to the corneal epithelium. The epithelium is invaded and the viral particles proliferate within the nucleus and cytoplasm. The epithelial nuclear DNA and nuclear membrane are used to form components of the replicating viral particles. Epithelial cells which have been killed detach from the surface.

Recurrent disease may lead to ulceration with destruction of Bowman's layer and viral invasion of keratocytes. Death of these cells releases collagenases (metalloproteinases) and stromal dissolution results (viral necrotising keratitis) with inflammatory cell infiltration. Descemetocoele formation and corneal perforation may ensue. Such severe sequelae may be prevented by fibrous tissue scarring. Vascular invasion leads to leakage of plasma lipids.

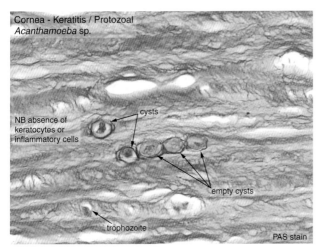

Figure 4.37

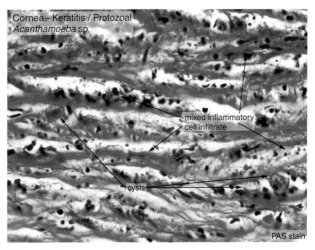

Figure 4.38

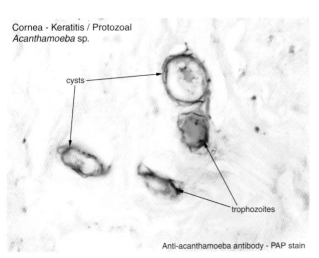

Figure 4.39

Figure 4.37 In a keratoplasty specimen viewed at a higher power, cysts may contain nuclei or be empty due to migration of the protozoa to form trophozoites. At the latter stage, it is difficult to identify the organism (PAS stain).

Figure 4.38 This is an example of bacterial superinfection in acanthamoebal keratitis. The presence of large numbers of inflammatory cells makes it difficult to identify trophozoites but cysts are still evident (PAS stain).

Figure 4.39 With the immunohistochemical technique, the organisms are stained with an anti-acanthamoebal antibody. The antibody labels the walls of the cyst and the cytoplasm of the trophozoites (PAP label).

An alternative non-necrotising form of damage involves the endothelium which is followed by localised stromal oedema (disciform oedema). Inflammatory cell infiltration in the anterior chamber is manifest on slit-lamp examination as flare and clusters of cells on the endothelium (keratic precipitates). A non-granulomatous iritis and trabeculitis with secondary glaucoma may also be present.

Possible modes of treatment
1 Antiviral medications including: acyclovir, trifluridine, vidarabine, and idoxuridine.
2 Steroids in chronic disciform oedema.
3 Cyanoacrylate glue, lamellar and penetrating keratoplasty for perforations and scarring.

Paradigm shifts
The advent of effective antiviral treatment has decreased the incidence of complications.

Polymerase chain reaction (PCR) and immunofluorescence microscopy (using a fluorescent HSV antibody label) provide rapid identification of the viral type.

Macroscopic
When presented to the pathologist, the specimen is usually in the form of a corneal disc that contains a descemetocoele (Figure 4.22) or extensive scarring (Figure 4.40).

Microscopic
In early cases, it is sometimes possible to identify intranuclear inclusions in the infected epithelial cells (Figure 4.41).

If the virus spreads into the stroma, the keratocytes are infected and the inflammatory cells enter the stroma via small blood vessels. These vessels leak plasma which contains lipids such as cholesterol, and a giant cell granulomatous reaction is induced by the residual lipids and the cholesterol crystals (Figure 4.42). The lamellae are replaced by fibrous tissue. Secondary lipid keratopathy is not confined to herpes simplex, but is also seen in herpes zoster, and after severe trauma and chemical injury. Primary lipid keratopathy is extremely rare (see below).

In the necrotising form of infection the stroma is destroyed by secondary inflammatory cell infiltration, although Descemet's membrane is frequently preserved (Figure 4.43). Leucocytes, macrophages, and lymphoplasmacytoid cells are found in the inflammatory infiltrate.

Special investigations/stains
1 Phloxine-tartrazine stains the intranuclear inclusions purple or red (Figure 4.41).
2 Giemsa and Papanicolaou stains may be preferred by some pathologists.
3 PCR to identify viral DNA is now in common usage, but in the past transmission electron microscopy was useful for identification of the viral particles (Figure 4.44).

Herpes zoster
The pathological features of herpes zoster infection of the cornea are very similar to those described for chronic herpes simplex. The features of varicella zoster ophthalmicus are described in the Chapter 8.

Syphilis
The corneal manifestation of syphilis is in the form of interstitial keratitis – refer to Chapter 8.

Non-infectious

Rheumatoid

The ocular complications of this common systemic collagen disorder are often serious and sight threatening. This section is restricted to a description of the corneal pathology but other features of rheumatoid disease include secondary Sjögren's syndrome, episcleritis, and scleritis.

Clinical presentation
Patients present with symptoms commonly associated with dry eye or keratoconjunctivitis sicca. Ulceration and stromal lysis can be paracentral or peripheral and can evolve rapidly. While there appears to be a multitude of clinical variations of corneal disorders associated with rheumatoid disease, in keratoplasty specimens there are two variants:
1 Stromal lysis in the presence of inflammatory cell infiltration.
2 Stromal lysis in the absence of inflammatory cell infiltration.

Pathogenesis
Various factors have been implicated in both variants of rheumatoid keratitis:
1 Unstable epithelium due to decreased tear production favours bacterial colonisation and/or migration of acute inflammatory cells.
2 Occlusive microangiopathy in limbal vessels (due to immune complex deposition) leads to tissue ischaemia.
3 Production of collagenases (metalloproteinases) and proteases by keratocytes initiates a collagenolytic cascade. A reduction in tissue inhibitors of metalloproteinases (TIMPs) also contributes to collagenolysis.
4 Release of interferon γ from T-helper 2 lymphocytes in the limbus stimulates macrophagic activity.

Genetics
Females predominate in this disease. There is also an increased frequency of HLA-DR1 and HLA-DR4.

Possible modes of treatment
Definitive treatments vary according to the institution and are beyond the scope of this text but involve the following principles:
1 Promotion of epithelial healing with improved lubrication of the eye using artificial tears, mucolytic agents, and procedures to reduce tear drainage.
2 Topical and systemic immunosuppressants with or without cytotoxic therapy.
3 Amniotic membrane or conjunctival grafts in impending perforation.
4 Surgery: cyanoacrylate glue and keratoplasty for perforation.

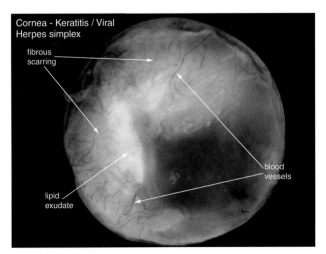

Figure 4.40

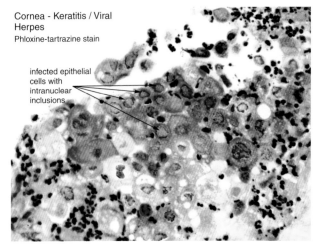

Figure 4.41

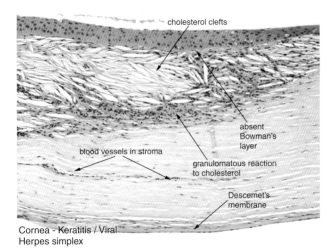

Figure 4.42

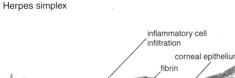

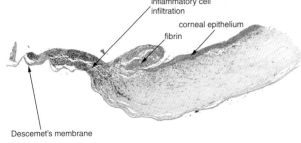

Figure 4.43

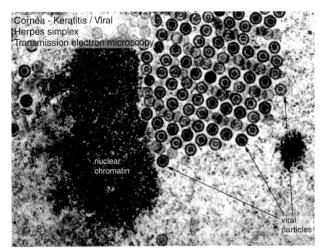

Figure 4.44

Figure 4.40 Prior to antiviral therapy, penetrating keratoplasties were often performed in the treatment of the complications of herpes simplex keratitis. Scarring is extensive and lipid leakage from the neovascularisation produces yellow deposits (secondary lipid keratopathy).

Figure 4.41 The disrupted infected cells in herpes simplex keratitis contain intranuclear inclusions. The nuclear chromatin is replaced by amorphous pink- or purple-staining material when demonstrated by using a special stain (phloxine-tartrazine stain).

Figure 4.42 Secondary lipid keratopathy from neovascular leakage is a common complication of advanced herpes simplex keratitis. The lipid is in the form of cholesterol crystals which are removed in tissue processing leaving needle-like spaces. The presence of these crystals induces a granulomatous reaction. In this example the adjacent lamellar architecture is preserved.

Figure 4.43 Herpes keratitis can be complicated by secondary bacterial infection leading to stromal lysis but with preservation of Descemet's membrane. Epithelial defects may be plugged by fibrin. Note the absence of an epithelium in the region of the ulcer bed which is in keeping with the initial epithelial damage in HSV keratitis. This should be compared with rheumatoid ulceration, in which the stroma is the initial focus of tissue destruction (see Figure 4.48).

Figure 4.44 Electron microscopy demonstrating the structure of the viral particles of herpes simplex. The central core is surrounded by a layer called a capsid.

Macroscopic

The most likely specimen would be in the form of a corneal disc from a penetrating keratoplasty (Figure 4.45).

In cases failing to respond to treatment, an enucleation specimen will be submitted.

Microscopic

In common with the two subsets described below, the epithelium is relatively unaffected by comparison with herpes simplex ulceration.

1 *Inflammatory:*
  (a) In paracentral ulcers, the inflammatory reaction is in close proximity to the ulcer and is of lymphoplasmacytoid type (Figures 4.46, 4.47).
  (b) In peripheral ulcerative keratitis (PUK), the inflammatory reaction is much more intense due to the adjacent vascular limbus which facilitates migration of inflammatory cells (Figure 4.48).
2 *Non-inflammatory:* this form of ulceration and perforation is usually paracentral and is characterised by minimal inflammatory cell infiltration. The presumed mechanism of damage is that of a collagenolytic cascade initiated by intrinsic corneal cells (Figures 4.49, 4.50).

Pathological evidence of treatment

Evidence of a cyanoacrylate glue plug (Figures 4.45, 4.46) or an amniotic membrane (see below) may be present.

Wegener's granulomatosis

This disease may present with peripheral corneal ulceration that is thought to be due to immune complex deposition in the limbal vessels (see Chapter 5). The appearances are similar to those shown for inflammatory rheumatoid peripheral ulcerative keratitis (Figure 4.48).

Degenerations

Non-specific degenerations are commonly encountered in the form of abnormal materials deposited within the corneal layers.

Band (calcium) keratopathy

This consists of a horizontal wing-shaped superficial opacity consisting of calcium hydroxyapatite crystals found in the Bowman's layer. See "How to examine a corneal specimen", p. 62 (Figures 4.9, 4.10).

Spheroidal degeneration (climatic droplet keratopathy/Labrador keratopathy)

Spheroidal degeneration is manifest clinically as a specific bilateral *primary* disease entity in which tiny yellow spherical bodies are scattered throughout the superficial stroma. One cause of this abnormality is overexposure to UV radiation as in arctic or desert environments. The precise biochemical nature of these deposits is unknown but keratin has been identified within the compound.

Deposits of keratin-containing material are also seen as a non-specific *secondary* change in chronic corneal inflammatory disease (Figure 4.51). These deposits are usually located within scar tissue and appear as discrete yellow/orange particles using a Masson stain (Figure 4.52).

The histological appearances of the primary and secondary types are identical.

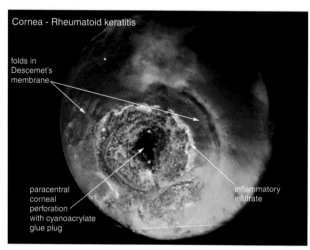

Figure 4.45

Figure 4.45 A rheumatoid patient developed a spontaneous paracentral inflammatory ulceration with perforation. The defect was temporarily occluded with a cyanoacrylate glue plug (pale purple) while awaiting penetrating keratoplasty.

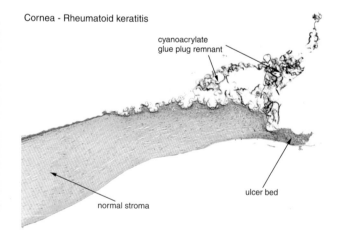

Figure 4.46

Figure 4.46 Low power micrograph from the same case shown in Figure 4.45. The ulcer bed contains inflammatory cells (lymphocytes) and contraction of the cyanoacrylate glue plug has caused undulations on the corneal surface. The adjacent corneal stroma is free from inflammation and neovascularisation.

Cornea - Rheumatoid keratitis

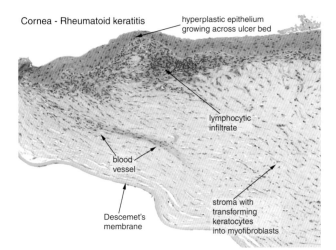

hyperplastic epithelium growing across ulcer bed

lymphocytic infiltrate

blood vessel

Descemet's membrane

stroma with transforming keratocytes into myofibroblasts

Figure 4.47

Cornea - Rheumatoid keratitis

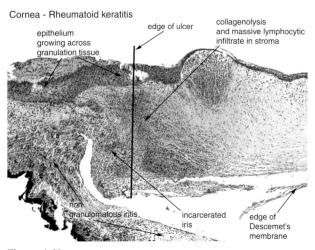

epithelium growing across granulation tissue

edge of ulcer

collagenolysis and massive lymphocytic infiltrate in stroma

non granulomatous iritis

incarcerated iris

edge of Descemet's membrane

Figure 4.48

Cornea - Rheumatoid keratitis Non inflammatory

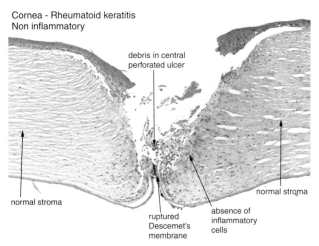

debris in central perforated ulcer

normal stroma

normal stroma

ruptured Descemet's membrane

absence of inflammatory cells

Figure 4.49

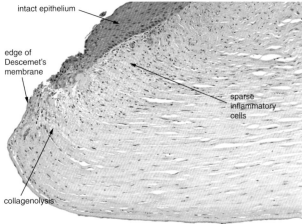

intact epithelium

edge of Descemet's membrane

sparse inflammatory cells

collagenolysis

Cornea - Rheumatoid keratitis / Non inflammatory

Figure 4.50

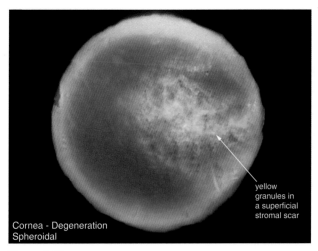

Cornea - Degeneration Spheroidal

yellow granules in a superficial stromal scar

Figure 4.51

Figure 4.47 The opposite edge of the ulcer (shown in Figure 4.46) is lined by hyperplastic epithelium and there is a dense lymphocytic infiltration in the underlying stroma. The keratocytes respond to the cytokines released by the inflammatory cells and transform into myofibroblasts. The delivery of inflammatory cells to the site is facilitated by neovascularisation.

Figure 4.48 In peripheral inflammatory ulcerative keratitis the vascular limbus provides ready access for inflammatory cells. The perforated ulcer in this example is plugged internally by the peripheral iris. As the pathological process is confined to the corneal stroma, the epithelial cells are less affected in comparison with a herpes keratitis.

Figure 4.49 In acute rheumatoid ulceration and perforation, the edges of the ulcer are straight and the defect is filled by necrotic cells. In this example, Descemet's membrane is ruptured. Inflammatory cell infiltration is often minimal in rheumatoid keratitis and the adjacent stroma is normal. The epithelium is detached at the edge of the ulcer, presumably due to aqueous egress.

Figure 4.50 At a later stage of rheumatoid ulceration, the epithelium grows across the defect. Inflammatory cells are sparse in the stroma. Descemet's membrane has rolled across the edge of the ulcer.

Figure 4.51 A non-specific change in the superficial corneal scar tissue is manifest as an accumulation of spherical yellow granules so that the term "spheroidal degeneration" is appropriate.

Cornea - Degeneration
Spheroidal

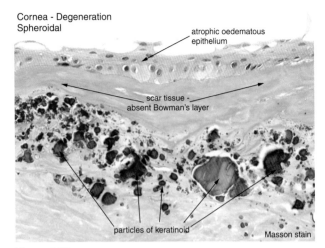

atrophic oedematous epithelium

scar tissue - absent Bowman's layer

particles of keratinoid

Masson stain

Figure 4.52

Cornea - Degeneration
Secondary amyloid deposit

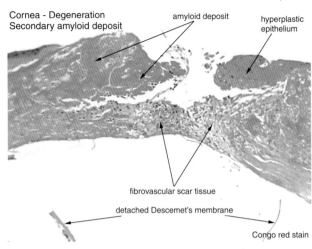

amyloid deposit

hyperplastic epithelium

fibrovascular scar tissue

detached Descemet's membrane

Congo red stain

Figure 4.53

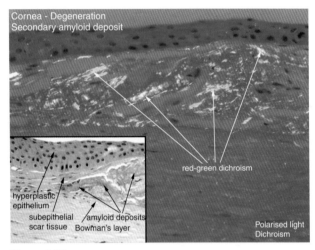

Cornea - Degeneration
Secondary amyloid deposit

red-green dichroism

hyperplastic epithelium

subepithelial scar tissue

amyloid deposits Bowman's layer

Polarised light
Dichroism

Figure 4.54

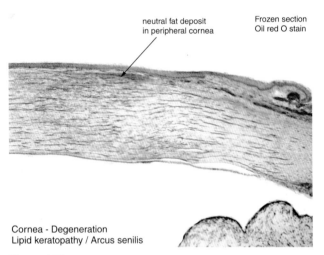

neutral fat deposit in peripheral cornea

Frozen section
Oil red O stain

Cornea - Degeneration
Lipid keratopathy / Arcus senilis

Figure 4.55

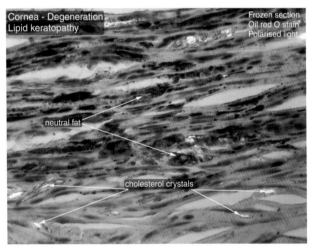

Cornea - Degeneration
Lipid keratopathy

Frozen section
Oil red O stain
Polarised light

neutral fat

cholesterol crystals

Figure 4.56

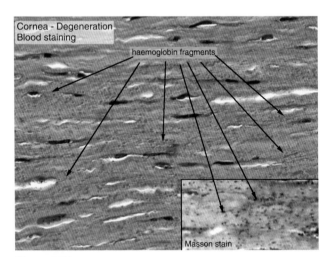

Cornea - Degeneration
Blood staining

haemoglobin fragments

Masson stain

Figure 4.57

Secondary amyloidosis

Although amyloid deposition is the primary abnormality in lattice dystrophy (see below), occasionally isolated amyloid deposits occur in corneal scar tissue (Figures 4.53, 4.54).

Lipid – primary and secondary

The most common form of lipid deposit is seen in arcus senilis (Figure 4.55), which is a primary condition. In an extremely rare primary lipoidal degeneration of the cornea (Schnyder's crystalline keratopathy), cholesterol crystals are deposited within keratocytes and the adjacent stroma.

Neutral fats and cholesterol are deposited as secondary lipid deposits during corneal inflammatory disease with vascularisation (Figures 4.42, 4.56).

Blood staining

When a prolonged hyphaema is associated with a high intraocular pressure, fragments of haemoglobin diffuse into the corneal stroma (Figure 4.57). Inflammatory cell infiltration is not a feature so that macrophages are not recruited to remove the red cell debris. This explains the persistence of corneal blood staining in the clinical setting.

Dystrophies

The term: "corneal dystrophies" is applied to a group of bilateral, inherited, and progressive disorders in which minor corneal opacification may lead ultimately to debilitating visual impairment.

It is conventional in describing corneal dystrophies to use anatomical subdivisions, i.e. epithelial, stromal, and endothelial. Stromal dystrophies are by far the commonest in pathological practice.

Epithelial dystrophies

The epithelial dystrophies are extremely rare. One example of an epithelial dystrophy would be Cogan's "map-dot-fingerprint" in which cystic spaces appear within the epithelium. Another is Meesmann's dystrophy, in which there is excessive basement membrane deposition within the layers of the epithelium.

Stromal dystrophies

The pathological classification of stromal dystrophies is supplemented by the use of special stains:
1 *Periodic acid-Schiff (PAS):* mucopolysaccharides – red/magenta. Pink background (stroma).
2 *Masson:* keratohyaline – red. Green background (stroma).
3 *Congo red/Sirius red:* amyloid – orange/red (with red-green dichroism in polarised light). Pink background (stroma).
4 *Hale's colloidal iron/Alcian blue:* mucopolysaccharides – blue/green. Pale green background (stroma) depending on the counterstain.

A useful mnemonic for stromal dystrophies is: "Marilyn Monroe Always Gets Her Man in LA City":

Marilyn	Macular
Monroe	Mucopolysaccharides
Always	Alcian blue stain
Gets	Granular
Her	Hyaline
Man in	Masson
L	Lattice
A	Amyloid
City	Congo red

Figure 4.52 The biochemical constituents of keratinoid particles are unknown. With the Masson stain, the particles are red or yellow in colour. The stain also highlights stromal fibrosis, which is the precursor of secondary spheroidal degeneration.

Figure 4.53 A large deposit of amyloid is present in scar tissue at the edge of a healed corneal perforation. The original defect is filled by fibrovascular tissue. Descemet's membrane is detached by an artefact.

Figure 4.54 The use of polarised light reveals that the amyloid deposits exhibit either red or green dichroism. The inset shows the equivalent area with Congo red staining (without the use of polarised light) – the amyloid deposits in the subepithelial scar tissue appear as irregular red clumps. In this case, there was a previous history of trauma.

Figure 4.55 In arcus senilis, a C-shaped band of lipid is deposited at the edge of the cornea. This section was taken from frozen tissue mounted in gelatin and was stained with Oil red O for fat.

Figure 4.56 In secondary lipid keratopathy, a frozen section was stained with Oil red O. The tissue was examined in polarised light which revealed tiny cholesterol crystals and red staining neutral lipids. In routine paraffin sectioning, cholesterol crystals are seen as clefts (see Figure 4.42).

Figure 4.57 When a hyphaema persists, the red cells break down in the anterior chamber and fragments which possess a granular appearance diffuse into the corneal stroma. The red cell fragments are demonstrated as blue spots by the Masson stain (inset). The iron atoms are bound within the haem molecule and staining for iron is negative.

Genetics (5q31)

The beta transforming growth factor-induced gene (βig-H3, also known as TGFβ1) located on chromosome 5q31 encodes the protein keratoepithelin which functions as an adhesion protein and is strongly expressed by the corneal epithelium.

The following stromal dystrophies are related to point mutations on the βig-H3 gene:
- Reis–Bückler dystrophy
- granular dystrophy
- lattice dystrophy
- avellino dystrophy
- Thiel–Behnke dystrophy.

The theory for the different appearances (phenotypes) of each dystrophy is based on the different diffusion properties of the mutated keratoepithelin proteins and their abilities to aggregate to form amyloid deposits.

The above dystrophies all have in common an *autosomal dominant* inheritance.

Reis–Bückler dystrophy

This is an autosomal dominant corneal dystrophy that presents in early adult life as fine reticular opacities in the superficial stroma. The histological features are non-specific and the diagnosis depends on the clinical appearance, identification of inheritance, and bilaterality. There is no evidence of inflammation or neovascularisation in the stroma and nodules of fibrous tissue proliferation project through gaps in Bowman's layer (Figure 4.58).

Granular dystrophy

This autosomal dominant dystrophy is often apparent clinically in childhood but visual impairment does not occur until past the fifth decade. Small opacities are scattered throughout the superficial and mid stroma (Figure 4.59). The intervening stroma between the opacities usually retains transparency until the late stages of the disease.

Microscopic identification depends on the use of the Masson stain, in which the keratohyaline deposits are red (Figure 4.60). The biochemical nature of keratohyaline deposits has not been precisely identified.

The condition is treated by penetrating keratoplasty but this is complicated by recurrence of deposits in the anterior stroma of the graft.

Lattice dystrophy

This is an autosomal corneal stromal dystrophy which appears in childhood and causes early visual impairment. Fine branching opacities are seen on slit lamp microscopy and by retroillumination of a penetrating keratoplasty (Figure 4.61).

Amyloid appears as a pink material in H&E preparations and orange in sections stained with Congo red. The deposits vary in size and shape, and localisation in Bowman's layer leads to epithelial separation (Figure 4.62).

This condition can also recur in a graft.

Avellino (combined granular/lattice) dystrophy

This dystrophy combines the appearances of both granular and lattice dystrophies. The vast majority of cases have ancestral origins from the Avellino region of Italy. This condition was first described in 1992.

The linear branching opacities of lattice dystrophy are overshadowed by the smaller hazy deposits of granular dystrophy located more superficially in the stroma.

At the microscopic level, the two types of deposit – keratohyaline and amyloid – are intermingled in the anterior stroma resulting in reduced epithelial adhesion (Figure 4.63).

Figure 4.58 Superficial corneal dystrophies are usually treated by lamellar keratoplasty, which explains the absence of the posterior part of the cornea. Subepithelial fibrous nodules and breaks in Bowman's layer lead to epithelial oedema and recurrent erosions. This is an example of Reis–Bückler dystrophy.

Figure 4.59 Granular dystrophy is treated with a full thickness penetrating keratoplasty. In pathological material, the disease will be at an advanced stage and there is little transparent stroma between the deposits.

Figure 4.60 In granular dystrophy, the deposits of keratohyaline distort the adjacent lamellae, but are well circumscribed so that the adjacent stroma is not disturbed. With the Masson stain, the keratohyaline granules are red (they are colourless in an H&E stained section).

Figure 4.61 Retroillumination of a repeat penetrating keratoplasty specimen demonstrates the fine branching strands characteristic of lattice dystrophy type 1 (the commonest variant).

Figure 4.62 The histological features of lattice dystrophy. The inset (H&E stain) shows that the distribution of amyloid in lattice dystrophy is greater in the anterior stroma. The upper and lower figures show the section stained with Congo red for amyloid, and by using polarised light, the colour of the deposits changes with the direction of polarisation. The deposits are also found in Bowman's layer and this leads to recurrent epithelial erosions.

Figure 4.63 In Avellino corneal dystrophy, two types of deposits can be identified: keratohyaline granules (similar to granular dystrophy) and amyloid deposits (similar to lattice dystrophy). The close proximity to the epithelium leads to destruction of Bowman's layer and recurrent erosions.

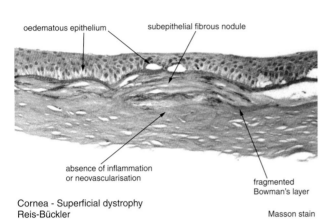

oedematous epithelium

subepithelial fibrous nodule

absence of inflammation
or neovascularisation

fragmented
Bowman's layer

Cornea - Superficial dystrophy
Reis-Bückler

Masson stain

Figure 4.58

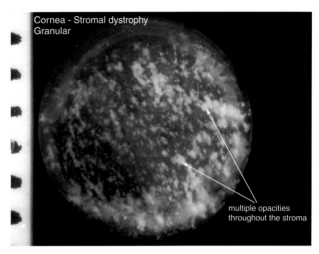

Cornea - Stromal dystrophy
Granular

multiple opacities
throughout the stroma

Figure 4.59

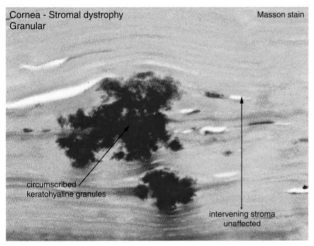

Cornea - Stromal dystrophy
Granular

Masson stain

circumscribed
keratohyaline granules

intervening stroma
unaffected

Figure 4.60

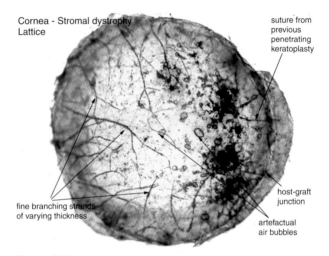

Cornea - Stromal dystrophy
Lattice

suture from
previous
penetrating
keratoplasty

host-graft
junction

fine branching strands
of varying thickness

artefactual
air bubbles

Figure 4.61

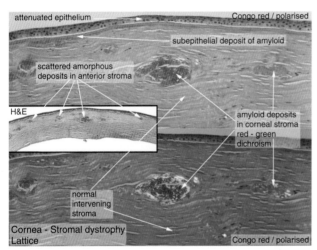

attenuated epithelium

Congo red / polarised

subepithelial deposit of amyloid

scattered amorphous
deposits in anterior stroma

H&E

amyloid deposits
in corneal stroma
red - green
dichroism

normal
intervening
stroma

Cornea - Stromal dystrophy
Lattice

Congo red / polarised

Figure 4.62

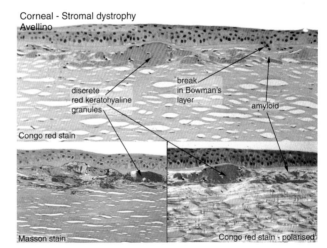

Corneal - Stromal dystrophy
Avellino

discrete
red keratohyaline
granules

break
in Bowman's
layer

amyloid

Congo red stain

Masson stain

Congo red stain - polarised

Figure 4.63

Macular dystrophy

Macular dystrophy differs from the other stromal dystrophies described above in many ways. All layers of the cornea with the exception of epithelium are affected by proteoglycan deposition. The current literature refers to the depositions as proteoglycans, but previously the terms "mucopolysaccharides" and "glycosaminoglycans" were used. The inheritance pattern is autosomal recessive and the genetic abnormality is located on chromosome 16q22.

There are two subtypes depending on the absence (type 1) or presence (type 2) of sulphated keratan sulphate (KS) in the serum. The phenotypes are identical. In type 1, abnormal unsulphated KS is localised to the corneal deposits.

In early childhood, faint white opacities appear initially in the stroma, and as the disease progresses these opacities become larger and the surrounding stroma becomes hazy. Visual impairment occurs early and treatment by a penetrating keratoplasty is often required. Recurrence in the graft is common.

Macroscopic examination of the corneal disc reveals indistinct white opacities against a diffuse haze (Figure 4.64).

In an H&E section, the proteoglycans do not stain. With stains for proteoglycans (i.e. Alcian blue and Hale's colloidal iron), there is deposition in every keratocyte with coalescence to form large clumps (Figures 4.65, 4.66).

Endothelial dystrophies

Fuchs' endothelial dystrophy

This condition is the most common indication for penetrating keratoplasty from a corneal dystrophy. It is bilateral and occurs in middle-aged to elderly patients irrespective of gender.

Clinical presentation

This abnormality is often detected during routine slit lamp examination which shows increased excrescences (guttata) on the central posterior corneal surface. Over time, the excrescences enlarge, increase in number, and coalesce.

With a sufficient decrease in the density of endothelial cells, decompensation in the form of stromal and epithelial oedema ensues.

Pathogenesis

As yet, there is no explanation for the abnormal deposition of collagen and glycosaminoglycans on the posterior surface of Descemet's membrane. The excrescences thus formed appear to lead to gradual loss of endothelial cells and progressive corneal oedema.

Genetics

Although some studies have suggested a genetic basis, the majority of patients do not have a confirmed family history.

Possible modes of treatment

Penetrating keratoplasty if the condition is visually debilitating. The progress of this disease may be accelerated following cataract surgery.

Macroscopic

The cornea is diffusely cloudy (Figure 4.67) and there may be evidence of bullous keratopathy (see above).

Microscopic

The hallmark appearance of this condition is the presence of central excrescences and an apparent thickening of Descemet's membrane. In H&E and PAS preparations, the excrescences are easily identified (Figure 4.68). In atypical examples, the excrescences may be buried by secondary membrane formation which requires PAS for confirmation (Figure 4.69).

In all examples, the endothelium becomes attenuated.

Figure 4.64 Penetrating keratoplasty for macular dystrophy is performed when the opacification of the cornea is advanced with diffuse haze and enlargement of the focal opacities.

Figure 4.65 Histologically, macular dystrophy is characterised by the deposition of proteoglycans in the keratocytes throughout the stroma and in the endothelium. As the keratocytes degenerate, larger deposits are formed in the superficial stroma (Hale's colloidal iron stain).

Figure 4.66 Detail of proteoglycan deposition in macular dystrophy (Hale's colloidal iron stain). In the anterior stroma there may be large deposits of proteoglycan (left). Proteoglycan accumulates in the corneal endothelial cells in addition to the keratocytes (right).

Figure 4.67 Penetrating keratoplasty was performed on a patient with long term Fuchs' endothelial dystrophy. This specimen was initially divided for research

purposes. There are no distinctive features and the stroma is hazy due to oedema and bullous keratopathy.

Figure 4.68 Histology of classic Fuchs' dystrophy. Upper: the excrescences on the original Descemet's membrane are slightly pinker and the endothelium is attenuated (H&E stain). Lower: the PAS stain demonstrates the glycosaminoglycan in the excrescences on Descemet's membrane. In this stain, the endothelial cells are no longer identifiable.

Figure 4.69 Histology of advanced Fuchs' dystrophy. In some cases, the endothelium recovers and forms a second membrane which buries pre-existing excrescences so that the surface appears relatively smooth (H&E stain, upper). The PAS stain demonstrates the excrescences buried by the formation of a secondary Descemet's membrane (lower).

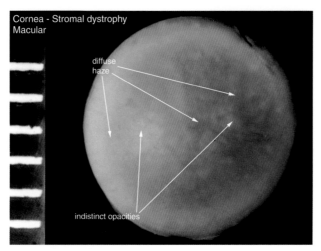

Cornea - Stromal dystrophy
Macular

diffuse
haze

indistinct opacities

Figure 4.64

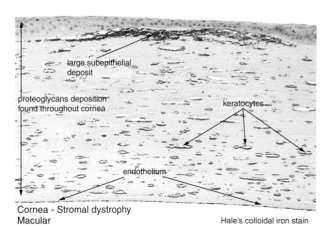

large subepithelial
deposit

proteoglycans deposition
found throughout cornea

keratocytes

endothelium

Cornea - Stromal dystrophy
Macular

Hale's colloidal iron stain

Figure 4.65

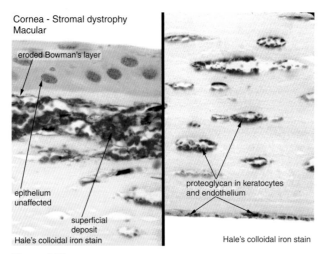

Cornea - Stromal dystrophy
Macular

eroded Bowman's layer

epithelium
unaffected

superficial
deposit

Hale's colloidal iron stain

proteoglycan in keratocytes
and endothelium

Hale's colloidal iron stain

Figure 4.66

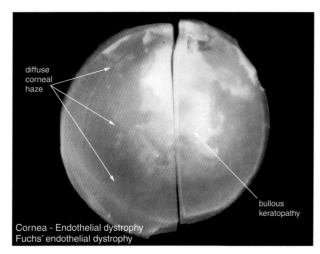

diffuse
corneal
haze

bullous
keratopathy

Cornea - Endothelial dystrophy
Fuchs' endothelial dystrophy

Figure 4.67

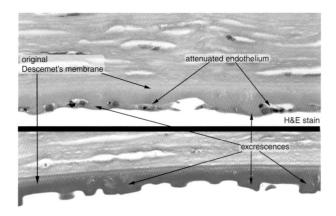

original
Descemet's membrane

attenuated endothelium

H&E stain

excrescences

Cornea - Endothelial dystrophy
Fuchs' endothelial dystrophy

PAS stain

Figure 4.68

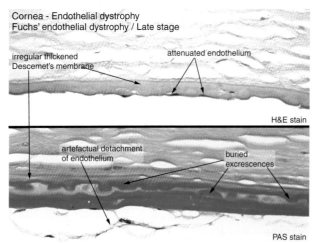

Cornea - Endothelial dystrophy
Fuchs' endothelial dystrophy / Late stage

irregular thickened
Descemet's membrane

attenuated endothelium

H&E stain

artefactual detachment
of endothelium

buried
excrescences

PAS stain

Figure 4.69

Table 4.1 Characteristic features of endothelial dystrophies.

Endothelial dystrophy	Clinical presentation	Genetics	Slit-lamp/specular microscopy	Histology
Congenital hereditary endothelial dystrophy (CHED)	Bilateral diffuse corneal cloudiness in infancy Increased corneal thickness Normal intraocular pressure and diameter	Chromosome 20p11 AD and AR variants have been described	Specular: orange skin appearance	A layer of fibrous tissue lines Descemet's membrane Endothelial cells are attenuated (Figure 4.71)
Posterior polymorphous dystrophy (PPD)	Bilateral circumscribed opacities or total opacification appearing in childhood Pathogenesis of this condition is not understood	Chromosome 20p11 AD and AR variants have been described	Slit lamp: snail track areas with scalloped edges Specular: vesicular structures with mottled centre (early stages)	Stratified squamous cells line the posterior cornea (Figures 4.72, 4.73) Descemet's membrane is of normal thickness
Irido-corneal endothelial syndrome (ICE)*	See below for details Unilateral	Positive family history More common in women	Slit lamp: speckled endothelial cells in swathes	Endothelial cells contain vesicles Descemet's membrane is of normal thickness (Figure 4.74)

* The acronym ICE also refers to a triad of abnormalities: (i) iris naevus (associated with glaucoma), (ii) Chandler's syndrome – corneal oedema and glaucoma, and (iii) essential iris atrophy.

Special investigations/stains

PAS is always required to show excrescences.

Scanning electron microscopy provides a three dimensional appreciation of the globular nature of these excrescences and identifies the surviving cells (Figure 4.70) – see Figure 4.6 for the appearance of normal endothelium.

Other endothelial dystrophies

These endothelial dystrophies are extremely rare and the definitions vary among authorities. The characteristic features are more conveniently described in the form of a table (Table 4.1).

Management is conservative initially, but usually a penetrating keratoplasty is required when endothelial decompensation and corneal oedema ensue. Recurrence in grafts is common.

Keratectasia

Keratectasia (corneal ectasia) is a term that characterises a group of disorders in which there is stretching and thinning of the corneal stroma leading to an alteration in shape. It may be primary as in keratoconus, or secondary as a non-specific response to previous inflammatory disease, trauma, or glaucoma (for example keratoglobus in congenital glaucoma). Keratectasia should be differentiated from a corneal staphyloma in which the thinned deformed cornea is lined by iris tissue.

Keratoconus

Keratoconus is a specific form of bilateral keratectasia in which the thinning is axial or paraxial and is of unknown aetiology. This disease is one of the commonest indications for a penetrating keratoplasty and the postoperative results are favourable. A second graft is rarely required.

Clinical presentation

The patient is often in the younger age group with a history of worsening myopia and irregular astigmatism. Refractive errors associated with this condition are difficult to correct with spectacles and soft contact lenses.

Numerous signs are described:

1 "Oil droplet" and "scissoring" reflexes in ophthalmoscopy and retinoscopy respectively.
2 Slit lamp microscopy may show a brown ring around the base of the cone due to iron deposits in the epithelium (Fleischer ring). Vogt lines from the vertical wrinkling of Descemet's membrane and prominent corneal nerves may also be evident.
3 Bulging of lower eyelid on downgaze (Munson's sign).

In advanced cases, hydrops and subsequent corneal scarring may occur (see below).

Investigations may include:

1 Keratometry and topographical analysis, which shows irregularity of the surface.
2 Pachymetry, used to measure central or paracentral thinning.

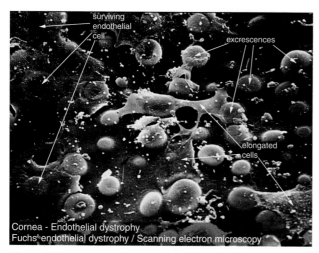

Figure 4.70

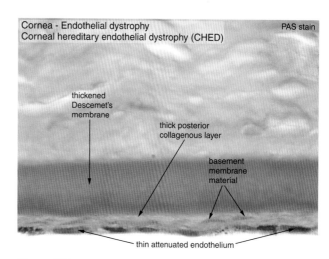

Figure 4.71

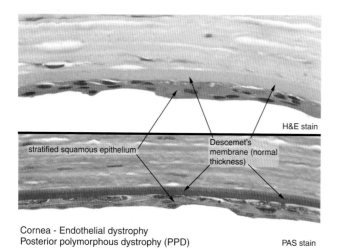

Figure 4.72

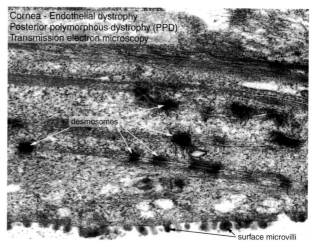

Figure 4.73

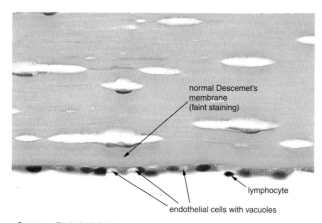

Cornea - Endothelial dystrophy
Iridocorneal endothelial (ICE) syndrome

Figure 4.74

Figure 4.70 Scanning electron microscopy of the posterior corneal surface in Fuchs' dystrophy illustrates the varying sizes of the globular excrescences. Surviving endothelial cells are elongated and stretched between the excrescences.

Figure 4.71 In late congenital hereditary endothelial dystrophy, the endothelial cells are attenuated and a thick layer of collagenous material containing basement membrane strands is deposited on the inner surface of Descemet's membrane (PAS stain).

Figure 4.72 In posterior polymorphous dystrophy, Descemet's membrane is of normal thickness and is lined by a multilayer of stratified cells (upper: H&E stain; lower: PAS stain).

Figure 4.73 Transmission electron microscopy reveals desmosomal attachments between the spindle cells on the posterior corneal surface in posterior polymorphous dystrophy. Desmosomes are a feature of a stratified squamous epithelium which implies endothelial metaplasia. Microvilli on the posterior surface are similar to those seen on the surface of the corneal epithelium.

Figure 4.74 In iridocorneal endothelial syndrome, the endothelium contains vacuoles, but persists as a monolayer. Descemet's membrane is of normal thickness. Occasional macrophages or lymphocytes are seen within the endothelium which raises the possibility of an infectious aetiology.

Pathogenesis

This disorder is poorly understood and is thought to be an interplay of genetic and environmental factors. An attractive hypothesis is that there are imbalances between collagenases secreted by epithelium and keratocytes with collagenase inhibitors within the surrounding stroma.

There is a link to chronic eye rubbing, as would be seen in allergic eye disease and trisomy 21 (Down's syndrome).

Genetics

Many links to different syndromes have been described but more commonly the incidence is increased in:
- trisomy 21
- vernal conjunctivitis and atopy
- collagen disorders: Ehlers–Danlos syndrome, Marfan's syndrome, osteogenesis imperfecta.

Possible modes of treatment

1 Treatment is mostly conservative by means of careful refraction and correction with contact lenses.
2 Penetrating keratoplasty is offered if spectacle or contact lens refraction is no longer effective.
3 Numerous other surgical procedures have been suggested including epikeratoplasty.

Macroscopic

A corneal disc with axial/paraxial thinning of varying degree (Figure 4.75).

Microscopic

The diagnostic hallmarks to be sought in the thinned region of a *classical keratoconus* are:
1 Epithelial atrophy or hyperplasia (Figures 4.76, 4.77 respectively).
2 Breaks in Bowman's layer with subepithelial scarring.
3 Hypercellularity of the stroma.
4 Usually an intact Descemet's membrane.
5 Irregular distribution of nuclei in the endothelium.

Special stains

The Masson stain is valuable for demonstrating breaks in Bowman's layer and PAS for the integrity of Descemet's membrane.

Secondary effects – hydrops

Corneal hydrops This occurs when Descemet's membrane ruptures in the region of the conus and an influx of aqueous into the stroma results in corneal oedema (Figures 4.78, 4.79). As an extreme rarity (Figure 4.80), a large corneal cyst may develop. As a sequel to the acute event, stromal scarring occurs and a secondary Descemet's membrane fills the original defect (Figures 4.81, 4.82). It is not common to perform a keratoplasty procedure in an acute hydrops secondary to keratoconus until scarring has occurred.

Fleischer rings These are due to iron deposition at the base of the conus – it is presumed that this is the location where tears pool and are stagnant so that iron salts are concentrated (Figure 4.83).

Malformations

Dermoid

A large fibrovascular mass may be present within the cornea at birth (Figure 4.84). The aetiology is based on a failure of surface ectoderm to differentiate to normal corneal epithelium. As a consequence, the ectoderm retains the properties of skin and forms pilosebaceous follicles and subepithelial fibrofatty dermal tissue. In association with bilateral limbal dermoids, the additional presence of preauricular skin tags, lid colobomas, and hemifacial microsomia may also be present; this constellation of signs is classified as Goldenhar's syndrome. The histology seen in a corneal dermoid is similar to that seen in a conjunctival dermoid (see Chapter 3).

Peters' anomaly

A well recognised malformation of the neonate in which there is a dense central white circular opacity in the centre of the cornea (leucoma). This disorder is considered in Chapter 6.

Miscellaneous

Trauma

Aspects of corneal trauma are dealt with in Chapter 9.

Treatment-related pathology

Postaphakic decompensation

This condition is becoming more frequent due to an ageing population and increasing demand for cataract surgery. It is currently the commonest indication for a penetrating keratoplasty.

Clinical presentation

A previous history of cataract surgery will be confirmed by clinical examination. The condition initially presents with visual disturbance from corneal oedema secondary to endothelial failure.

At an advanced stage, bullous keratopathy develops with its associated complications (see above).

Pathogenesis

An accelerated loss of endothelial cells due to previous intraocular surgery is the basis for the onset of corneal oedema. At birth, there are 6000 cells/mm^2. This population gradually declines with age, and at a level of 800 cells/mm^2 aqueous retrograde transport is not sufficient to keep the cornea in relative dehydration.

Possible modes of treatment

1 Conservative measures for bullous keratopathy.
2 Penetrating keratoplasty.

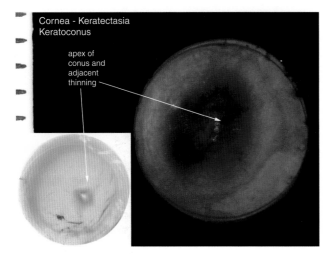

Cornea - Keratectasia
Keratoconus

apex of conus and adjacent thinning

Figure 4.75

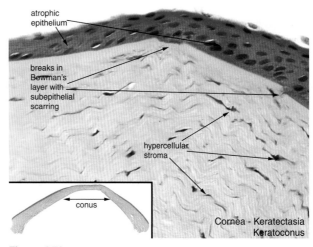

atrophic epithelium

breaks in Bowman's layer with subepithelial scarring

hypercellular stroma

conus

Cornea - Keratectasia
Keratoconus

Figure 4.76

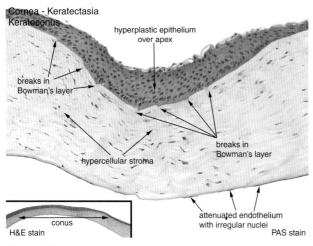
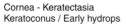

Cornea - Keratectasia
Keratoconus

hyperplastic epithelium over apex

breaks in Bowman's layer

hypercellular stroma

breaks in Bowman's layer

attenuated endothelium with irregular nuclei

conus

H&E stain

PAS stain

Figure 4.77

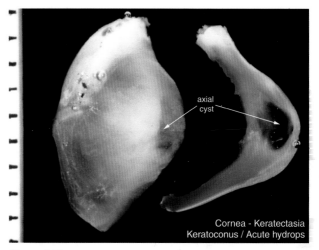

axial cyst

Cornea - Keratectasia
Keratoconus / Acute hydrops

Figure 4.78

Cornea - Keratectasia
Keratoconus / Early hydrops

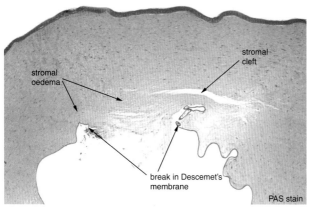

stromal oedema

stromal cleft

break in Descemet's membrane

PAS stain

Figure 4.79

Figure 4.75 A keratoplasty disc for keratoconus is often flat or even concave after fixation. The conus may be paraxial and there is thinning around the apex of the conus, which is best identified by retroillumination (inset).

Figure 4.76 In keratoconus, the atrophic epithelium over the apex overlies breaks in Bowman's layer. The stroma in the region of the conus is hypercellular and the lamellar architecture is disorganised. The inset is a low power view of the cornea in classic keratoconus.

Figure 4.77 In some cases, the epithelium is markedly thickened but the other basic abnormalities are similar to those described in Figure 4.75. The thinning of the conus may be more diffuse (inset). In this example, Descemet's membrane is thin but intact, although the endothelium is attenuated and the nuclei are irregular in distribution (PAS stain; inset, H&E stain).

Figure 4.78 This keratoplasty specimen has been divided to show the cut surface of an axial cyst in keratoconus complicated by acute hydrops.

Figure 4.79 When Descemet's membrane ruptures in keratoconus, there is initially an elastic recoil; aqueous seeps into the stroma and clefts form (PAS stain).

Cornea - Keratectasia
Keratoconus / Late hydrops

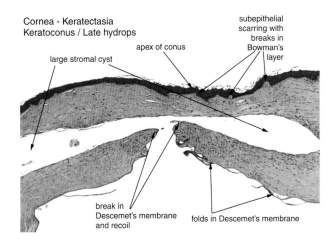

large stromal cyst

apex of conus

subepithelial scarring with breaks in Bowman's layer

break in Descemet's membrane and recoil

folds in Descemet's membrane

Figure 4.80

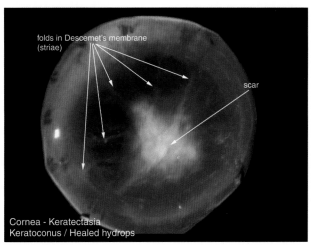

folds in Descemet's membrane (striae)

scar

Cornea - Keratectasia
Keratoconus / Healed hydrops

Figure 4.81

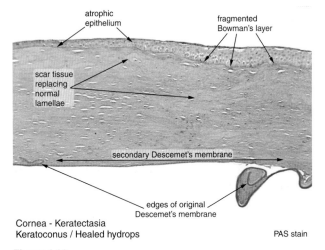

atrophic epithelium

fragmented Bowman's layer

scar tissue replacing normal lamellae

secondary Descemet's membrane

edges of original Descemet's membrane

Cornea - Keratectasia
Keratoconus / Healed hydrops

PAS stain

Figure 4.82

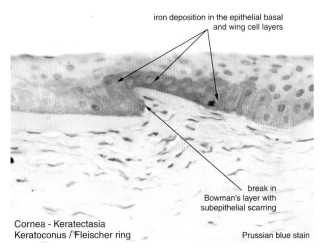

iron deposition in the epithelial basal and wing cell layers

break in Bowman's layer with subepithelial scarring

Cornea - Keratectasia
Keratoconus / Fleischer ring

Prussian blue stain

Figure 4.83

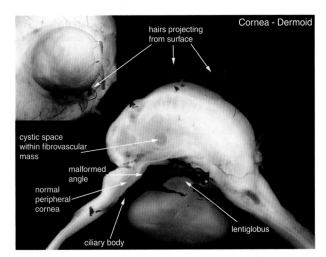

Cornea - Dermoid

hairs projecting from surface

cystic space within fibrovascular mass

malformed angle

normal peripheral cornea

ciliary body

lentiglobus

Figure 4.84

Figure 4.80 In advanced hydrops due to keratoconus, as a rarity, a distinct cyst may form within the corneal stroma (PAS stain).

Figure 4.81 The macroscopic appearance of the scar which forms after healing of an acute hydrops. The location of the scar depends on the site of rupture of Descemet's membrane. Secondary elastic recoil of Descemet's membrane accentuates lines on the corneal posterior surface (striae).

Figure 4.82 In this case of healed hydrops, the presence of a pre-existing keratoconus is revealed by fragmentation of Bowman's layer and epithelial atrophy. Healing takes place when the endothelium covers the bare stroma at the site of rupture and a secondary Descemet's membrane is formed. The fluid within the stroma is removed after the endothelium resurfaces the defect. The original oedematous lamellae of the cornea are replaced by disorganised scar tissue (PAS stain).

Figure 4.83 If a stain for iron salts (Prussian blue reaction) is used, a well circumscribed sector of iron deposition can be identified in the basal and lower wing cell layers at the base of the conus (Fleischer ring).

Figure 4.84 An infant was born with a large hairy mass projecting from the corneal surface (inset). A section through the anterior segment reveals cystic spaces within the fibrofatty mass and extensive destruction of the cornea. These are the features of a corneal dermoid confirmed histologically. The chamber angle is malformed and there is an anterior bulge in the lens (lentiglobus).

Macroscopic

Diffusely cloudy cornea (similar appearance to Fuchs' endothelial dystrophy, Figure 4.67).

Microscopic

The important diagnostic features include a preserved Bowman's layer, absence of vascularisation in the stroma, and an intact Descemet's membrane. Epithelial oedema may be present and endothelial attenuation is pronounced (Figure 4.85). There may be evidence of concurrent (pyogenic) infection secondary to bullous keratopathy or previous infection, for example replacement of Bowman's layer by scar tissue

Graft rejection/immunosuppression

Corneal grafts are the most successful form of transplantation due to the immune privilege of the anterior segment of the eye. However, graft rejection can occur if the host tissue possesses an activated immune system against the foreign antigens of the donor cornea.

Clinical presentation

In the acute event, the patient presents with a red eye and a previous history and the clinical findings of a penetrating keratoplasty. Photophobia and decreased vision are associated features.

The clinical appearance of corneal graft rejection varies according to which level of the anatomical plane of the cornea (epithelial, stromal, and endothelial) is affected. Rejection at the level of the epithelium is characterised by a line in which the donor epithelium is replaced by host cells. At a deeper level, subepithelial infiltrates derived from host epithelium and inflammatory cells are present. Vascularisation of the stroma provides a route for lymphocytic infiltration seen as a haze. The most serious type of rejection occurs at the level of the endothelium and is characterised by a Khodadoust line, in which there is a wave of advancing lymphocytes against a receding front of donor endothelium.

At the late stage, with gradual loss of endothelial cells, stromal neovascularisation, and inflammatory cell infiltration, there is loss of corneal transparency.

With injudicious usage of topical steroids, microbial colonisation can occur resulting in bacterial crystalline keratopathy or fungal infection (see above).

Pathogenesis

Langerhans cells in the epithelium and the intrinsic corneal cells can be upregulated to recognise foreign antigens. This is particularly so when the cornea is vascularised and provides ingress of T lymphocytes and macrophages.

Genetics

HLA typing is not regarded as valuable in some corneal units.

Possible modes of treatment

Prevention through the use of topical and systemic immunosuppression is important to avoid sensitisation of the immune system.

Penetrating keratoplasty may be repeated in cases of end-stage graft failure in which transparency is lost. The chances of graft survival are reduced with each subsequent graft.

Macroscopic

A corneal disc containing evidence of a previous penetrating keratoplasty (host–graft junction and suture scars) will be submitted. The corneal opacification is non-specific.

Microscopic

The stroma and endothelium are infiltrated by T lymphocytes and macrophages (Figures 4.86–4.89). The presence of T lymphocytes in the endothelium leads to endothelial cell degeneration and death.

Immunohistochemistry

Various markers for T-cells subsets (CD2–CD8), B cells (CD19, CD20, CD22), and macrophages (CD68) are valuable in identifying the specific characteristics of the immune response.

Pathological evidence of treatment

A marked reduction in lymphocytic infiltration suggests intensive immunosuppression.

Retrocorneal membranes

Before microsurgical techniques for corneal grafts became established, it was difficult to make a precise apposition of the edges between the donor and host cornea. As a consequence, a gap between the interfaces stimulated the host keratocytes to proliferate behind the edge of the graft and an opaque crescent of tissue developed at the graft–host junction. Histologically, this process was manifest as a layer of fibrous tissue behind the donor Descemet's membrane. In some cases, subsequent migration of host endothelium was followed by the formation of a secondary Descemet's membrane (Figure 4.90).

Amniotic membrane

Commercially prepared amniotic membrane is sutured onto the corneal surface in emergency treatment of corneal ulceration with a threat of perforation. On histological examination, the membrane is amorphous and stains pink in H&E/PAS sections (Figures 4.91, 4.92). The epithelium may grow over or under the membrane depending on the surgical technique. Over time, the membrane fragments.

Cornea - Treatment related pathology
Postaphakic decompensation

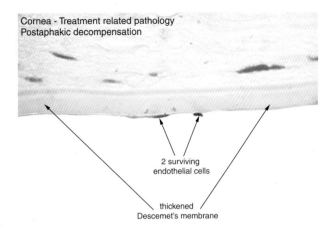

2 surviving
endothelial cells

thickened
Descemet's membrane

Figure 4.85

Cornea - Treatment related pathology
Graft failure / Rejection

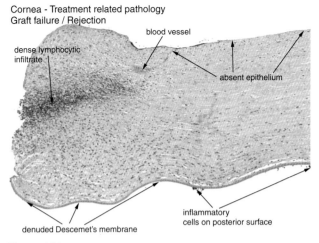

dense lymphocytic
infiltrate

blood vessel

absent epithelium

denuded Descemet's membrane

inflammatory
cells on posterior surface

Figure 4.86

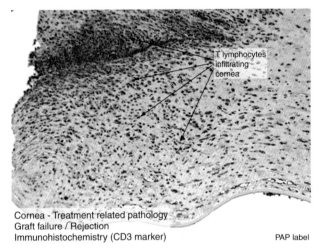

T lymphocytes
infiltrating
cornea

Cornea - Treatment related pathology
Graft failure / Rejection
Immunohistochemistry (CD3 marker)

PAP label

Figure 4.87

Cornea - Treatment related pathology
Graft Failure / Endothelial rejection

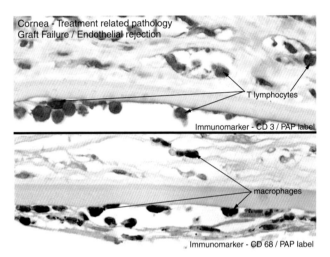

T lymphocytes

Immunomarker - CD 3 / PAP label

macrophages

Immunomarker - CD 68 / PAP label

Figure 4.88

Cornea - Graft failure
Endothelial rejection

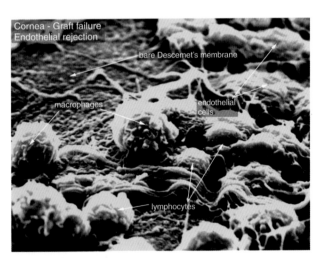

bare Descemet's membrane

macrophages

endothelial cells

lymphocytes

Figure 4.89

Figure 4.85 This elderly patient had uncomplicated extracapsular cataract surgery 5 years before corneal oedema developed. The pathological features of postaphakic decompensation are banal. Apart from epithelial oedema, the only other significant abnormality is a marked reduction in the number of endothelial cells. Thickening of Descemet's membrane is a feature of ageing and is non-specific.

Figure 4.86 Corneal graft rejection is characterised by vascularisation with lymphocytic and macrophagic infiltration. The endothelium is destroyed leaving a denuded Descemet's membrane. The epithelium is detached, presumably due to bullous keratopathy.

Figure 4.87 In this example of graft rejection, immunohistochemistry using a CD3 marker labelled with PAP demonstrates the presence of T lymphocytes. In this specimen, numerous macrophages were also identified using the CD68 marker.

Figure 4.88 The immune attack against endothelial cells includes lymphocytes (upper) and macrophages (lower). Sections from this cornea were stained with CD3 for T lymphocytes, and CD68 for macrophages. In the lower figure, the macrophages are infiltrating a layer of spindle cells which could be fibroblasts or attenuated endothelial cells.

Figure 4.89 Scanning electron microscopy reveals the relationships between lymphocytes, macrophages, and endothelial cells in endothelial rejection. The endothelial cells are shrinking and the intercytoplasmic processes are extended.

Refractive surgery

Radial keratotomy

Radial cuts in the peripheral cornea cause scarring and contraction. This technique was once popular and was used to correct refractive errors such as myopia or astigmatism. Macroscopically, radial and circular scars are easily identified (Figure 4.93). Histologically, this appears as a thin scar extending almost to Descemet's membrane (Figure 4.94).

Photorefractive keratectomy (PRK)

PRK is the procedure in which an excimer laser is used to ablate the superficial corneal tissue in order to alter the curvature and improve refraction. When the procedure was first introduced, the ablation took the form of concentric rings so that in section the epithelium was undulating (Figure 4.95 upper). Later developments of laser techniques produced a gentler curve (Figure 4.95 lower).

Laser-assisted *in situ* keratomileusis (LASIK)

In a similar principle to PRK as described above, the anterior surface curvature of the cornea is altered by means of reducing the thickness of the stroma. Using a mechanised microtome, a split is created along the plane of the cornea, and laser ablation is carried out on the posterior surface of the split. The anterior flap is then replaced.

The many recognised complications of LASIK will not require further excision of corneal tissue, hence, pathological material is scarce.

In an intact cornea, a LASIK procedure can be recognised by an apparent interface shift in the stroma, with minimal scarring at the edge of the flap where the epithelial cover is intact (Figure 4.96).

Cornea - Treatment related pathology
Graft failure / Retrocorneal fibrous ingrowth

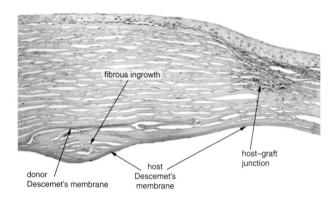

Figure 4.90

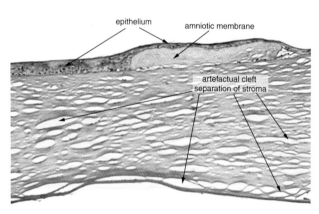

Cornea - Treatment related pathology
Amniotic membrane graft

Figure 4.91

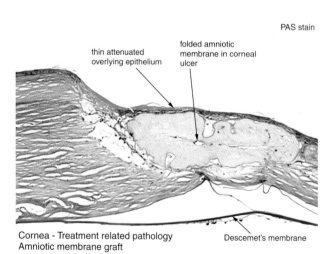

Cornea - Treatment related pathology
Amniotic membrane graft

Figure 4.92

Figure 4.90 If the edge of a donor disc is not in accurate apposition with the host cornea, fibrous tissue grows behind the donor Descemet's membrane. The host endothelium then slides across the retrocorneal fibrous membrane and subsequently a secondary Descemet's membrane is formed.

Figure 4.91 Amniotic membrane appears as a layer of amorphous pink material. In this example, the membrane is located on the surface of Bowman's layer external to an ulcer. A thin layer of epithelium covers the membrane.

Figure 4.92 Within a corneal ulcer, a strip of folded amniotic membrane is lined by attenuated epithelium. It is possible that the membrane was folded to fill an imminent descemetocoele (PAS stain).

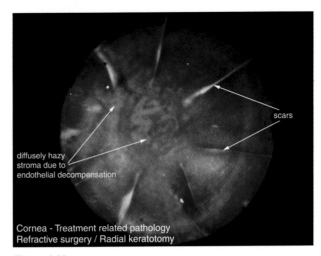

Cornea - Treatment related pathology
Refractive surgery / Radial keratotomy

Figure 4.93

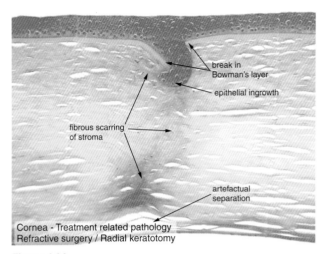

Cornea - Treatment related pathology
Refractive surgery / Radial keratotomy

Figure 4.94

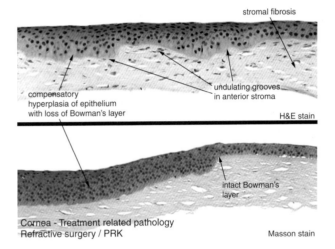

Cornea - Treatment related pathology
Refractive surgery / PRK   Masson stain

Figure 4.95

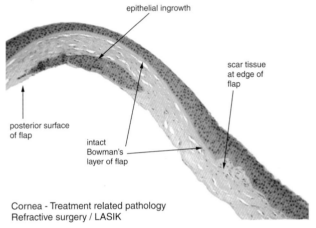

Cornea - Treatment related pathology
Refractive surgery / LASIK

Figure 4.96

Figure 4.93 Penetrating keratoplasty was performed on a patient with postaphakic corneal decompensation. This patient had a history of radial keratotomy. Note the radial scars and the hazy stroma.

Figure 4.94 In this histological example of a radial keratotomy, there is a full thickness scar and an epithelial ingrowth through a defect in Bowman's layer.

Figure 4.95 Loss of corneal transparency after photorefractive keratectomy (PRK) is often treated by lamellar keratoplasty and these are two such examples. Upper (H&E stain): the laser was used to produce concentric rings so that in section there are undulating grooves in the stroma with compensatory

epithelial hyperplasia. Loss of transparency in this example was due to fibrous replacement of the corneal lamellae (compare with Figure 4.1 in which there is a regular arrangement of lamellae). Lower (Masson stain): the laser was designed to create a flatter surface. The epithelium undergoes compensatory hyperplasia.

Figure 4.96 After a LASIK procedure, an opacity developed in the interface between the flap and the stromal bed. To improve vision, a lamellar keratoplasty was performed at approximately the same depth as the flap to remove the opaque area. Histological examination showed that this opacity was caused by an epithelial ingrowth. In this example, the edge of the flap was demarcated by scar tissue.

Chapter 5
Orbit and optic nerve

Orbital tissue pathology

Clinical diagnosis has been refined by various imaging techniques which often lead to an accurate diagnosis without biopsy. Nonetheless, it is important that the reader should have some appreciation of the commoner pathological entities which might be encountered.

Normal anatomy

The orbit contains the following structures which may be involved in pathological processes:
- globe and optic nerve
- muscles – extraocular striated and smooth (Müller's)
- lacrimal gland
- nerves
- blood vessels
- connective tissue and fat.

Types of specimens

Recognition of an orbital specimen is described below.

Biopsy

The types of biopsies submitted range from fine needle aspirations to complete excision of an orbital tumour.

In a biopsy, epithelium would not be present unless the conjunctiva is involved. Inflammatory or neoplastic tissue may contain fibrofatty tissue or possibly part of an extraocular muscle. Pathological processes involving the lacrimal gland will bear some resemblance to normal histology. Tumours derived from connective tissue retain basic histogenetic features, but diagnosis in this situation is rightly the province of the pathologist who will utilise modern technology including immunohistochemistry and electron microscopy.

Exenteration

Exenteration specimens are easily recognised and include globe, optic nerve, and extraocular muscle with attached eyelids. The eyelids will be spared in some surgical procedures and in the autopsy room, where it is not acceptable to disfigure a corpse.

Inflammatory

Infective

Orbital cellulitis

Orbital cellulitis is a metastatic infection that is more common in children. This condition responds well to broad spectrum antibiotics and therefore biopsies are rarely indicated. A common source of infection is from an adjacent periorbital structure such as a paranasal sinus. However, endogenous (for example bacteraemia or septic embolisation) and exogenous (for example trauma) sources of infections have been described. The most common organisms identified by culture are *Staphylococcus aureus, Streptococcus* sp.,

Haemophilus influenzae, and other Gram negative rods. Fungal infections may also occur in immunocompromised patients and have the poorest prognosis: of the fungal infections, the most important is mucormycosis (see below).

Fungal infection

In comparison to bacteria, fungal elements are much larger.

Mucormycosis
Other names: zygomycosis, phycomycosis.

Mucor sp. is a ubiquitous fungus that may opportunistically infect the orbit, classically in patients in diabetic ketoacidosis or those who are immunocompromised. This disease is characterised by rapid tissue destruction from direct invasion, but occlusive arteritis leads to a more extensive necrosis of the orbital contents, nasal passages, and sinuses. The eye may also be infected, usually in the form of a choroiditis.

A confirmatory biopsy and culture of this condition is important in the prompt diagnosis and treatment, which consists of intravenous amphotericin B and aggressive tissue clearance (for example exenteration – Figure 5.1). The prognosis was invariably grave but survival rates are improving due to clinical awareness and early diagnosis.

The biopsy specimen may be taken from the orbit, nasal mucosa, or oropharynx. The main histological feature is the presence of non-septate branching hyphae which are considerably larger than any other fungal pathogen (Figure 5.2). There is extensive infarction of orbital and ocular tissues due to the predilection of the organism to invade blood vessels which become thrombosed. Special stains such as PAS or methenamine-silver may be useful in diagnosis but are usually unnecessary owing to the large size of the organism.

Aspergillosis
Aspergillosis is also an opportunistic infection in the orbit. Invasion is usually via the paranasal sinuses and there is extensive tissue destruction. Large colonies of fungi are present within the abscesses (Figure 5.3). Treatment is by systemic antifungal agents and surgical clearance if necessary.

Non-infective

Idiopathic orbital inflammatory disease (pseudotumour)

An orbital pseudotumour is a term which describes a chronic diffuse inflammatory disease of the orbit in the absence of systemic disease. "Pseudotumour" is a diagnosis of exclusion and the term is a misnomer since the inflammatory mass that forms within the orbit has serious consequences. Patients from teenage to elderly present with a painful proptosis and restricted extraocular movements. The conjunctiva and sclera are often involved and the globe may show evidence of chronic exposure secondary to proptosis. Ocular involvement is possible with conjunctivitis and scleritis. This condition may occasionally be bilateral. Orbital imaging using CT and MRI most commonly reveals a mass with a ragged indistinct outline: this is mirrored by the appearance in a macroscopic specimen (Figure 5.4).

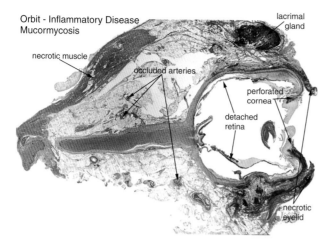

Figure 5.1

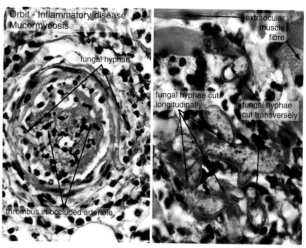

Figure 5.2

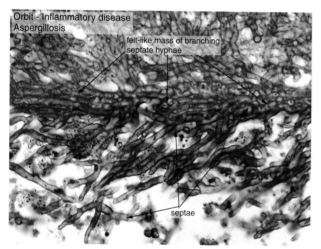

Figure 5.3

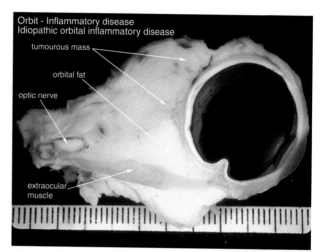

Figure 5.4

Figure 5.1 In the past, exenteration (sometimes bilateral) was attempted to extirpate a mucor infection. This is an exenteration specimen in which there is widespread tissue necrosis due to thrombosis within the posterior ciliary arteries (see Figure 5.2). (Specimen by courtesy of Professor F. Stefani.)

Figure 5.2 In fungal infection due to *Mucor* sp. the organism invades the vessel walls with resultant thrombotic occlusion (left). The organism also invades tissue directly and can be identified by its relatively large size, branching pattern, and absence of septae (shown in outline). The organism may be cut longitudinally or in transverse section (right).

Figure 5.3 An immunocompromised patient developed proptosis which was due to an orbital cellulitis. Biopsy of an intraorbital abscess revealed numerous branching septate fungal hyphae. Septae are best identified at the edge of the mass.

Figure 5.4 Autopsy material from a patient with longstanding idiopathic orbital inflammatory disease. The disease invests the globe and extends as far as the optic nerve. The cut surface is somewhat darker in colour than orbital fat, but the appearances are not diagnostic at the macroscopic level.

Similar pathological processes occur within the neck, thorax, and abdomen (for example Riedel's thyroiditis, mediastinal fibrosis, and retroperitoneal fibrosis) and the aetiology is unknown.

Idiopathic orbital inflammatory disease is very sensitive to steroid treatment in the early stages, although cytotoxic agents are sometimes employed.

Pathology

Previously a biopsy was used to confirm the diagnosis before treatment, but currently diagnosis is aided by advanced imaging and the rapid response to a treatment trial with steroids. Without treatment, the disease progresses from inflammatory cell infiltration (early) to dense fibrosis (late/sclerosing).

The main histological features of idiopathic orbital inflammatory disease are:

1 *Early stage:* lymphocytes, plasma cells, macrophages, and fibroblasts form a polymorphous infiltrate (Figure 5.5) which distinguishes this process from lymphoid neoplasia (see below for comparison). In some cases, uniform mature lymphocytes predominate and plasma cells are less obvious (Figure 5.6).
2 *Late stage:* inflammatory cell infiltration is followed by fibrosis (Figure 5.7). Finally, exenteration may be required to treat a decompensated globe with extensive proptosis (Figure 5.8).

Sarcoidosis

The orbit may be involved in systemic sarcoidosis, but more commonly the disease is located within the lacrimal gland. This condition presents as a non-tender mass usually in the upper orbit. Histologically numerous non-caseating granulomas are present within the excised tissue (Figure 5.9).

Amyloidosis/amyloid tumour

Nodules in the orbit formed by deposition of amyloid may or may not be part of a systemic disease. This condition is usually unilateral, can involve any orbital tissue, and may be combined with conjunctival amyloid. Extraocular muscle involvement results in motility disorders.

Amyloid appears as a pink acellular mass in a conventional H&E stain and brick-red with Congo red stain (Figure 5.10). Polarised light is used to demonstrate dichroism.

Systemic autoimmune vasculitides

There are many known causes for vasculitis (for example syphilitic, mycotic, pyogenic bacterial, and viral infections), but the following idiopathic autoimmune entities are included due to their clinical importance. These conditions have multiorgan involvement but the following description is limited only to the ophthalmic manifestations.

Giant cell arteritis (GCA) is by far the commonest vasculitic disease encountered in ophthalmology, and the pathology in this condition will be fully illustrated. All the autoimmune vasculitides cause ischaemic damage to the retina, but unlike GCA, the three other entities listed below may also be complicated by sclerokeratitis.

Giant cell arteritis (GCA)

This is a systemic condition with inflammation within the walls of blood vessels leading to thrombosis and distal infarction. The process of thrombus formation and recanalisation explains the premonitory symptoms of occlusive disease (transient visual loss) due to intermittent occlusion of the branches of the ophthalmic artery. The most important ophthalmic consequence is blindness from anterior ischaemic optic neuropathy.

Wegener's granulomatosis

Within the orbit, Wegener's granulomatosis is characterised by a necrotising granulomatous inflammation of the arterioles and venules.

Systemic lupus erythematosus (SLE)

This disorder is restricted to a non-granulomatous vasculitis mainly involving retinal vessels.

Polyarteritis nodosa (PAN/PN)

Ophthalmic manifestations are extremely rare.

Table 5.1 summarises the ophthalmic features of the vasculitides (the clinical and systemic features are not described).

Figure 5.5 If a biopsy is taken at an early stage in the evolution of a "pseudotumour", various inflammatory cell types can be identified. In this example, the process involves extraocular muscle.

Figure 5.6 As the disease progresses, lymphocytic infiltration predominates and plasma cells are less evident. The inflammatory cells infiltrate the orbital fat.

Figure 5.7 The orbital fat is destroyed by the inflammatory cell infiltrate and this stimulates reactionary fibrosis.

Figure 5.8 Ultimately, the orbit is filled by fibrous tissue and extraocular movements are so restricted that the clinical description is a "frozen orbit". The dense fibrous tissue distorts the globe and chronic exposure results in conjunctivitis and corneal ulceration.

Figure 5.9 Sarcoid granulomas are compact (inset) and consist of a central mass of histiocytes with occasional multinucleate giant cells and are surrounded by lymphocytes and plasma cells. Note the pointed cytoplasmic projections of the giant cells, which contrasts with the smooth surface of Langhans' giant cells in tuberculosis (see Chapter 8).

Figure 5.10 Amyloid deposits are brick-red with stains such as Congo red and Sirius red (left). When such stained sections are viewed in polarised light, parts of the deposit appear red and parts appear green (characteristic dichroism).

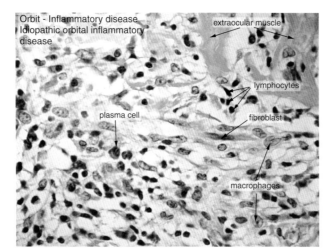

Orbit - Inflammatory disease
Idiopathic orbital inflammatory
disease

extraocular muscle

lymphocytes

plasma cell

fibroblast

macrophages

Figure 5.5

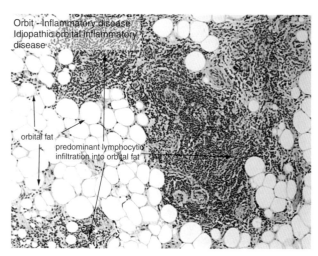

Orbit - Inflammatory disease
Idiopathic orbital inflammatory
disease

orbital fat

predominant lymphocytic
infiltration into orbital fat

Figure 5.6

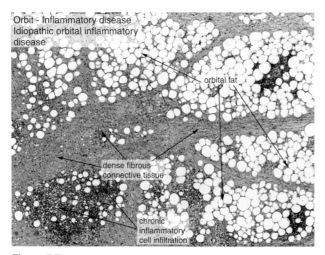

Orbit - Inflammatory disease
Idiopathic orbital inflammatory
disease

orbital fat

dense fibrous
connective tissue

chronic
inflammatory
cell infiltration

Figure 5.7

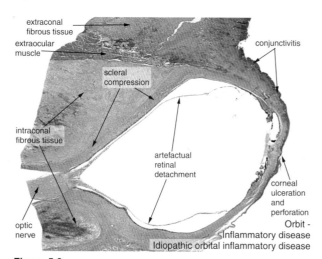

extraconal
fibrous tissue

extraocular
muscle

scleral
compression

conjunctivitis

intraconal
fibrous tissue

artefactual
retinal
detachment

optic
nerve

corneal
ulceration
and
perforation

Orbit -
Inflammatory disease
Idiopathic orbital inflammatory disease

Figure 5.8

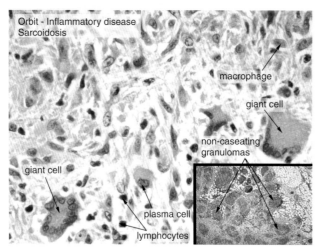

Orbit - Inflammatory disease
Sarcoidosis

macrophage

giant cell

non-caseating
granulomas

giant cell

plasma cell

lymphocytes

Figure 5.9

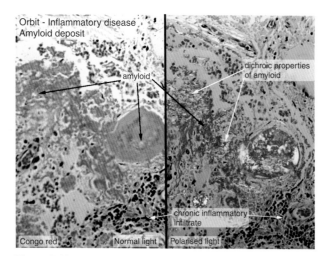

Orbit - Inflammatory disease
Amyloid deposit

amyloid

dichroic properties
of amyloid

chronic inflammatory
infiltrate

Congo red

Normal light

Polarised light

Figure 5.10

Table 5.1 The ophthalmic features of the vasculitides.

Disease	Types of vessels affected	Pathology	Orbital/ocular involvement	Laboratory investigation
Giant cell arteritis	Branches of carotid and ophthalmic arteries and the temporal arteries (Figure 5.11)	Giant cell granulomatous reaction within the media adjacent to the internal elastic lamina (Figures 5.12–5.15)	Ocular: thrombotic occlusion of the posterior ciliary and ophthalmic arteries. Infarction of the optic nerve (Figure 5.16)	Often raised serum ESR and CRP. Temporal artery biopsy is often performed in suspected cases
Wegener's granulomatosis	Small arteries within the orbit	Granulomatous vasculitis of small arteries and veins with fibrinoid necrosis (Figures 5.17, 5.18)	Orbit: apperance of a mass in the orbit that may simulate a malignancy Ocular: anterior necrotising scleritis due to episcleral vasculitis (Figure 5.19)	Test for: c-ANCA
Systemic lupus erythematosus	Arterioles within the retina	Immune complex deposition in small vessels with damage to subendothelial connective tissue	Ocular: retinal microinfarction and haemorrhage. Peripheral ulcerative keratitis and scleritis	Test for: ANA, dsANA
Polyarteritis nodosa	Medium muscular arteries	Non-granulomatous vasculities with fibrinoid necrosis	Ocular: peripheral ulcerative keratities and retinal microinfarcts	Test for: p-ANCA

ANA = antinuclear antibodies, ANCA = antineutrophil cytoplasmic antibodies, CRP = C-reactive protein, ESR = erythrocyte sedimentation rate.

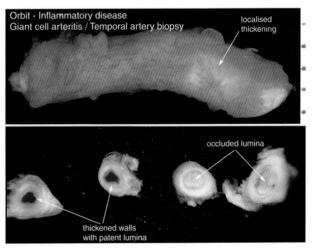

Figure 5.11

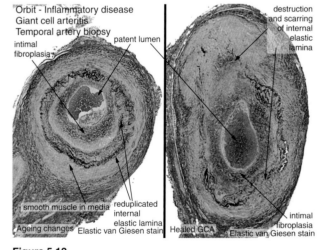

Figure 5.12

Figure 5.11 An excised temporal artery is irregularly thickened in giant cell arteritis (upper). When the vessel is sliced into blocks, it is often evident that the disease is patchy and only some parts of the vessel are occluded (skip lesions) (lower).

Figure 5.12 A stain for elastic tissue is useful in demonstrating intimal fibroplasia as part of the ageing process (left) and healed inflammatory destruction of the elastica in giant cell arteritis (GCA, right). The inflammatory process has destroyed sectors of the multilayered internal elastic lamina and this was followed by fibrous replacement (right). The elastic van Gieson stain identifies smooth muscle as yellow and elastic tissue as black.

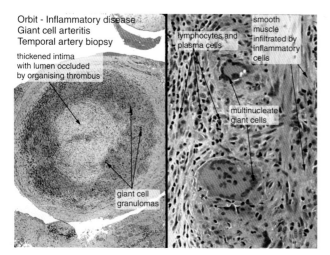

Orbit - Inflammatory disease
Giant cell arteritis
Temporal artery biopsy

thickened intima
with lumen occluded
by organising thrombus

lymphocytes and
plasma cells

smooth
muscle
infiltrated by
inflammatory
cells

multinucleate
giant cells

giant cell
granulomas

Figure 5.13

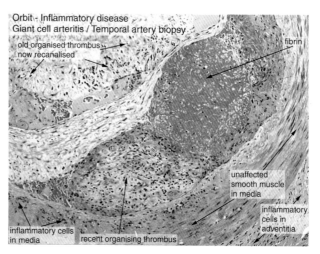

Orbit - Inflammatory disease
Giant cell arteritis / Temporal artery biopsy

old organised thrombus
now recanalised

fibrin

unaffected
smooth muscle
in media

inflammatory
cells in
adventitia

inflammatory cells
in media

recent organising thrombus

Figure 5.14

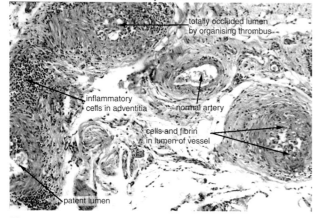

Orbit - Inflammatory disease
Giant cell arteritis / Posterior ciliary arteries

totally occluded lumen
by organising thrombus

inflammatory
cells in adventitia

normal artery

cells and fibrin
in lumen of vessel

patent lumen

Figure 5.15

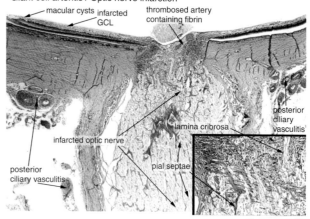

Orbit - Inflammatory disease
Giant cell arteritis / Optic nerve infarction

macular cysts infarcted
GCL

thrombosed artery
containing fibrin

posterior
ciliary
vasculitis

lamina cribrosa

infarcted optic nerve

pial septae

posterior
ciliary vasculitis

Figure 5.16

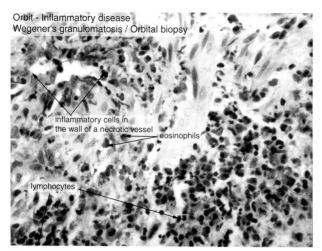

Orbit - Inflammatory disease
Wegener's granulomatosis / Orbital biopsy

inflammatory cells in
the wall of a necrotic vessel

eosinophils

lymphocytes

Figure 5.17

Figure 5.13 In a routine H&E section, inflammatory cells are present in the muscular layer (left) and multinucleate giant cells are located in the region of the internal elastic lamina (right). This example is typical of advanced giant cell arteritis with a markedly thickened intima and an organising thrombus in the lumen.

Figure 5.14 The process of vascular occlusion in the temporal artery is initiated by fibrin thrombus formation in the presence of extensive vessel wall inflammation. The thrombus eventually recanalises and this channel may become re-occluded by a fibrin thrombus at a later date. In this example, the fibrin is invaded by fibrovascular tissue which is an example of early organisation of a thrombus.

Figure 5.15 In giant cell arteritis, there is patchy inflammation and occlusion of the posterior ciliary arteries. Many of the vessels remain patent, which explains sparing of the outer retina.

Figure 5.16 The ophthalmic artery and the posterior ciliary arteries supply the optic nerve via the meninges. In this autopsy case of giant cell arteritis, the ophthalmic artery and the posterior ciliary arteries were occluded by the inflammatory process and this resulted in a retrolaminar infarction of the optic nerve. The ganglion cell layer (GCL) is atrophic. The inset shows some preservation of cells in the lamina cribrosa and total loss of neural tissue between the pial septae.

Figure 5.17 An orbital biopsy in Wegener's granulomatosis is characterised by extensive necrosis in the arterioles, venules, and the adjacent tissue. The inflammatory infiltrate includes lymphocytes, plasma cells, eosinophils, and polymorphonuclear leucocytes.

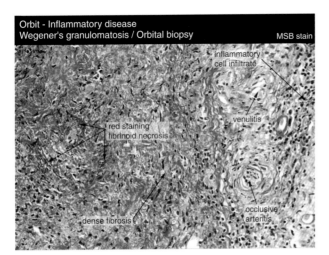

Orbit - Inflammatory disease
Wegener's granulomatosis / Orbital biopsy   MSB stain

inflammatory
cell infiltrate

venulitis

red staining
fibrinoid necrosis

dense fibrosis

occlusive
arteritis

Figure 5.18

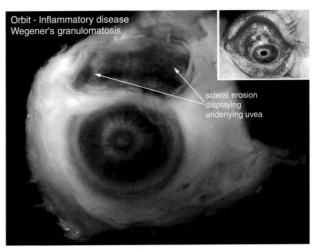

Orbit - Inflammatory disease
Wegener's granulomatosis

scleral erosion
displaying
underlying uvea

Figure 5.19

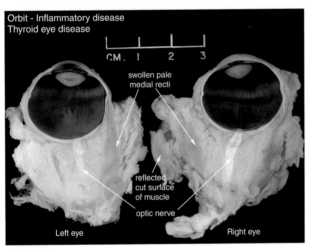

Orbit - Inflammatory disease
Thyroid eye disease

CM.   1   2   3

swollen pale
medial recti

reflected
cut surface
of muscle

optic nerve

Left eye   Right eye

Figure 5.20

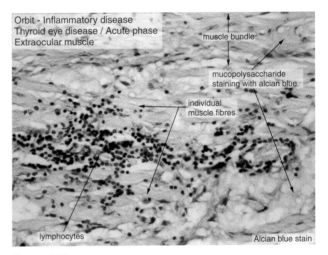

Orbit - Inflammatory disease
Thyroid eye disease / Acute phase
Extraocular muscle

muscle bundle

mucopolysaccharide
staining with alcian blue

individual
muscle fibres

lymphocytes   Alcian blue stain

Figure 5.21

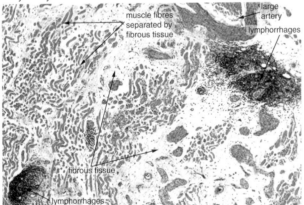

Orbit - Inflammatory disease
Thyroid eye disease

muscle fibres
separated by
fibrous tissue

large
artery

lymphorrhages

fibrous tissue

lymphorrhages

Figure 5.22

Figure 5.18 Vasculitis with fibrinoid necrosis is best demonstrated with a Martius–scarlet–blue (MSB) stain. Dense fibrosis and inflammatory cell infiltration are responsible for producing an orbital mass in Wegener's granulomatosis.

Figure 5.19 This illustration is included to emphasise the importance of Wegener's granulomatosis in the differential diagnosis of necrotising sclerokeratitis. This is an autopsy specimen and the inset shows the appearance of the same eye 6 years before death from secondary renal failure.

Figure 5.20 A patient suffering from thyroid eye disease for many years died from unrelated causes. Both globes and orbital tissues were removed at autopsy and were dissected to demonstrate pale and thickened extraocular muscles. Compare with Figures 5.4 and 5.43 for the appearance of normal extraocular muscle.

Figure 5.21 Thickening of the extraocular muscle in the congestive phase of thyroid eye disease is due to an accumulation of mucopolysaccharides in the extracellular matrix and infiltration by lymphocytes. Mucopolysaccharides stain with alcian blue.

Figure 5.22 In advanced thyroid eye disease, the individual muscle fibres are separated and distorted. Broader bands of fibrovascular tissue are found between the muscle bundles. Dense aggregates of lymphocytes (lymphorrhages) are characteristic of thyroid eye disease.

Thyroid eye disease (TED)

Other names: dysthyroid eye disease, endocrine exophthalmos, Graves' dysthyroid ophthalmopathy, thyroid related orbitopathy.

TED is the most common cause of unilateral and bilateral exophthalmos in adults. Although often referred to as an "eye disease", ocular and optic nerve involvement is secondary to inflammatory enlargement of extraocular muscle and subsequent scarring.

Clinical presentation

The disease has acute and chronic stages and there is marked variation in severity ranging from conjunctival congestion to severe proptosis with secondary exposure keratitis. The acute stage of TED occurs on average 2.5 years following the diagnosis of systemic or localised thyroid disease, although diagnosis of TED does not rely on a prior history of thyroid disease. The stage of disease does not correlate with thyroid function tests.

Diagnosis

One of the more popular methods for describing the clinical features of this disease is to use Werner's NOSPECS mnemonic:

- **N**o signs or symptoms.
- **O**nly upper lid signs: retraction, lag, and stare.
- **S**oft tissue: resistance to retropulsion, oedema of conjunctiva, caruncle and eyelids, lacrimal gland enlargement, and injection over rectus muscle insertions.
- **P**roptosis.
- **E**xtraocular muscle involvement (motility disorders).
- **C**orneal involvement (exposure).
- **S**ight loss due to optic nerve compression.

The mnemonic does not necessarily represent a stepwise progression of TED.

The diagnosis of TED relies on accurate CT/MRI orbital imaging. The characteristic finding is the enlargement of the rectus muscles with sparing of the tendinous insertions.

The important differential diagnoses to consider are: orbital lymphomas and idiopathic orbital inflammatory disease.

A biopsy is rarely indicated (see below).

Pathogenesis

Both humoral and cell mediated immunity mechanisms have been implicated, but, as yet, the specific abnormalities have not been identified.

As a result of accumulations of T cells and B cells within the muscle, there is an excessive mucopolysaccharide deposition which attracts fluid with resultant swelling. Chronic inflammation is then followed by fibrosis.

Genetics

Women are 3–10 times (according to different authors) more likely to be affected by TED (mean age of onset is 41 years). The condition occurs at a later age in men (later than 50 years), but is more severe.

Possible modes of treatment

Treatment for TED is controversial. Topical lubricants are used to treat exposure symptoms. Systemic steroids and low dose radiotherapy can control the acute disease. Orbital decompression may be carried out if there is severe proptosis which is refractory to medical treatment. In chronic disease, when there is a greater problem with orbital fibrosis, treatment includes eyelid surgery (lid lowering) and strabismus surgery for diplopia.

Macroscopic

Due to advances in orbital imaging technology, tissue biopsy for the diagnosis of TED is rare and unnecessary. However, specimens are occasionally encountered in autopsy material (Figure 5.20) which reveals thickened and pale extraocular muscles with sparing of the tendinous insertions.

Glaucoma, compressive optic atrophy, and exposure keratopathy may be evident due to uncontrolled proptosis.

Microscopic

The individual extraocular muscle fibres are separated initially by mucopolysaccharide accumulation and infiltration by lymphocytes and plasma cells (Figure 5.21). This is followed by fibrous tissue replacement (Figure 5.22). The orbital fat is of normal appearance.

Tumours

Cysts

Dermoid

Dermoid cysts are located in the upper orbit and are often adjacent to the lacrimal gland. Excision should be complete as release of the cysts contents (keratin and hairs) into the orbit induces a granulomatous inflammatory reaction.

The pathology is described in Chapter 2.

Mucocoele

A mucocoele is an expansion of the paranasal space secondary to drainage obstruction from chronic sinusitis, trauma, or a tumour. The mucosa expands, in turn thinning and even obliterating the orbital wall. The frontal and sphenoidal sinuses are most commonly affected. The treatment ranges from observation to complete excision.

Pathologically, the cystic cavity is lined by a columnar epithelium occasionally containing goblet cells (Figure 5.23). Accumulation of mucoid material within the lumen of the cyst leads to atrophy of the epithelium.

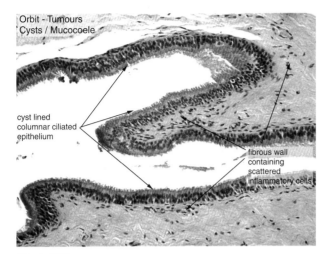

Figure 5.23

Orbit - Tumours
Cysts / Mucocoele

cyst lined
columnar ciliated
epithelium

fibrous wall
containing
scattered
inflammatory cells

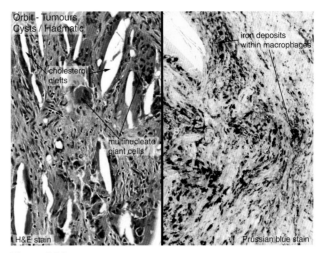

Figure 5.24

Orbit - Tumours
Cysts / Haematic

cholesterol
clefts

iron deposits
within macrophages

multinucleate
giant cells

H&E stain

Prussian blue stain

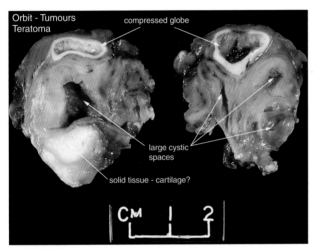

Figure 5.25

Orbit - Tumours
Teratoma

compressed globe

large cystic
spaces

solid tissue - cartilage?

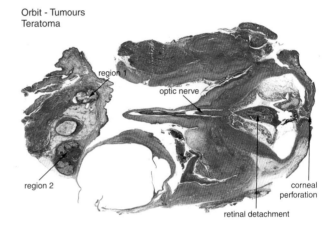

Figure 5.26

Orbit - Tumours
Teratoma

region 1

optic nerve

region 2

corneal
perforation

retinal detachment

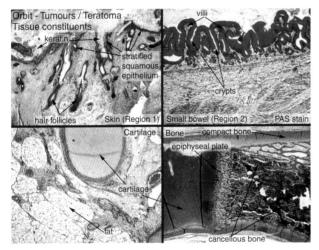

Figure 5.27

Orbit - Tumours / Teratoma
Tissue constituents

keratin

stratified
squamous
epithelium

villi

crypts

hair follicles

Skin (Region 1)

Small bowel (Region 2)

PAS stain

Cartilage

Bone

compact bone

epiphyseal plate

cartilage

fat

cancellous bone

Figure 5.23 A cyst formed by a mucosal projection (mucocoele) into the orbit is identified by the presence of columnar epithelium typical of the mucosa in the sinuses. An epithelium of this type is characterised by nuclei in the basal half of the cell and a layer of cilia (requiring high magnification for identification) on the apical surfaces. The epithelium is surrounded by dense fibrovascular tissue containing scattered inflammatory cells.

Figure 5.24 The wall of a haematic cyst in an orbit often contains the breakdown products of blood. Cholesterol crystals are removed during processing but their pre-existing location is identified by multinucleate giant cells encircling cleft-like spaces (left). The demonstration of haemoglobin breakdown into iron salts is traditionally performed with the Prussian blue stain, which produces a blue reaction product within macrophages (right).

Figure 5.25 After delivery, a unilateral large mass was found in the orbit of an infant. Proptosis led to corneal ulceration and the mass was removed *in toto*. The illustration shows two levels through the orbital tissue and collapsed globe. Large cystic cavities suggest the presence of a teratoma (see Figure 5.26).

Figure 5.26 A section through the centre of the specimen shown in Figure 5.25 reveals the presence of a collapsed globe due to corneal perforation complicated by lens expulsion and retinal detachment. The cysts in the orbit are lined by dermal (region 1) and intestinal tissue (region 2) (see Figure 5.27).

Figure 5.27 Examples of the types of tissue which may be found in different parts of an orbital teratoma. Upper left: skin; upper right: small bowel; lower left: cartilage and fat; lower right: immature bone.

Table 5.2 An outline of tumours occurring in the orbit.

Tissue origin	Benign	Malignant	Notes
Embryonic tissue	Orbital teratoma	Malignant teratoma of the orbit*	Pluripotential embryonic tissue: endoderm, mesoderm, ectoderm
Vascular	**Cavernous haemangioma (adults)** **Capillary haemangioma (children)** **Lymphangioma** (adults)	Angiosarcoma	The benign variants increase in size due to haemorrhage Capillary haemangiomas occur in children and are extensions from an eyelid tumour
Nerves	Central (optic nerve): **glioma, meningioma** Peripheral: **schwannoma, neurofibroma (plexiform/ solitary neurofibroma)**	Malignant schwannoma*, neurofibrosarcoma*	See section on optic nerve pathology in this chapter See below
Fibrous connective tissue	Fibroma – includes solitary fibrous tumour* and ossifying fibroma*	Fibrosarcoma*	
Fat	Lipoma	Liposarcoma	
Muscle	Rhabdomyoma, leiomyoma*	**Rhabdomyosarcoma,** leiomyosarcoma*	Rhabdomyosarcoma is extremely important in the differential diagnosis of orbital myositis in a child
Bone	Osteoma, fibrous dysplasia	Osteosarcoma	Postirradiation of the orbit after radiotherapy for retinoblastoma
Lymphoid tissue	**Benign reactive lymphoid hyperplasia** **Atypical lymphoid hyperplasia**	**Malignant lymphoma – B or T cell** **Lymphocytic leukaemia**	
Langerhans cell histiocytosis	Benign*	Malignant*	Previously considered as separate entities (eosinophilic granuloma, Letterer–Siwe, Hand–Schüller–Christian)
Lacrimal gland	**Pleomorphic adenoma**	**Adenoid cystic carcinoma** **Adenocarcinoma** **Lymphoma**	
Metastasis	—	**Spread from paranasal sinuses** **Blood borne (breast, lung, gastrointestinal tract, kidney)** **Neuroblastoma**	

Haematic cyst

A blood filled cyst in the orbit can form spontaneously or follow blunt trauma. Histology reveals that the fibrous wall contains the breakdown products of blood with a giant cell granulomatous reaction to cholesterol (Figure 5.24).

Neoplasias including hamartomas, teratomas, and choristomas

Table 5.2 describes the wide variety of tumours that can arise in the orbit. The tumours which are considered to be important or common are marked in **bold** print and will be described in further detail below. Tumours marked with an asterix (*) are excessively rare.

Important orbital tumours

Teratoma

A unilateral congenital tumour derived from all germ cell layers (ectoderm, mesoderm, and endoderm). Teratomas are present at birth and may increase in size due to the enlargement of cystic spaces lined by secretory epithelium. Complete excision including the globe is the usual form of management.

Macroscopic examination reveals a globe compressed by cystic spaces and solid tissue within the orbit (Figure 5.25). Histological examination will reveal a wide variety of structures including dermal, neural, gastrointestinal, cartilaginous and osseous tissue (Figures 5.26, 5.27).

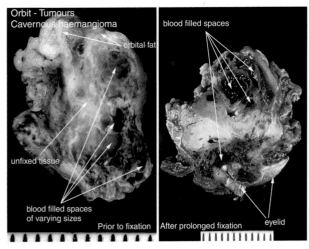

Figure 5.28

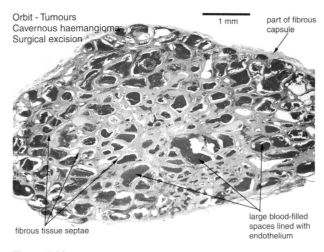

Figure 5.29

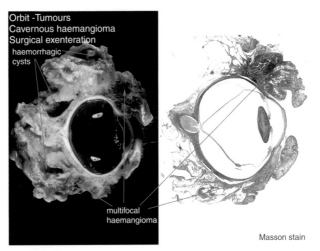

Figure 5.30

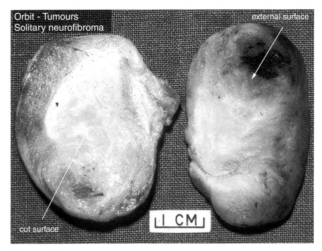

Figure 5.31

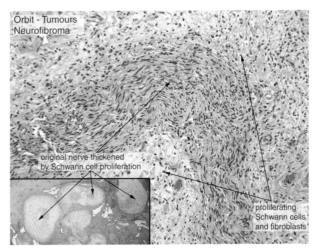

Figure 5.32

Figure 5.28 This figure illustrates two different cavernous haemangiomas. On the left is a partially fixed excision of a tumour which measures 10 × 20 mm. On the right, a much larger specimen was fixed for several days so that the blood-filled spaces are brown in colour. Haemorrhage within the tumour leads to the formation of large spaces and explains why the tumours appear to grow in size, sometimes rapidly.

Figure 5.29 A low power histological view of a relatively small tumour in which the haemorrhage is less pronounced. The small blood filled spaces (0.5–1 mm diameter) spaces are separated by thin fibrous septae lined by endothelium.

Figure 5.30 Cavernous haemangiomas may be multifocal within the orbit and haemorrhage within the tumours may cause severe proptosis and require surgical treatment by exenteration as is shown in this example. The left figure is a complete exenteration specimen to show the difference between the primary cavernous haemangioma and the complication of haemorrhagic cyst formation. The low power histology (right; Masson stain for connective tissue: green) does not include the entire macroscopic specimen but shows the multifocal nature of this hamartoma.

Figure 5.31 A solitary neurofibroma is ovoid with a smooth surface and is solid when divided. The appearance is non-specific – this tumour could be any variant of a fibrous tumour.

Figure 5.32 The diagnosis of a neurofibroma is easier when a structure resembling a nerve is present – this may not be readily apparent without special staining, especially in the case of a solitary tumour. The remainder of the tumour is formed by spindle cells which are identified as Schwann cells and fibroblasts. The inset shows a typical plexiform neurofibroma with thickening of multiple nerves.

Table 5.3 Summary of the salient features of neurofibromatosis.

	NF1	NF2
Genetics – autosomal dominant	Chromosome 17	Chromosome 22
Diagnostic criteria	Any two of the following: • Neurofibromas: solitary (>2) or plexiform • Café-au-lait spots(>5) • Axillary/inguinal freckling • Iris (Lisch) nodules (>2) • Dysplasia of the greater wing of sphenoid • Optic nerve glioma • First degree relative with NF1	• Bilateral 8th nerve tumours (acoustic neuromas) Or any two of the following: • Unilateral 8th nerve tumour • Neurofibroma • Meningioma • Glioma • Schwannoma • Juvenile posterior subcapsular lens opacity (PSCC) • First degree relative with NF2
Clinical findings	Skin: café-au-lait, axillary/groin freckling, neurofibromas CNS: astrocytomas, meningiomas Visceral: phaeochromocytoma, rhabdomyoma of heart Osseous: dysplasia of greater wing of sphenoid	
Ocular findings	Neurofibromas: in lid, choroid, or orbit Cornea: thickened nerves Iris: Lisch nodules – proliferation of melanocytes in the anterior stroma Retina: astrocytic hamartoma – tumour formed by proliferation of astrocytes in the inner retina Choroid: diffuse thickening from neurofibromatous tissue Glaucoma: secondary to neurofibromatous tissue covering trabecular meshwork or neovascularisation	Lens: PSCC Ocular hamartomas Optic nerve: meningioma

Vascular tumours

The most common vascular tumour encountered in the orbit of adults is a cavernous haemangioma. These are benign slow growing hamartomas which are often well circumscribed within the orbit. Treatment can be conservative although surgical excision may be required for the complications of proptosis.

Macroscopically, the tumour is reddish-purple in colour and the surface is nodular. The cut surface reveals areas where the angioma is intact and the blood filled spaces measure 0.5–1 mm. Bleeding within the mass creates large blood filled cysts (Figure 5.28). Microscopically in a small tumour, the blood filled spaces are relatively uniform in size and are separated by fibrous tissue (Figure 5.29). In rare cases, cavernous haemangiomas are multifocal, and intraorbital haemorrhage may require radical surgery such as an exenteration (Figure 5.30).

Neural tumours

Neurofibroma

Two variants are encountered:

1 *Solitary:* isolated findings in individuals are common and are not part of the syndrome of neurofibromatosis.
2 *Plexiform:* multiple abnormalities which are usually part of a syndrome such as neurofibromatosis (Table 5.3).

When present in the eyelid, the tumour is described as "bag of worms".

Neurofibromatosis

Although rare, an awareness of this condition is essential for ophthalmologists. Two forms of neurofibromatosis are recognised: NF1 and NF2.

Pathological features of solitary neurofibroma and neurofibromatosis

The histopathological characteristics of the two variants are very similar, consisting of proliferating Schwann cells and fibroblasts within and around peripheral nerves. A solitary neurofibroma appears as an isolated, solid, well circumscribed mass (Figure 5.31), which contains spindle shaped Schwann cells and fibroblasts. When the tumour is formed within a number of closely associated nerves, the term plexiform neurofibroma is applied (Figure 5.32). In orbital neurofibromatosis, there is diffuse infiltration of normal tissues: the histological appearance is similar to that seen in a neurofibroma (Figure 5.33).

The ocular features of neurofibromatosis differ from those in the orbit in that the uveal tract is thickened by Schwann cell and melanocytic proliferation, with less fibrous tissue formation (Figure 5.34). Involvement of the chamber angle leads to secondary glaucoma (Figure 5.35). Isolated melanocytic proliferations within the iris are known clinically as Lisch nodules.

Schwannoma

Other name: neurilemmoma.

This tumour may be found in isolation or in association with neurofibromatosis type 2. When a schwannoma occurs in the eighth cranial nerve, the term acoustic neuroma is applied. In ophthalmology, schwannomas must be considered in the differential of solid slowly growing orbital tumours.

All the cells within this tumour are of Schwann cell origin which differentiates it from a neurofibroma (see above). The Schwann cells have a characteristic mixed pattern with both pallisading arrangement of nuclei (Antoni type A) or loosely dispersed in a myxoid matrix (Antoni type B – Figures 5.36, 5.37).

Musculoskeletal tumours

Rhabdomyosarcoma

Rhabdomyosarcoma is the most common mesenchymal soft tissue malignancy in childhood, representing approximately 3% of all childhood malignancies, with 70% occurring in the first decade of life. The male to female relative preponderance is 3 to 2. Rarely this tumour can occur in the elderly.

This disease presents as a rapidly growing irregular orbital mass leading to proptosis, lid and conjunctival oedema, chemosis, motility restrictions, and ptosis. Orbital imaging is helpful in recognising the extent of involvement but a biopsy is essential. Previously the metastatic mortality rate was high (70%) when exenteration was the only treatment available, but currently with radiotherapy and adjuvant chemotherapy survival rates reach 95%.

The tumour appears as a pale tan coloured mass within and extending from an extraocular muscle (Figure 5.38).

Prior to immunohistochemistry, the diagnosis in some cases of rhabdomyosarcoma was challenging due to the poor differentiation of the tumour. Three categories were used according to histological differentiation (starting from the least): embryonal, alveolar, and (adult) pleomorphic. The pleomorphic subtype is the easiest to identify because the rhabdomyoblasts closely resemble striated muscle fibres (Figure 5.39). These malignant cells possess abundant eosinophilic cytoplasm containing fibrillary material: this type of tumour is commoner in adults. In children, the embryonal tumour consists of bizarrely shaped rhabdomyoblasts with only scanty evidence of cross-striations (Figure 5.40).

Alveolar rhabdomyosarcomas are so called because the malignant cells are confined by circular fibrous septae which resemble alveoli in the lung (Figure 5.41). Only 50–60% of embryonal-type lesions and 30% of alveolar-type tumours display cross-striations.

Immunohistochemistry utilises antibodies (for example Myo-D, actin, desmin) which will identify the myoglobin constituent within the suspect tumour cells (Figure 5.42).

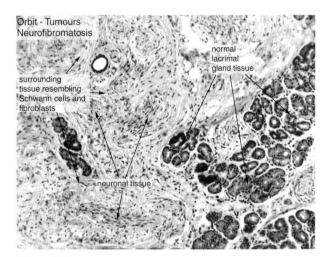

Figure 5.33

Figure 5.33 In neurofibromatosis, the histology seen is similar to that in neurofibromas but there is more extensive infiltration of normal tissue, in this case the lacrimal gland.

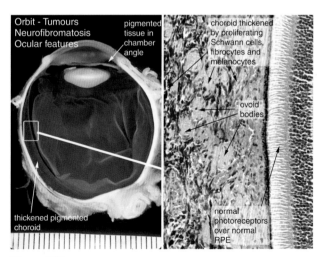

Figure 5.34

Figure 5.34 The principal ocular feature in neurofibromatosis is thickening of the uveal tract, which may cause diagnostic confusion with a diffuse melanoma (left). Histology from the thickened choroid reveals Schwann cells and melanocytic proliferation. Ovoid bodies are a characteristic feature and are formed by Schwann cell proliferation (right). RPE = retinal pigment epithelium.

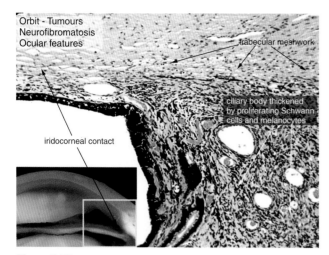

Orbit - Tumours
Neurofibromatosis
Ocular features

trabecular meshwork

ciliary body thickened
by proliferating Schwann
cells and melanocytes

iridocorneal contact

Figure 5.35

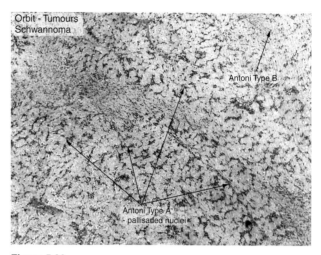

Orbit - Tumours
Schwannoma

Antoni Type B

Antoni Type A
- pallisaded nuclei

Figure 5.36

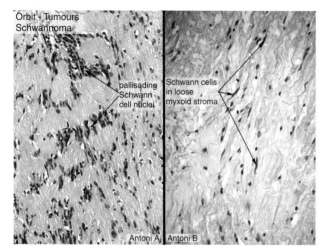

Orbit - Tumours
Schwannoma

pallisading
Schwann
cell nuclei

Schwann cells
in loose
myxoid stroma

Antoni A | Antoni B

Figure 5.37

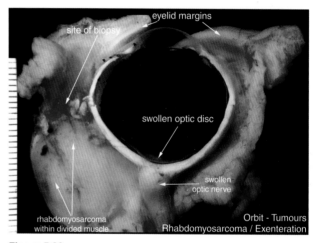

eyelid margins

site of biopsy

swollen optic disc

swollen
optic nerve

rhabdomyosarcoma
within divided muscle

Orbit - Tumours
Rhabdomyosarcoma / Exenteration

Figure 5.38

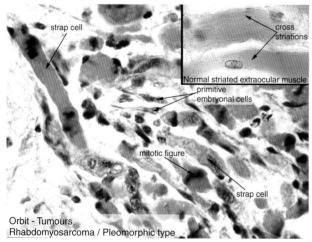

strap cell

cross
striations

Normal striated extraocular muscle
primitive
embryonal cells

mitotic figure

strap cell

Orbit - Tumours
Rhabdomyosarcoma / Pleomorphic type

Figure 5.39

Figure 5.35 The inset shows part of the anterior segment of the globe illustrated in Figure 5.34. The high power histology corresponds to the box outlined in the inset. The stroma of the ciliary body and iris is extensively infiltrated by spindle cells, mainly Schwann cells and melanocytes. The trabecular meshwork is compressed and there is a secondary angle closure.

Figure 5.36 A low power illustration of a schwannoma demonstrates the two types of tissue (Antoni types A and B) which are diagnostic of this tumour (see Figure 5.37).

Figure 5.37 Antoni type A tissue is recognised by the pallisading arrangement of Schwann cell nuclei (left). In type B, the nuclei are scattered and surrounded by a loose myxoid matrix (right).

Figure 5.38 An archival specimen illustrates the appearance of a rhabdomyosarcoma in an extraocular muscle. A previous biopsy, complicated by secondary haemorrhage, confirmed the diagnosis. The tumour was not responsive to radiotherapy or chemotherapy, and radical surgery was required. Optic disc swelling is evident due to compression of the optic nerve and is also secondary to radiotherapy. Note that there is a localised swelling in the distal portion of the optic nerve secondary to radiation and infarction.

Figure 5.39 The marked variation in nuclear size and shape and the prominent pink (eosinophilic) cytoplasm indicate a malignant tumour derived from striated muscle. Strap cells within the tumour recapitulate normal striated muscle fibres (inset) but cross-striations are less conspicuous. Many of the cells (rhabdomyoblasts) resemble primitive mesenchymal cells.

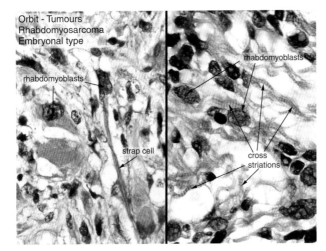

Orbit - Tumours
Rhabdomyosarcoma
Embryonal type

rhabdomyoblasts

rhabdomyoblasts

strap cell

cross striations

Figure 5.40

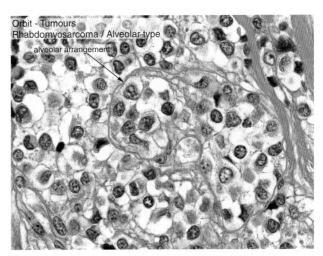

Orbit - Tumours
Rhabdomyosarcoma / Alveolar type

alveolar arrangement

Figure 5.41

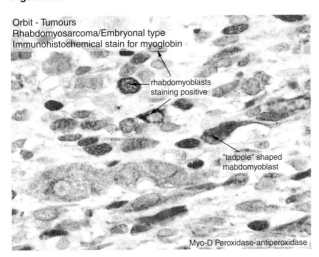

Orbit - Tumours
Rhabdomyosarcoma/Embryonal type
Immunohistochemical stain for myoglobin

rhabdomyoblasts staining positive

"tadpole" shaped rhabdomyoblast

Myo-D Peroxidase-antiperoxidase

Figure 5.42

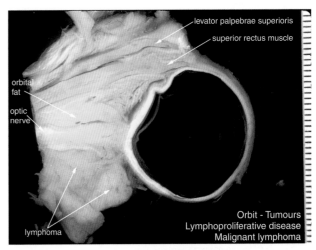

levator palpebrae superioris

superior rectus muscle

orbital fat

optic nerve

lymphoma

Orbit - Tumours
Lymphoproliferative disease
Malignant lymphoma

Figure 5.43

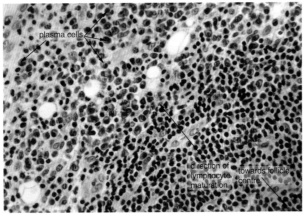

plasma cells

direction of lymphocyte maturation

towards follicle centre

Orbit - Tumours / Lymphoproliferative disease
Benign reactive lymphoproliferative hyperplasia

Figure 5.44

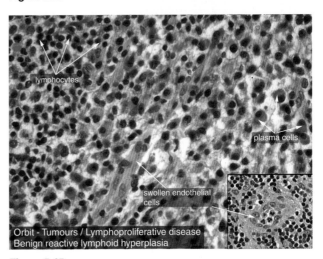

lymphocytes

plasma cells

swollen endothelial cells

Orbit - Tumours / Lymphoproliferative disease
Benign reactive lymphoid hyperplasia

Figure 5.45

Figure 5.40 In the embryonal rhabdomyosarcoma of childhood, the majority of cells are of primitive embryonal type and helpful features are strap cells and cells which have plentiful eosinophilic cytoplasm (rhabdomyoblasts – left). The identification of cross-striations within the cytoplasm of the tumour cells provides a definitive diagnosis (right).

Figure 5.41 In an alveolar rhabdomyosarcoma, the rhabdomyoblasts appear to fill circular spaces which resemble pulmonary alveoli (shown in outline).

Figure 5.42 Immunohistochemistry using an antibody (for example Myo-D in this case) against myoglobin simplifies the diagnosis of poorly differentiated malignant tumours derived from smooth and striated muscles.

Figure 5.43 A vertical section through an autopsy exenteration specimen reveals an intraconal mass moulded around the optic nerve and the posterior portion of the globe. The specimen also illustrates the normal appearance of extraocular muscle and fat.

Figure 5.44 Benign reactive lymphoid hyperplasia (BRLH) is characterised by the presence of lymphoid follicles with maturation to mature lymphocytes at the periphery of the follicle. The tissue adjacent to the follicle contains numerous plasma cells.

Figure 5.45 BRLH is also diagnosed by the presence of intermingled *mature* lymphocytes and plasma cells. In many cases it is possible to demonstrate swelling of the vascular endothelial cells commonly termed high endothelial venules.

Lymphoid tumours

Lymphocytic proliferations of the conjunctiva and globe are discussed in Chapters 2 and 11. A continuous spectrum exists in the classification of lymphoid tumours ranging from benign reactionary lymphoid hyperplasia to malignant lymphoma. One of the problems in the classification of lymphoid tumours is that, over time, a tumour previously classified as benign can transform to a more malignant form (multistep neoplasia). *Note that, apart from the lacrimal gland, the retroseptal orbital tissue does not contain lymphoid tissue or lymphatics – therefore, the presence of any lymphoid tissue in this space is an indication of lymphoproliferative disease.*

Lymphoproliferative disease affects mainly the elderly and presents with an insidious onset of proptosis, ocular motility restriction, or a palpable mass – 25% of cases occur bilaterally. The lacrimal gland can be involved in isolation or as part of an orbital infiltration. Orbital imaging reveals a mass that is classically described as "moulding" around the globe. The corresponding appearance in an exenteration specimen is shown in Figure 5.43.

In all cases of orbital lymphoproliferative disease, it is extremely important to detect or exclude systemic involvement by appropriate screening.

Precise classification of lymphoid constituents is the responsibility of the pathologist and the following is a brief outline of the three major subgroups:

Benign reactive lymphoid hyperplasia

The presence of lymphoid follicles (Figure 5.44) and a polyclonal colonisation (T and B lymphocytes and plasma cells) are the major diagnostic criteria (Figure 5.45). Mitotic activity is relatively sparse.

An important differential diagnosis is idiopathic orbital inflammatory disease (see above) in which polymorphonuclear leucocytes and fibrous connective tissue are more prominent.

Atypical lymphoid hyperplasia

This group is a diagnostic challenge for the pathologist. The tumour consists of sheets of lymphocytes (and an absence of plasma cells), the majority of which are mature and there is minimal mitotic activity (Figure 5.46). Both T and B lymphocytes can be identified by immunohistochemistry (mixed cellular infiltrate) in this subgroup.

Malignant lymphoma

The histopathological features which indicate malignancy in a lymphoma are as follows: nuclear irregularity at high power, mitotic activity, and loss of follicular architecture (Figure 5.47). The majority of malignant orbital lymphomas are of B-cell type and monoclonality is demonstrated by immunohistochemistry or PCR. Hodgkin's disease does not occur in the orbit as a primary tumour, but orbital involvement may be a part of systemic disease. Tumours of plasma cells (plasmacytoma and multiple myeloma) are excessively rare tumours.

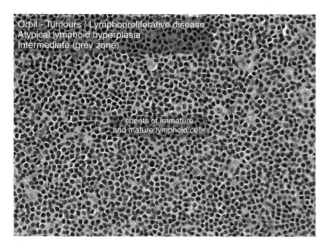

Figure 5.46

Figure 5.46 Atypical lymphoid hyperplasia is characterised by sheets of mature lymphocytes with occasional immature lymphoid cells. The nuclei tend to be regular in shape and mitotic figures are sparse.

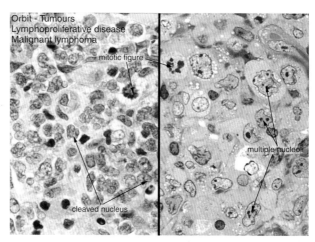

Figure 5.47

Figure 5.47 Malignant lymphocytes have markedly irregular nuclei and mitotic figures are evident. The cells appear to crowd and overlap each other in an H&E paraffin section (left). A thin plastic section provides much greater detail of nuclear irregularity: note the presence of multiple nucleoli (right).

Pathological classification of orbital lymphoproliferative disease

Currently a pathologist may require fresh unfixed tissue in order to apply modern techniques such as immunophenotyping, messenger RNA by *in situ* hybridisation, or DNA abnormalities (Southern blot, PCR, fluorescence *in situ* hybridisation (FISH), and gene sequencing). This is required for better classification of lymphoid tumour subgroups in relation to prognosis following treatment.

Lymphoproliferative disease is usually well controlled by radiotherapy if localised and by chemotherapy if systemic.

Lacrimal gland

Normal lacrimal gland

In order to appreciate the morphology of primary tumours of the lacrimal gland, histology of the normal gland is illustrated (Figure 5.48). Neoplasms can arise from acini (adenocarcinoma) or ducts (pleomorphic adenomas/adenocarcinomas). The term "pleomorphic" is applied because tumours which arise from ducts can contain cells which have arisen in epithelial cells and mesenchymal cells (myoepithelium – Figure 5.49). The normal presence of lymphoid tissue around the acini explains the relatively high incidence of primary lymphoid neoplasms in the lacrimal gland.

Inflammatory diseases of the lacrimal gland

Enlargement of the lacrimal gland may be due to various inflammatory processes and these are rare. Biopsies are occasionally performed on acute inflammations that do not resolve. Important inflammatory conditions are described below.

Dacryoadenitis

There have been many reports of infection by bacteria and viruses which can lead to unilateral or bilateral swellings of the gland.

Sarcoidosis

Non-caseating granulomas within the lacrimal gland have been described in systemic sarcoidosis – see Figure 5.9.

Mikulicz's syndrome

Consists of bilateral swellings of both salivary and lacrimal glands secondary to sarcoidosis, lymphoid neoplasia, and leukaemia.

Sjögren's syndrome (keratoconjunctivitis sicca with dry mouth)

A systemic autoimmune disease affecting mainly elderly women in whom there is idiopathic chronic inflammatory destruction of salivary and lacrimal gland tissue leading to deficiency in saliva and tear production (see Chapter 3 for changes in the conjunctival epithelium). Labial gland biopsies are preferred over the lacrimal gland (Figure 5.50) due to convenience of access. Serological investigations include ANA, rheumatoid factor, SS-A, and SS-B as part of the work-up.

Tumours of the lacrimal gland

Most lacrimal gland tumours present by mass effect within the orbit. The diagnosis and management of lacrimal tumours are heavily dependent on high resolution orbital imaging. The remainder of this section will be confined to epithelial tumours of the lacrimal gland. Lymphoid malignancies, inflammatory and metastatic diseases in the lacrimal gland are identical to those occurring in the orbit. Lacrimal gland tumours are summarised in Table 5.4.

Benign

Pleomorphic adenoma

Other name: benign "mixed" tumour of the lacrimal gland – this term was used to account for the variable histology as described below.

A pleomorphic adenoma presents as a painless exophthalmos that has been slowly progressive over 12 months. CT scans show a well circumscribed tumour in the lacrimal fossa and, if sufficiently large, remoulding of the adjacent orbital bone without infiltration. The incidence is between the second and fifth decades (peak in the fourth) with a sex ratio of 1.5 : 1 (male : female).

Although classified as benign, the surgical treatment for pleomorphic adenoma relies on a complete excision (including the pseudocapsule) by means of a lateral orbitotomy. If the surgical procedure leaves residual tumour within the orbit there is a high risk of recurrence with the possibility of malignant transformation.

Macroscopic examination reveals a single solid pale-grey mass with a bosselated surface. The cut surface shows solid tumour with mucoid cystic spaces and areas of haemorrhage (Figure 5.51).

Table 5.4 Summary of lacrimal gland tumours.

Tissue origin	Conditions
Epithelial (20–25%)	Benign mixed tumour: pleomorphic adenoma (50% of epithelial tumours) Adenoid cystic adenoma Adenocarcinoma
Lymphoid	Benign reactionary lymphoid hyperplasia Atypical lymphoid hyperplasia Malignant lymphoma
Metastatic	

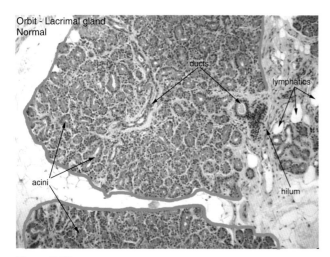

Orbit - Lacrimal gland
Normal

ducts

lymphatics

acini

hilum

Figure 5.48

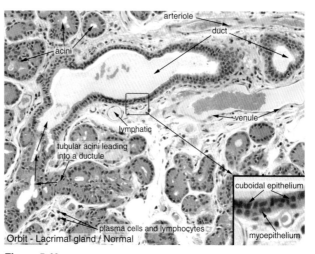

arteriole

duct

acini

venule

lymphatic

tubular acini leading
into a ductule

cuboidal epithelium

myoepithelium

plasma cells and lymphocytes

Orbit - Lacrimal gland / Normal

Figure 5.49

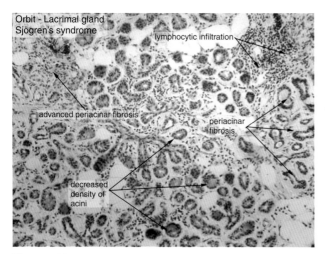

Orbit - Lacrimal gland
Sjögren's syndrome

lymphocytic infiltration

advanced periacinar fibrosis

periacinar
fibrosis

decreased
density of
acini

Figure 5.50

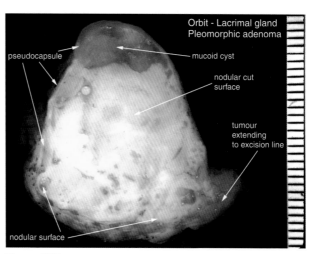

Orbit - Lacrimal gland
Pleomorphic adenoma

pseudocapsule

mucoid cyst

nodular cut
surface

tumour
extending
to excision line

nodular surface

Figure 5.51

Figure 5.48 The primary unit within a lacrimal gland is a lobule (shown in outline), which contains acini, ductules, lymphatics, and nerves. The hilum is the central core which connects the lobules. The larger lacrimal ducts which drain into the fornix are present in the hilum.

Figure 5.49 Acini are circular structures formed by cuboidal cells with a central lumen – these are the secretory units for tears and the cells also transport immunoglobulins produced by the adjacent plasma cells. The tear fluid is passed into ductules and ducts which are lined by cuboidal epithelial cells and a surrounding contractile cell layer (myoepithelium, inset) resembling a sweat gland duct. Contraction of the ducts is responsible for reflex tearing. Benign and

malignant tumours may be derived from both types of cells in the ducts and, therefore, they contain two or more cell types, i.e. epithelial and mesenchymal cells.

Figure 5.50 At a late stage of Sjögren's syndrome, there is extensive periacinar fibrosis and a marked reduction in the number of acini (compared with Figures 5.48, 5.49). A lymphocytic infiltration is present within the fibrous tissue.

Figure 5.51 In this excision of a pleomorphic adenoma, the tumour was not adequately cleared. The surface of the tumour is in part covered by a pseudocapsule, but elsewhere tumour tissue extends to the excision line. The surgeon and patient were fortunate that the tumour did not recur.

Microscopic examination shows the tumour to consist of two different components:

1 *Epithelial:* the tumour cells adopt a glandular pattern in which cords and ducts resemble the ducts in a normal lacrimal gland (Figures 5.52, 5.53). The lumen of some of the ducts may be filled with an eosinophilic proteinaceous secretion.

2 *Stromal:* this tissue is formed by myoepithelial cells which break away from ducts and proliferate to form connective tissue (Figures 5.52, 5.53). The components are primarily fibrous with myxoid areas but the tumour may also contain fat and cartilage (Figure 5.54).

It is important to note that the pseudocapsule in a pleomorphic adenoma is merely a fibrous condensation which contains infiltrating tumour. It is the responsibility of the pathologist to take multiple samples of the pseudocapsule to ascertain the possibility of incomplete clearance, which implies that there is residual tumour in the orbit.

Malignant

Malignant tumours of the lacrimal gland differ clinically from the benign by a relatively faster onset of growth (less than 12 months) and an often painful proptosis. Orbital imaging often shows destruction of adjacent bone with reactionary ossification.

Malignant pleomorphic adenoma

This tumour usually arises after several incomplete excisions and the most malignant component is a squamous carcinoma or an adenocarcinoma.

Adenoid cystic carcinoma

Adenoid cystic carcinoma is the most common malignant variant of lacrimal gland carcinoma with a peak incidence in the fourth decade.

The macroscopic appearance of this tumour is that of a pale-grey mass similar to a pleomorphic adenoma, although the capsule may not appear to be formed or be intact.

Microscopic examination shows solid cords of hyperchromatic cuboidal cells with a high mitotic rate, proliferating around cystic spaces containing myxoid material – hence the "Swiss cheese" appearance (Figure 5.55). This classical cribriform pattern is only one of several different patterns described, but these are in the province of the pathologist.

This tumour has a propensity for perineural invasion which explains the common symptom of pain and leads to considerable difficulties in assessing clearance margins. Treatment is by total excision or exenteration with adjunctive radiotherapy, but the prognosis is poor.

Adenocarcinoma

The cellular constituents of an adenocarcinoma are the same as those seen in an adenoid cystic carcinoma but the pattern is that of solid masses of tumour tissue (Figure 5.55 inset).

Metastases

A careful history and a thorough general examination are mandatory to ascertain the possibility of metastatic disease when an orbital tumour is identified. Metastases usually present with rapid proptosis. Note that a metastatic scirrhous carcinoma of the breast (Figure 5.56) or stomach may result in an enophthalmos due to orbital fibrous tissue contraction.

Other primary sources for metastatic disease include: lung, prostate, gastrointestinal tract, and kidney, but occasionally no source is found.

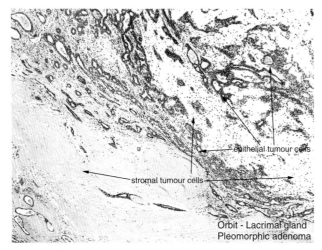

Figure 5.52

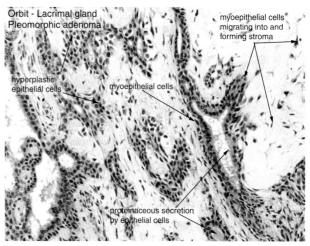

Figure 5.53

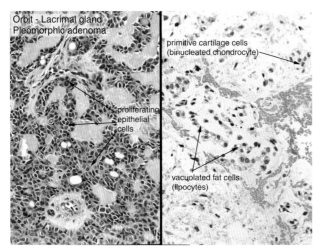

Figure 5.54

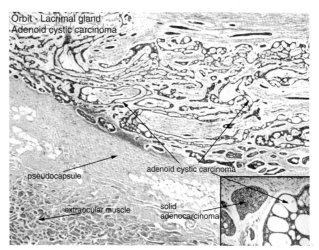

Figure 5.55

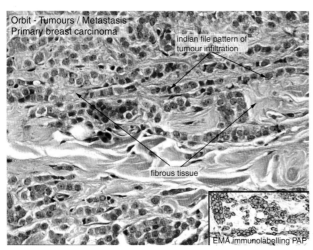

Figure 5.56

Figure 5.52 A low power illustration of the wide variation in cell morphology in a pleomorphic adenoma. The tumour is formed by the proliferation of epithelial cells and stromal cells (connective tissue including fibrocytes, chondrocytes, and lipocytes). The stromal cells are derived from myoepithelial cells in the ducts.

Figure 5.53 A higher magnification from the specimen shown in Figure 5.52 illustrates the proliferation of myoepithelial cells to form the stromal component in a pleomorphic adenoma. The epithelial component is hyperplastic and is also proliferating as nests of cells. Note the resemblance to normal ducts of the lacrimal gland (see Figure 5.49).

Figure 5.54 Pleomorphic adenomas display wide variations in cellular morphology. In the left example, epithelial cells predominate, while in the right example, the myoepithelial cells have formed mesenchymal tissue (resembling cartilage and fat).

Figure 5.55 Malignant tumours derived from the epithelial cells of acini and ducts may form solid masses (adenocarcinoma) or may form cystic and duct-like structures (adenoid cystic carcinoma). The inset shows a solid adenocarcinoma adjacent to the cystic variant.

Figure 5.56 In a metastatic scirrhous carcinoma of the breast, enophthalmos is due to contraction of the fibrous tissue proliferation which accompanies tumour cell infiltration. In this example, the cancer cells adopt a single "Indian-file" pattern within the fibrous tissue. By immunohistochemistry (inset), the tumour is identified as being of epithelial origin by the epithelial membrane antigen (EMA) marker.

Optic nerve pathology

Normal anatomy

The normal optic nerve contains 1.2 million axons with supporting glial cells and blood vessels. The surrounding layers are formed by the pia mater, the arachnoid mater, and the dura mater (Figure 5.57). The pathologist relies on the H&E stain for the identification of glial cell replacement of atrophic myelinated axons (Figure 5.58). Special stains for the identification of axons and myelin are also employed (Figures 5.59, 5.60).

Optic disc swelling/optic atrophy

The numerous causes of unilateral and bilateral optic disc swellings and atrophy are comprehensively documented in clinical textbooks. In this prioritised account of the relevant

pathology (clinicopathological incidence), optic disc swelling in pathological specimens is mostly observed in the *acute* phase of a disease process. Disc swelling will be followed by loss of myelinated axons in the optic nerve if treatment (for example for acute glaucoma) is unsuccessful – it is at this stage that the majority of pathological specimens are encountered. Often there is total loss of myelinated axons with replacement gliosis, but in some conditions the geographical pattern of axonal loss is diagnostic:

- *Glaucoma:* swelling occurs in acute glaucoma (see Figure 7.53). Atrophy in chronic forms is characterised by *posterior cupping of the lamina cribrosa and loss of prelaminar neural tissue* (see Figures 7.54–7.57).
- *Trauma:* mechanical, for example swelling in hypotonia following penetrating injury (Figure 5.61). Optic atrophy follows any process which leads to extensive retinal atrophy, for example post-traumatic pseudoretinitis pigmentosa (see Chapter 9).

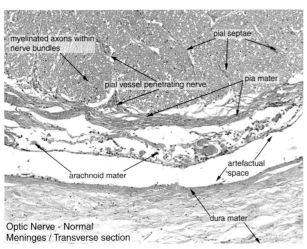

Figure 5.57

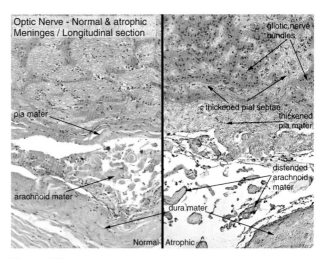

Figure 5.58

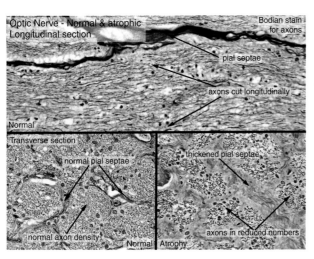

Figure 5.59

Figure 5.57 This transverse section of an optic nerve is from a young patient who died from pneumococcal meningitis – polymorphonuclear leucocytes are present in the arachnoid layer. Note that the thin pial septae surround the nerve bundles and contain capillaries (derived from the network within the pia mater).

Figure 5.58 In a longitudinal section through an optic nerve, the myelinated axons are parallel to the pia mater (left). Advanced optic atrophy (right) is characterised by gliotic replacement of the nerve bundles and fibrous thickening of the pial septae. The atrophic nerve shrinks away from the dura so that the arachnoid space becomes enlarged.

Figure 5.59 A stain which demonstrates axons, in this example the Bodian stain, can be useful in demonstrating the normal density (upper and lower left) and axonal loss in optic atrophy (lower right).

- *Ischaemic neuropathy:* any vascular disease, degenerative or inflammatory, can lead to an insufficient blood supply to the optic nerve, for example giant cell arteritis, anterior ischaemic optic neuropathy, ophthalmic artery occlusion, diabetes, and radiation vasculopathy. A total infarction of the optic nerve in GCA has been illustrated earlier in Figure 5.16. Two branches from the ophthalmic artery form the posterior ciliary arteries. Occlusion of one of these branches leads to hemi-infarction of the optic nerve. The clinical manifestation is that of an altitudinal hemianopia which is mirrored in a pathological specimen (Figure 5.62).
- *Inflammatory/demyelinating disease:* optic neuritis, multiple sclerosis, sarcoidosis, syphilis, and tuberculosis. Chronic inflammation within the optic nerve results in focal or generalised demyelination and atrophy (Figure 5.63). In some cases, as in multiple sclerosis, there is survival of axons.
- *Compressive lesion:* orbital or intracranial masses (see Tables 5.2, 5.3) may directly compress the optic nerve or chiasm. Mechanical pressure can cause atrophy by direct compression, or by interference with the blood supply of the nerve (Figure 5.64). *Optic nerve/disc drusen* are included in this section because the retrolaminar masses interfere with axoplasmic flow and cause disc swelling. On clinical examination, drusen appear as localised refractile masses which autofluoresce within the optic disc. The pathogenesis is thought to be the result of abnormalities in axoplasmic flow leading to calcification. The histological appearance is that of an irregular basophilic mass within the nerve (Figure 5.65). This condition is associated with an abnormal central retinal vasculature and a predisposition to central retinal vein occlusion. Drusen are also found in association with angioid streaks and pseudoxanthoma elasticum.
- *Toxic/nutritional:* alcohol and many drugs (for example ethambutol, chloramphenicol), toxins (for example cyanide), combined with nutritional deficiencies (vitamins B_1, B_2, B_{12}, and folate) produce a characteristic pattern of atrophy of the papillomacular bundle within the optic nerve (Figure 5.66). Visual field investigations detect a characteristic bilateral centrocaecal scotoma. The common pathway that is theorised is a disturbance of mitochondrial metabolism, which is thought to be more sensitive within the papillomacular bundle.
- *Metabolic:* for example Leber's hereditary optic neuropathy. Identical clinical and pathological findings described for toxic amblyopia occur in young males in the second and third decades: females are unaffected. This condition is maternally inherited (via mitochondrial DNA) and is included as an example of an inherited disorder of mitochondrial enzyme systems. The point mutations in mitochondrial DNA have been identified. The abnormality presents initially as a unilateral acutely progressive loss of central vision. This is followed within weeks by involvement of the second eye. The major clinical feature is an apparent swelling of the nerve fibre layer surrounding the disc, with radiating telangiectatic vessels. Pathologically at a later stage, there is atrophy of the papillomacular bundle (Figure 5.67).

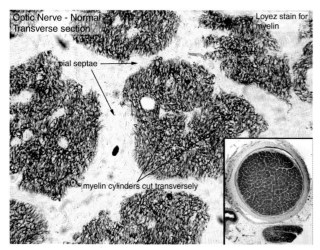

Figure 5.60

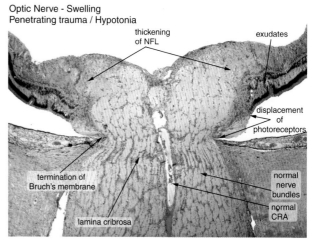

Figure 5.61

Figure 5.60 A stain for myelin (Loyez stain) at low power reveals a uniform distribution of myelinated axons in the normal optic nerve (inset). At higher magnification, myelinated axons appear as black circles surrounding the non-staining axons.

Figure 5.61 In a case of penetrating trauma, there may be severe hypotonia which interferes with the blood supply of the prelaminar part of the optic nerve and results in the interruption of axoplasmic flow. Swelling of the nerve fibre layer (NFL) is such that the photoreceptors are displaced away from the termination of Bruch's membrane. The central retinal artery (CRA) is patent. Note the normal architecture of the retrolaminar part of the optic nerve. (Compare with Figure 7.53.)

Optic Nerve - Atrophy
Hemi-infarct   pathologist's notch to indicate superior dura

total infarction of
superior half
of nerve

central vessels

surviving myelinated axons
in inferior half of nerve

widening of subarachnoid
space

Bodian stain   Loyez stain

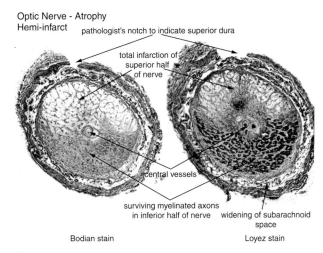

Figure 5.62

Optic Nerve - Atrophy   Loyez stain for myelin
Focal demyelination
Multiple sclerosis   plaque of demyelination

thickened
dura

widened
subarachnoid
space due to
nerve atrophy

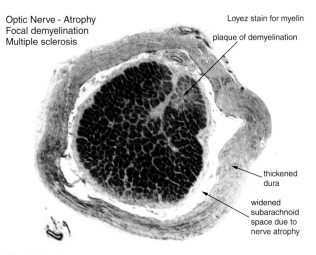

Figure 5.63

Optic Nerve - Infarction
Acute ischaemia from tumour compression
mild optic
disc swelling

artefactual
retinal
detachment

retolaminar
infarction

tumour
mass

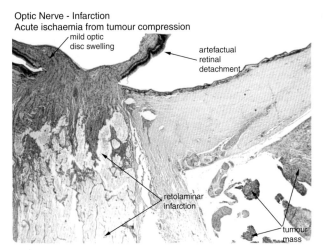

Figure 5.64

Optic Nerve - Disc drusen   white
masses
swollen NFL

macula

drusen

lamina cribrosa

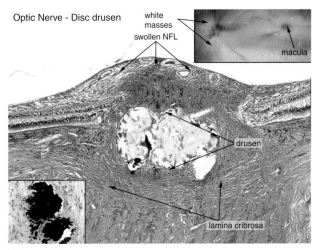

Figure 5.65

Optic Nerve - Atrophy
Toxic Amblyopia
Alcohol/Nutritional

normal nerve
bundles

atrophy of nerve fibres
in papillomacular
Bodian stain bundle located centrally Loyez stain

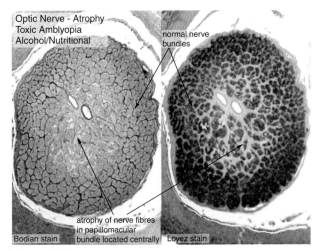

Figure 5.66

Figure 5.62 A patient died following cerebral infarction after he had complained of a unilateral altitudinal inferior field defect. The nerve was removed at autopsy and a transverse section revealed an infarction in the superior half (left: Bodian stain for axons; right: Loyez stain for myelin). Compare with the normal optic nerve in Figure 5.60 (note that the Loyez stain in this case does not have a yellow counterstain).

Figure 5.63 Focal areas of demyelination are characteristic of plaques in multiple sclerosis.

Figure 5.64 A patient developed optic disc swelling due to compression from a large malignant fibrous tumour of the orbit which was subsequently treated by an exenteration. Histology showed that the retro-ocular tumour had caused thrombosis of the ophthalmic artery and its posterior ciliary branches (not illustrated). This resulted in an infarction of the retrolaminar part of the optic nerve.

Figure 5.65 In an autopsy specimen, optic disc drusen appeared as pale nodules within the optic disc (upper inset). Because drusen are heavily calcified, the material is hard and even small drusen fragment on microtomy (lower inset). Decalcification exposes the underlying undisturbed matrix of a drusen in the prelaminar portion of the optic nerve. NFL = nerve fibre layer.

Figure 5.66 An autopsy specimen from a patient with end-stage liver failure due to chronic alcoholism. Atrophy of the macular ganglion cells is followed by retrograde atrophy of the papillomacular bundle, which is central at this level of the optic nerve. At the periphery of the nerve, the myelinated axons are present within bundles of normal size. In the centre, the nerve bundles are atrophic (left: Bodian stain; right: Loyez stain).

- *Raised intracranial pressure* with transfer of pressure to the subarachnoid space around the nerve produces bilateral optic disc swelling (papilloedema). Papilloedema may be either primary (for example benign idiopathic intracranial hypertension – BIIH) or secondary (for example space occupying lesion, inflammation, infection). The mechanism is assumed to be the combined effects of both *mechanical* pressure and *ischaemia* (due to interference with vasculature) impeding axoplasmic flow at the level of the lamina cribrosa. Pathological examination reveals widening of the subarachnoid space and atrophy of the optic nerve and disc (Figure 5.68).
- *Primary optic nerve tumours:* for example glioma/meningioma (see below).

Primary optic nerve tumours

Glioma

The term glioma refers to a group of tumours derived from the supporting cells in neural tissue, for example astrocytomas grades I–IV, oligodendroglioma, and glioblastoma multiforme. In the optic nerve, the gliomas in children are equivalent to intracranial astrocytoma type I and are low grade.

Therefore in ophthalmic practice, gliomas of the optic nerve are usually low grade, unilateral, and are most common in children. Bilateral cases are almost pathognomonic for neurofibromatosis type 1.

The clinical presentation will depend on the *location* of this tumour. Most cases have decreased vision, altered colour perception, and a relative afferent pupillary defect. The optic disc may be normal, exhibit swelling or atrophy (see above), and with sufficient compression result in a central retinal vein occlusion. Intraorbital gliomas present with proptosis, whereas those in the chiasm may have bilateral visual field disturbances or symptoms due to secondary effects on the central nervous system.

High resolution orbital imaging (CT or MRI) demonstrates a fusiform enlargement of the nerve with axial proptosis along the line of the optic nerve, and this is important in diagnosis and treatment planning.

A meningioma should be considered in the differential diagnosis.

Surgery appears to be the only effective treatment as the tumour is unresponsive to radiotherapy and chemotherapy, and this creates much controversy, especially with regards to the risks and morbidity of surgery for those tumours located in the optic chiasm or the intracranial part of the optic nerve. It is for this reason that most cases of resection encountered by an ophthalmic pathologist would be in the intraorbital location.

Previously, the specimens took the form of a globe and nerve containing a glioma (Figure 5.69). Currently attempts are made to excise the tumour, leaving behind the globe if possible. Microscopically, gliomas consist of neoplastic astrocytes with oval or spindle shaped nuclei and branching cytoplasmic processes (Figures 5.70, 5.71). Neoplastic proliferation of astrocytes destroys myelinated axons within the nerve bundles.

Gliomas in adults are rarer, but are more aggressive in behaviour and their histopathological characteristics are those of a poorly differentiated astrocytoma.

Meningioma

These slowly growing neoplastic proliferations of meningothelial cells occur as primary tumours within the meninges of the optic nerve. Alternatively a meningioma in the skull may spread into the orbit. Unlike optic nerve gliomas, meningiomas more commonly present in middle-aged adults, usually women.

Symptoms will depend on the location of the tumour – an orbital location would result in a posterior mass effect with proptosis and corneal exposure. Location within the optic canal may result in visual loss, altered colour perception, or an afferent pupillary defect, and the initial optic disc swelling is followed by atrophy.

Diagnosis is very much dependent on high resolution CT/MRI.

Management of orbital meningiomas is usually conservative with serial imaging and visual fields to assess growth and tumour extension. Active treatment depends on the severity of optic nerve compression and the location of the tumour. Although the tumour is partially responsive to radiotherapy and hormonal therapy, surgery is still the treatment of choice and can vary from local excision to exenteration combined with craniotomy for intracranial extension.

The tumour usually surrounds the optic nerve, but there may also be an eccentric mass which distorts the orbital tissues (Figure 5.72). Histologically, the commonest form of *orbital* meningioma is the *meningothelial type* (Figure 5.73). In this tumour, fibrous septae surround small spindle cells which do not have prominent cytoplasm – these cells resemble those in the normal arachnoid mater. Psammomatous meningiomas contain numerous pink-staining "psammoma" bodies (Figure 5.73). Within the cranial cavity, meningiomas have a variety of appearances – this classification is in the province of the neuropathologist.

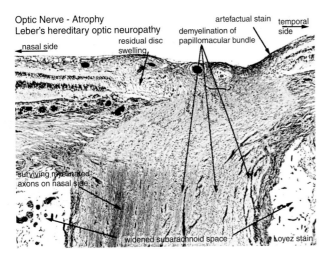

Optic Nerve - Atrophy
Leber's hereditary optic neuropathy

nasal side →

← temporal side

artefactual stain

demyelination of papillomacular bundle

residual disc swelling

surviving myelinated axons on nasal side

widened subarachnoid space

Loyez stain

Figure 5.67

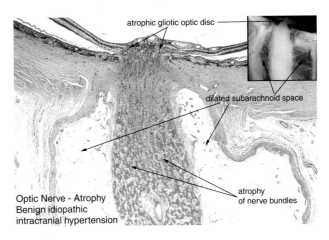

atrophic gliotic optic disc

dilated subarachnoid space

atrophy of nerve bundles

Optic Nerve - Atrophy
Benign idiopathic
intracranial hypertension

Figure 5.68

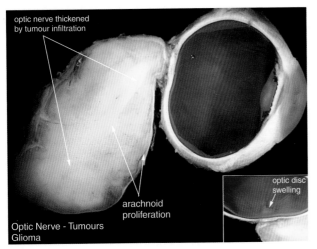

optic nerve thickened by tumour infiltration

arachnoid proliferation

optic disc swelling

Optic Nerve - Tumours
Glioma

Figure 5.69

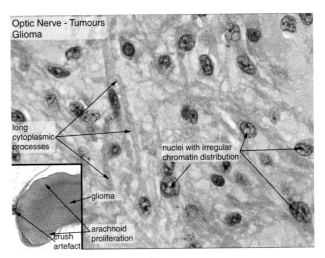

Optic Nerve - Tumours
Glioma

long cytoplasmic processes

nuclei with irregular chromatin distribution

glioma

crush artefact

arachnoid proliferation

Figure 5.70

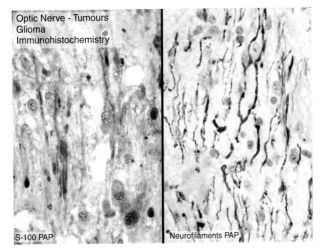

Optic Nerve - Tumours
Glioma
Immunohistochemistry

S-100 PAP

Neurofilaments PAP

Figure 5.71

Figure 5.67 In the retrolaminar part of the optic nerve, the papillomacular bundle is on the temporal side. In this example of Leber's hereditary optic neuropathy, there is extensive loss of myelinated axons in the papillomacular bundle with some survival on the nasal side. The arachnoid space is widened because the optic nerve is atrophic (Loyez stain).

Figure 5.68 A patient suffering from benign idiopathic intracranial hypertension died from meningitis after an infection of a ventriculo-peritoneal shunt. The case serves to illustrate the pathology of the effects of longstanding raised intracranial pressure. The subarachnoid space is widened, and the optic nerve is atrophic. At this stage, the optic disc is also atrophic and gliotic. The peripapillary retina is drawn inwards (in contrast with the initial outward displacement of photoreceptors seen in optic disc swelling).

Figure 5.69 An optic nerve glioma is ovoid or fusiform in shape, in this case, measuring 20 mm in diameter and 35 mm in length. The cut surface reveals indistinct enlargement of the optic nerve surrounded by arachnoidal proliferation. A superficial biopsy containing only arachnoidal proliferation can be deceptive for the pathologist who might consider the diagnosis of a meningioma. In this specimen, the tumour extends to the excision line which implies the risk of spread into the optic foramen and chiasm. The inset shows optic disc swelling.

Figure 5.70 In a glioma of the optic nerve, myelinated axons are replaced by proliferating astrocytes which are recognised by their long cytoplasmic processes. Mitotic figures are only rarely found. The inset shows a low power view of a glioma which was clamped behind the globe: note the diffuse infiltration within the optic nerve and the reactionary arachnoidal proliferation.

Figure 5.71 Immunohistochemistry confirms the presence of neoplastic astrocytes which react positively with S-100 antibody (left). S-100 labels any cells of neural crest origin and a more specific marker is the antibody against intermediate contractile filaments (neurofilaments) which are present in astrocytes (right). Note the branching cytoplasmic processes.

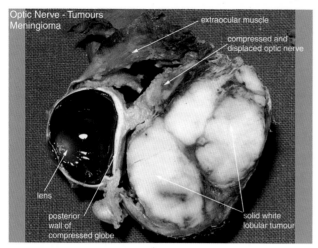

Figure 5.72

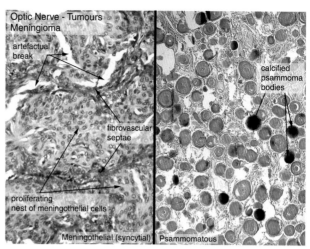

Figure 5.73

Figure 5.72 Meningiomas within the orbit can grow to a large size and cause severe distortions of the optic nerve and globe requiring exenteration. The solid pale grey lobules in close proximation to the nerve hint at the diagnosis of a meningioma.

Figure 5.73 The commonest histological subtypes of intraorbital meningiomas are meningothelial or syncytial (left) and psammomatous (right). The meningothelial tumour is formed by neoplastic arachnoidal cells which do not have extended cytoplasmic processes. The tumour cells are surrounded by fibrovascular septae. A tumour which contains several spherical pink bodies is classified as a psammomatous meningioma – similar pink bodies may be seen in the normal arachnoid mater.

Chapter 6
Development and malformation

The following description is restricted to those malformations which are encountered in clinical ophthalmology.

Normal development/embryology of the anterior segment

The eye develops as an outpouching from the forebrain and this forms the optic vesicle (day 26 – Figure 6.1a). An invagination occurs to form the optic cup (day 36 – Figure 6.1b), but this is not total and there is an infero-medial fissure which closes progressively to leave a gap through which the hyaloid artery penetrates to provide a blood supply to the developing lens (tunica vasculosa lentis – Figure 6.1c). The primary vitreous is derived from mesenchyme, while the secondary vitreous is formed by the cells of the retina. The tertiary adult vitreous is formed by cells of the ciliary epithelium (Figure 6.1d).

The inner layer of the optic cup forms the neural retina, the inner non-pigmented layer of the ciliary epithelium and, initially, the posterior layer of the iris pigment epithelium. The outer layer of the optic cup forms the retinal pigment epithelium, the outer layer of the ciliary epithelium, and the anterior layer of the iris (Figure 6.1d). The lens forms as a placode in the surface ectoderm (Figure 6.1a) and this invaginates and separates from the ectoderm to migrate into the optic cup (Figure 6.1b,c).

The cornea forms after lens migration and initially consists of a surface layer of ectoderm and a posterior layer of neural crest cells (first wave) which become endothelium. The stroma develops by migration of the second wave of neural crest cells between the two surface layers (Figures 6.2, 6.3). The iris stroma migrates with the anterior lip of the optic cup to separate the anterior and posterior chambers. The iris stroma is formed from the third wave of neural crest and mesenchymal tissue. Note that the two epithelial layers of the iris are derived from both layers of the optic cup (Figure 6.4). The outflow system develops from neural crest cells in the chamber angle (Figure 6.4). The central part of the lens contains elongated cells (primary lens fibres) which degenerate. The cells at the equator form new lens fibres which extend to the anterior and posterior poles (Figure 6.3).

The neuroblastic cells in the inner layer of the optic vesicle form a single layer initially but then divide and migrate to form the three neural layers of the retina. Axons from the ganglion cells pass through the scleral canal to synapse with cells in the lateral geniculate body. Myelination of axons in the optic nerve is not complete until birth. See p. 129 for normal retinal development.

In the following text, normal histology will be provided to illustrate the mechanisms of failure in development.

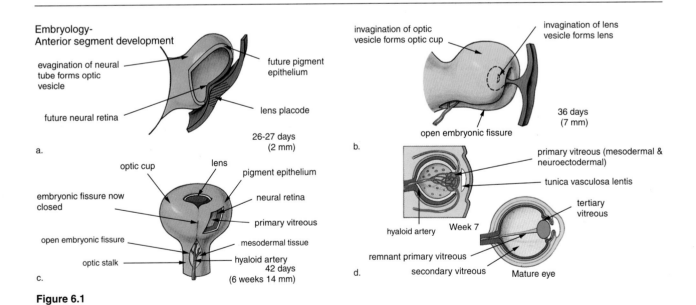

Figure 6.1

Figure 6.1 Diagrams to show the stages of ocular development during the first trimester. Colour scheme: pink = optic vesicle and outer layer of optic cup, blue = neural retina, dark green = tissue derived from ectoderm, yellow = mesenchyme. For a detailed explanation, see text.

Embryology - Week 7
Anterior segment formation

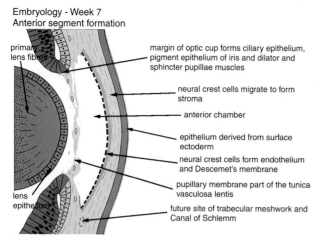

primary
lens fibres

lens
epithelium

margin of optic cup forms ciliary epithelium,
pigment epithelium of iris and dilator and
sphincter pupillae muscles

neural crest cells migrate to form
stroma

anterior chamber

epithelium derived from surface
ectoderm

neural crest cells form endothelium
and Descemet's membrane

pupillary membrane part of the tunica
vasculosa lentis

future site of trabecular meshwork and
Canal of Schlemm

Figure 6.2

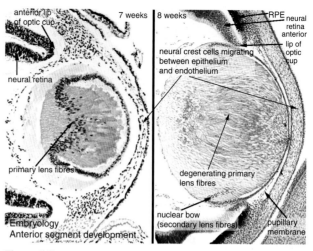

anterior lip
of optic cup   7 weeks

neural retina

primary lens fibres

8 weeks   RPE
                                               neural
                                               retina
                                               anterior
neural crest cells migrating   lip of
between epithelium   optic
and endothelium   cup

degenerating primary
lens fibres

nuclear bow
(secondary lens fibres)

pupillary
membrane

Embryology
Anterior segment development

Figure 6.3

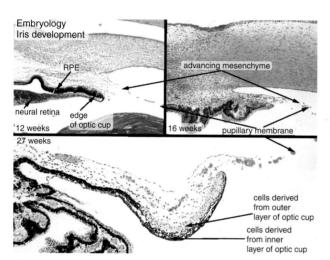

Embryology
Iris development

RPE

advancing mesenchyme

neural retina   edge
                      of optic cup
12 weeks   16 weeks   pupillary membrane

27 weeks

cells derived
from outer
layer of optic cup

cells derived
from inner
layer of optic cup

Figure 6.4

Figure 6.2 The cornea and lens are formed before the iris and ciliary body, which are derived from the third wave of neuroectoderm and mesenchyme. The colour scheme is identical to that in Figure 6.1.

Figure 6.3 The embryological features of the anterior segment around 7–8 weeks help in understanding the malformations which can occur. The failure of migration of neural crest cells (second wave, differentiating to stromal keratocytes) into the central cornea can give rise to corneal opacities (Peters' anomaly, type 1). Disturbance in the development of the primary and secondary lens fibres can result in a congenital cataract. RPE = retinal pigment epithelium.

Figure 6.4 The iris develops after the cornea and lens are fully formed, i.e. at a comparatively later stage of gestation. Neural crest and mesenchymal cells extend into the space between the lens and cornea to serve as a substrate for migrating cells from the optic cup: these migrating cells form the future anterior and posterior pigmented epithelial layers and the iris musculature.

Anterior segment anomalies

Cornea

Although most of the corneal anomalies can be diagnosed easily by clinical examination, on occasion there may be a constellation of anterior segment abnormalities. Currently there is much interest in the usage of the ultrasonic biomicroscope which allows accurate imaging of the anterior segment in complicated cases.

Peters' anomaly

Peters' anomaly represents a spectrum of anterior segment malformations, although essentially it is characterised by a central corneal opacity (leucoma) at birth due to a failure of formation of the posterior axial stroma and endothelium.

Clinical presentation

The neonate presents with a central avascular corneal opacity that may be unilateral or bilateral. The opacity can improve with time if the posterior defect is covered with endothelium (see description of pathology below).

Other ocular findings may include irido-corneal adhesions and an anteriorly displaced cataractous lens. Patients have a high risk of glaucoma (30–70%) despite treatment.

The corneal opacity in Peters' anomaly may occur in isolation, as part of a wider ocular malformation (for example microphthalmia or aniridia), or as part of a systemic syndrome (for example Peters' plus syndrome with numerous associated abnormalities including CNS/cardiac/genitourinary anomalies, and skeletal deformities).

Some authors subclassify Peters' anomaly (Figure 6.5):
- *Type 1:* without lens involvement although iris strands may be attached at the periphery of the posterior corneal defect.
- *Type 2:* as with type 1 but with lenticulocorneal contact.

An ultrasonic biomicroscopic (UBM) examination is extremely useful and is found to have a high correlation with pathological findings.

Genetics

This condition is not usually heritable, although in some cases the gene defects *PAX6* and *CYP1B1* (for congenital glaucoma) have been associated.

Possible modes of treatment

Treatment will depend on the severity of the malformation. Penetrating keratoplasty may be required for dense opacities that may otherwise threaten amblyopia. Involvement of the lens may require a lensectomy.

In all cases, the patients are monitored regularly for amblyopia, refractive error, and glaucoma. The visual prognosis is invariably poor despite treatment.

Pathogenesis and pathology: type 1

Pathogenesis Failure of migration of the first wave of neural crest cells to form the endothelium and Descemet's membrane leads to a posterior corneal stromal defect (Figures 6.3, 6.5a). This is associated with a failure in the normal formation of the iris in the third wave of neural crest and mesenchymal migration with the end result being iris fragments adherent to the cornea at the edge of the defect.

Macroscopic Most specimens would therefore be in the form of a host corneal disc following penetrating keratoplasty. The corneal disc will contain a dense white central (or paracentral) opacity and iris tissue may be adherent to the posterior edges of the leucoma (Figure 6.6).

Microscopic The key feature is a defect in the posterior stroma, Descemet's membrane, and endothelium (Figure 6.7). Depending on the timing of surgery following birth, the original defect may be covered by migration of endothelium from the periphery and formation of new Descemet's membrane.

Pathogenesis and pathology: type 2

Pathogenesis Incomplete separation of the lens vesicle from the overlying surface lens placode of the developing cornea may interfere with the first wave of neural crest cells and this causes a defect in the posterior stroma, Descemet's membrane, and endothelium (Figure 6.5b). The lens may not move into the optic cup and this is one explanation for the apparent lenticulocorneal contact.

Macroscopic Type 2 Peters' anomaly is most commonly seen by the pathologist in an enucleated globe. Lenticulocorneal contact with obvious cataractous changes in the lens are the most important diagnostic feature (Figure 6.8 inset).

Microscopic Apart from lenticulocorneal contact, the appearances can be variable. The iris may be adherent to the cornea or may be hypoplastic (Figures 6.8, 6.9).

Complications/secondary effects

Glaucoma is common with possible signs of corneal enlargement and buphthalmos. This condition is difficult to control and usually requires surgery.

Other conditions that may follow are postoperative keratoplasty cataract (type 1), retinal detachment, and phthisis (about a third of cases – type 2).

Malformation - Peters' anomaly

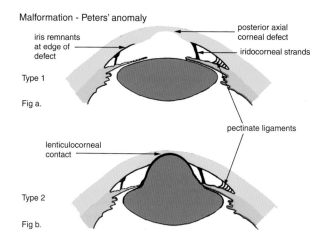

Figure 6.5

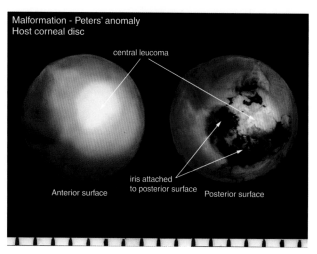

Figure 6.6

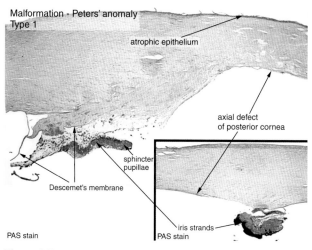

Figure 6.7

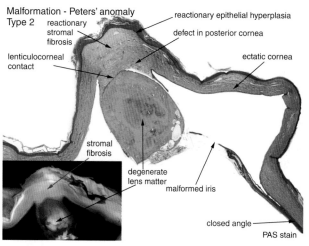

Figure 6.8

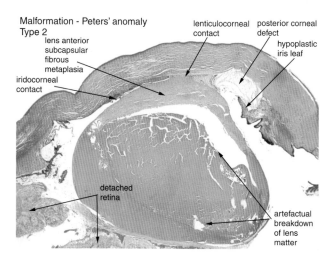

Figure 6.9

Figure 6.5 A diagram to show the features of Peters' anomaly type 1 (a) and type 2 (b). These illustrate the extreme ends of the spectrum and in reality there is considerable variation in individual cases.

Figure 6.6 The macroscopic features of Peters' anomaly include a central leucoma with iris tissue adherent to the posterior surface of the cornea around the leucoma.

Figure 6.7 In this case of Peters' anomaly, the PAS stain demonstrates the absence of Descemet's membrane at the site of a posterior corneal stromal defect. In the anterior part of the defect, the lamellar architecture is lost, possibly due to oedema, which explains the clinical opacity. The strands of iris tissue attached to the edge of the defect contain part of the sphincter pupillae. The inset shows the opposite edge of the defect with adherent iris at the periphery.

Figure 6.8 Type 2 Peters' anomaly is often complicated by malformations of the chamber angle. In this example, secondary angle closure glaucoma was followed by buphthalmos, and enucleation was required for cosmetic reasons in an end-stage eye. The inset shows the macroscopic appearance of iridolenticular contact with cataractous changes. Microscopically, a degenerate lens is fused with the posterior corneal surface at the site of a defect in Descemet's membrane. Many secondary changes in the cornea are present – keratectasia, epithelial metaplasia, and stromal fibrosis (PAS stain).

Figure 6.9 There may be a broad spectrum of anterior segment malformations in type 2 Peters' anomaly. In this example, the posterior corneal deficit is eccentric and the adjacent iris leaf is hypoplastic. The opposite iris leaf is adherent to the cornea as far as the point of lenticulocorneal contact. Retinal detachment was probably secondary to disorganisation of the anterior segment.

Sclerocornea

The term sclerocornea is derived from the apparent scleral appearance of an opaque vascularised cornea.

The patient usually presents at birth with bilateral diffuse or peripheral corneal opacities. Glaucoma is common and there may be associations with other anterior segment malformations. Systemically, there is an association with deafness, CNS, and skeletal abnormalities.

The pathogenesis is attributed to an apparent failure of differentiation of keratocytes in the second wave of mesenchymal migration leading to formation of a collagen of scleral type. Most cases are sporadic, although variable inheritance patterns have been described including autosomal dominant and autosomal recessive.

Treatment involves glaucoma control if necessary followed by penetrating keratoplasty.

Pathology

Most specimens are in the form of an opaque corneal disc following penetrating keratoplasty. In an enucleated globe, there may be other anterior segment anomalies and the secondary effects will include glaucoma.

An epithelium is present but Bowman's layer and Descemet's membrane are absent. The lamellar architecture is lost and the collagen bundles are similar in the arrangement to those in the sclera (Figure 6.10).

Congenital hereditary endothelial dystrophy (CHED)

See Table 4.1.

Angle

See Chapter 7, section "Congenital/infantile/juvenile".

Iris

Aniridia

Aniridia is a rare bilateral congenital ocular condition that is characterised by maldevelopment of the iris. Aniridic patients require careful follow up from birth due to associated ocular and systemic complications.

Clinical presentation

Despite the term aniridia (suggesting "absent iris"), an iris stump is evident in the majority of cases. Related ocular symptoms and signs may be present:

1 Poor vision with pendular nystagmus, photophobia, strabismus, and amblyopia.
2 Superficial corneal pannus and keratopathy.
3 Glaucoma – high incidence (50%).
4 Lens abnormalities, for example cataract and microphakia.
5 Foveal hypoplasia and optic nerve hypoplasia.

The inheritance pattern determines the systemic associations:

1 *Autosomal dominant (85%):* no associated systemic conditions.
2 *Sporadic (13%):* Miller's/WAGR syndrome (WAGR: **W**ilm's tumour, **a**niridia, **g**enitourinary abnormalities, and mental **r**etardation).
3 *Autosomal recessive (2%):* Gillespie's syndrome with cerebellar abnormalities.

It is therefore important that any sporadic cases of aniridia undergoes a full family history and medical evaluation for systemic involvement.

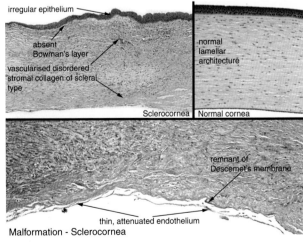

Malformation - Sclerocornea

Figure 6.10

Figure 6.10 In sclerocornea, the absence of the Bowman's layer and an abnormal scleral collagen provide an irregular substrate for the epithelium which has a corrugated appearance (upper left). An endothelium is present but Descemet's membrane is imperfectly formed (lower). The upper right illustration is a normal cornea for comparison.

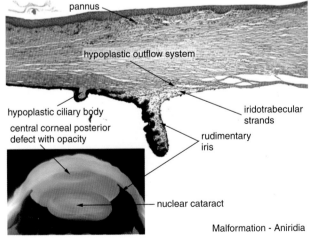

Malformation - Aniridia

Figure 6.11

Figure 6.11 In aniridia, a rudimentary iris stump is characteristic and is associated with hypoplasia of the trabecular meshwork and the formation of iridotrabecular strands. A corneal pannus is a frequent finding in aniridia. The inset illustrates the macroscopic features of aniridia in association with a type I Peters' anomaly.

Pathogenesis

Arrestment of the third neural crest wave with subsequent maldevelopment of the iris and chamber angle. With increasing age of the patient, contraction of the iris tissue straddling the angle may be such that an obstruction to outflow leads to increasing severity of glaucoma.

Genetics

Aniridia is associated with alterations in the *Pax6* gene which is a paired box sequence with the role of regulating the expression of other genes, presumably in regulating embryogenesis of the eye. The *Pax6* gene, located at the short arm of chromosome 11 (11p13), is of considerable research interest especially as it is commonly expressed in different species including the insectivores. It is accepted that point mutations or partial deletions of a copy of the *Pax6* gene will result in many phenotypic expressions of congenital ocular disorders, including aniridia and Peters' anomaly. Deletions of both copies are not compatible with life.

The *Pax6* locus is close to the gene for nephroblastoma, which may explain the associations in the WAGR syndrome.

Possible modes of treatment

Glaucoma surgery is invariably required as resistance to medication increases usually during adulthood. A clinically significant cataract may require lensectomy.

Macroscopic

As a rarity, an enucleated globe will be presented for pathological investigation as a consequence of complicated secondary glaucoma. An iris stump is usually evident fusing or obscuring the chamber angle (Figure 6.11, inset).

Microscopic

The sphincter pupillae and dilator pupillae are absent from the iris stump (Figure 6.11). There may also be associated maldevelopment of the angle and cortical cataracts.

Keratopathy is often an undocumented feature of aniridia; this is due to an apparent stem cell deficiency with metaplasia of corneal epithelium to resemble conjunctival epithelium containing goblet cells (Figure 6.12).

Persistent pupillary membrane

This structure appears as a consequence of incomplete resolution of the vascular tissue which provides a scaffold for the pigmented cells at the tip of the optic cup (see Figure 6.4). The membrane appears as a thin atrophic fibrovascular structure straddling the pupillary space (Figure 6.13). The membrane is innocuous, is identified at birth, and may persist through adulthood.

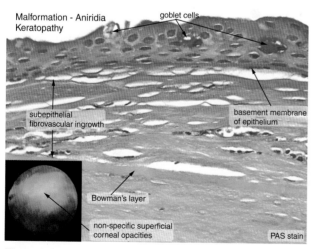

Figure 6.12

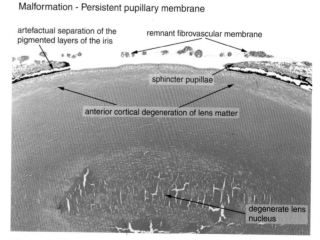

Figure 6.13

Figure 6.12 In aniridic keratopathy, "conjunctivalisation" of the surface epithelium of the cornea can be identified by the presence of goblet cells. An unstable epithelium promotes the fibrovascular ingrowth between Bowman's layer and epithelium (PAS stain). The superficial opacification is non-specific (inset).

Figure 6.13 In a persistent pupillary membrane, strands of fibrovascular tissue extend across the pupil. This was an incidental finding in an adult globe in which there were degenerative changes in the lens.

Lens

Congenital cataract

Congenital cataracts occur when there is maldevelopment of fetal lens tissue. The aetiology is often unknown but, especially in bilateral cases, may be the result of systemic disease or maternal infection (TORCH syndrome: **t**oxoplasma, **o**ther infections – syphilis and viruses, **r**ubella, **c**ytomegalovirus, and **h**erpes simplex).

Primary hereditary congenital cataracts may also occur and are usually autosomal dominant in transmission.

The descriptions and classifications of congenital cataracts are well documented in clinical texts (for example polar, sutural, nuclear, lamellar, and capsular). These variations depend on the stage of lens development at which the injurious agent was introduced. Congenitally deformed lenses (for example lentiglobus) are occasionally encountered. Whereas extracapsular cataract surgery is required for visually significant cataracts, intact lens specimens are rare in pathology (Figure 6.14).

Posterior segment anomalies

Vitreous

Persistent hyperplastic primary vitreous (PHPV)

Early in embryonic life (Figures 6.1, 6.15) the lens is surrounded by embryonic vascular tissue (tunica vasculosa lentis), which in turn merges with the primary vitreous containing fibrovascular mesodermal tissue. Regression of this tissue may fail leaving *proliferating* fibrovascular remnants either behind the lens (persistent anterior hyperplastic primary vitreous) or on the inner surface of the peripapillary retina (persistent posterior hyperplastic vitreous). In some cases both variants may be present.

Clinical presentation

The hallmark features of PHPV are leucocoria, centripetal traction of the ciliary processes, and microphthalmia.

The wide spectrum of presentation of PHPV depends on the amount of residual primary vitreous and hyaloid vasculature:

1 *Anterior PHPV* presents as a retrolental mass. A Mittendorf dot represents the mildest manifestation and appears as a small white axial nodule. More severe variants appear as large plaques that span the posterior surface of the lens, and draw in the ciliary processes centripetally. Prior to diagnostic imaging, the retrolental plaque posed an important differential diagnosis in a suspected case of retinoblastoma (see Chapter 11 for complete differential diagnosis). Further contraction of the retrolental tissue may distort the iris and chamber angle with resultant angle closure glaucoma.

2 *Posterior PHPV* represents persistent hyaloid vasculature on the optic disc. A Bergmeister's papilla is an isolated white mass containing hyaloid artery remnants on the optic disc. Residual primary vitreous may form epiretinal membranes which contract to produce a range of appearances from falciform folds to tractional retinal detachment. Optic nerve hypoplasia may be a feature. Both anterior and posterior PHPV can occur simultaneously.

Possible modes of treatment

There is much controversy with regard to surgical treatment of PHPV as it is usually a unilateral condition and the post-surgical visual outcome is poor with amblyopia and pre-existing ocular maldevelopment. Vitrectomy and detachment surgery may be the treatment of choice if there is retinal involvement.

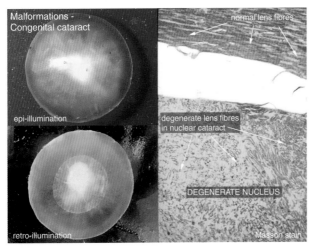

Figure 6.14

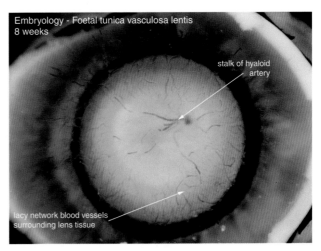

Figure 6.15

Figure 6.14 It is rare for a lens to be removed *in toto* and this is a valuable example of a congenital nuclear cataract. When viewed from above, the nuclear opacity is irregular (upper left) but retroillumination reveals a sharply demarcated zone between the cataractous nucleus and the normal cortex (lower left). Histology from this lens (right) shows normal cortical fibres adjacent to severely disrupted lens fibres in the nuclear cataract.

Figure 6.15 In a normal fetal eye at 8 weeks, the tunica vasculosa lentis and the feeder vessel (hyaloid artery) are beginning to regress and will be absent at full term.

Macroscopic and microscopic

In the past it was impossible to distinguish between a retinoblastoma and a large retrolental mass secondary to PHPV, and this has led to diagnostic errors. Currently enucleation is far less frequent with the advent of advanced diagnostic imaging.

1 *Anterior:* a large retrolental fibrovascular mass with a persistent hyaloid artery is diagnostic (Figure 6.16). In a severe case, contraction of the retrolental mass distorts the lens and pulls in the ciliary processes – this was a traditional diagnostic feature (Figure 6.17).

2 *Posterior:* enucleation specimens were also submitted if there was a large mass on the optic nerve head simulating a neoplasm (Figure 6.18).

The distortion of the disc and peripapillary retina may be relatively minor (Figure 6.19) and currently would be treated conservatively. However, occasionally such minor abnormalities may be encountered in globes enucleated for suspected malignancy when a coexisting anterior PHPV is present (Figures 6.16, 6.19, 6.20).

Retina

Normal retinal development

The normal neural retina develops in the inner layer of the optic cup as a thick layer of neuroblastic cells (Figure 6.21). Some of these cells migrate inwards to form the inner nuclear layer and subsequently the ganglion cell layer of the retina (Figure 6.21).

Axons migrate from the ganglion cells through the scleral foramen to form synapses within the lateral geniculate body.

Dysplasia

This histological feature is usually observed in stillborn infants with major chromosomal disorders such as trisomy D (chromosomes 13–15) and trisomy E (chromosomes 16–18).

In a zone of retinal dysplasia, the rosette-like formations retain the layered pattern which distinguishes them from neoplastic rosettes (Figure 6.22; see also "Retinoblastoma" in Chapter 11).

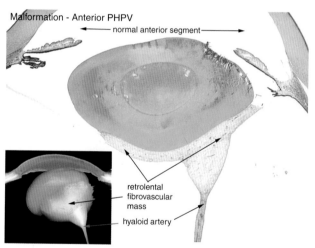

Figure 6.16

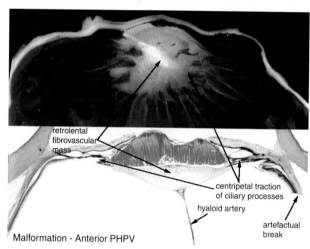

Malformation - Anterior PHPV

Figure 6.17

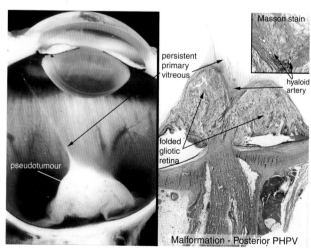

Figure 6.18

Figure 6.16 In less severe examples of anterior persistent hyperplastic primary vitreous (PHPV), a mass of fibrovascular tissue, supplied by a persistent hyaloid artery, is adherent to the posterior surface of the lens. The ciliary body and chamber angle are unaffected. In this archival case enucleation was performed because the leucocoria that presented in this patient could not be differentiated from a retinoblastoma (prior to availability of diagnostic ultrasound). The inset shows the macroscopic appearance of the same specimen.

Figure 6.17 Two examples of anterior persistent hyperplastic primary vitreous (PHPV) (upper macroscopic, lower microscopic) to illustrate a clinical pathognomonic feature, which is centripetal traction on the ciliary processes by a retrolental fibrous mass.

Figure 6.18 A child presented with a mass on the optic nerve head. The media were clear and neoplasia could not be excluded. In the enucleated globe (left), a large tumour expansion from the optic disc was in continuity with the vitreous strands. Histology shows marked distortion of the peripapillary retina, which is thrown into folds by contraction of a fibrous mass derived from hyperplastic primary vitreous (right). A hyaloid artery is identified within fibrovascular tissue which is best demonstrated in a Masson stain (right inset).

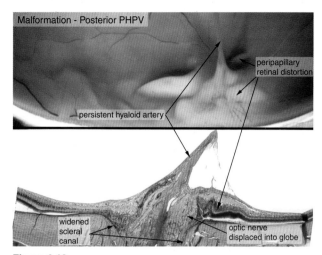

Malformation - Posterior PHPV

peripapillary retinal distortion

persistent hyaloid artery

widened scleral canal

optic nerve displaced into globe

Figure 6.19

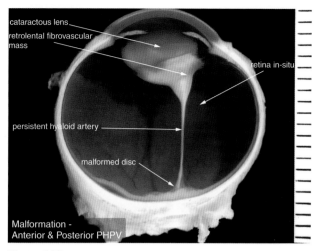

cataractous lens

retrolental fibrovascular mass

retina in-situ

persistent hyaloid artery

malformed disc

Malformation - Anterior & Posterior PHPV

Figure 6.20

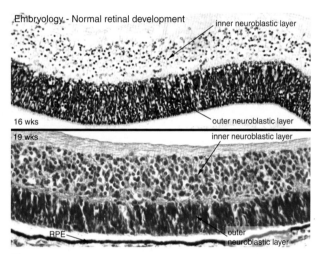

Embryology - Normal retinal development

inner neuroblastic layer

outer neuroblastic layer

16 wks

19 wks

inner neuroblastic layer

RPE

outer neuroblastic layer

Figure 6.21

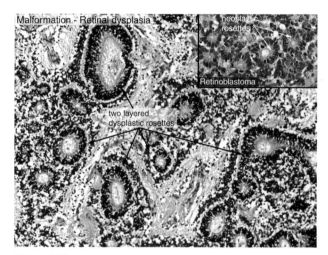

Malformation - Retinal dysplasia

neoplastic rosettes

Retinoblastoma

two layered dysplastic rosettes

Figure 6.22

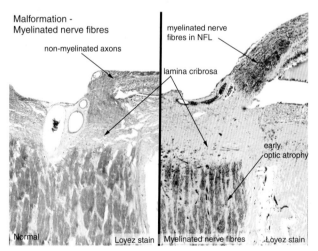

Malformation - Myelinated nerve fibres

non-myelinated axons

myelinated nerve fibres in NFL

lamina cribrosa

early optic atrophy

Normal   Loyez stain

Myelinated nerve fibres   Loyez stain

Figure 6.23

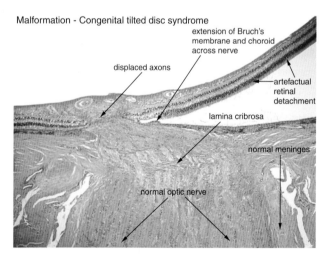

Malformation - Congenital tilted disc syndrome

extension of Bruch's membrane and choroid across nerve

displaced axons

artefactual retinal detachment

lamina cribrosa

normal meninges

normal optic nerve

Figure 6.24

Myelinated nerve fibres

Myelination (a function of oligodendrocytes) proceeds distally towards the eye and may be incomplete at birth. Myelinated nerve fibres in the retina represent an abnormal migration of oligodendrocytes into the retina resulting in abnormal myelination of the axons in the nerve fibre layer. Clinically, most patients are asymptomatic and the anomaly would only be discovered on routine fundus examination which reveals white feathery patches in the nerve fibre layer that may be discontinuous from the optic nerve head. In 20% of affected individuals, the abnormality is bilateral.

Unless specifically mentioned clinically or detected on macroscopic examination, myelinated nerve fibres may be missed on routine H&E sections. Stains specific for myelin (for example Loyez) will reveal the myelination of axons in the nerve fibre layer (Figure 6.23).

Optic disc

Malformations of the optic disc, for a variety of reasons, are of great clinical importance due to the numerous systemic associations. However, none require surgical intervention and are, therefore, rare in pathological experience.

Congenital tilted disc

The mildest form of malformation in the optic disc is a distortion of the shape of the disc due to an oblique entry of the optic nerve through the scleral canal. The resultant distortion gives the impression of "tilting" or "choking" and the visual consequence is a scotoma or a large field defect, which can be corrected to some extent by refraction. Myopic astigmatism is a common feature as well as thinning of the inferonasal retinal pigment epithelium (RPE) and choroid. Usually bilateral, tilted discs are found in 3% of the population and can occur in any direction, although a superotemporal orientation is commonest.

The anomaly is based on a failure of supporting tissues to shape the direction of nerve fibres in the pre- and retrolaminar part of the optic nerve.

Microscopic examination reveals an extension of Bruch's membrane over the lamina cribrosa with an apparent compression of the nerve fibres (Figure 6.24). Congenital tilted discs should be compared with the histology of a myopic disc (see Figures 10.93, 10.94), because both are regarded clinically as "tilted discs".

Figure 6.19 A minor disc malformation due to posterior persistent hyperplastic primary vitreous (PHPV) would not be presented to the pathologist ordinarily. This example is taken from the globe shown in Figure 6.20 in which there was a leucocoria (see Figure 6.16, which is also from the same case). Traction on the disc has displaced the optic nerve and distorted the peripapillary retina. In such cases there is widening of the scleral canal – a possible theory to explain this finding is that the malformation occurs several months before the lamina cribrosa is formed at 20 weeks.

Figure 6.20 The complete globe illustrated in Figures 6.16 and 6.19.

Figure 6.21 At an early stage in normal retinal development, there is one layer of neuroblastic cells derived from the inner layer of the optic cup (upper). Subsequently some of these cells migrate and mature in the inner retina to form the inner nuclear layer from which the ganglion cells are derived (lower). At this stage, the photoreceptors are not formed.

Figure 6.22 In retinal dysplasia, the arrangement of the cells is reminiscent of the early stages of retinal development with a clear zone between two layers of

neuroblastic cells (see Figure 6.21). A failure in the process of migration and maturation of the neuroblastic cells in the inner layer of the optic cup is responsible for this malformation. In a retinoblastoma (inset), there is never a tendency to form two layers of tumour cells.

Figure 6.23 The presence of myelinated axons is best demonstrated with a stain for myelin (e.g. Loyez – left). In this example (right), myelinated nerve fibres in the retina were a chance finding in a globe in which the pathology was complicated and there was a reduction in myelinated axons in the nerve bundles (secondary optic atrophy). It is of interest that the myelination is discontinuous between the retrolaminar portion of the optic nerve and the abnormal retinal myelination. NFL = nerve fibre layer.

Figure 6.24 The demonstration of a tilted disc depends on the correct selection of the plane of section, i.e. vertical compared with horizontal in myopic disc tilting. The optic nerve is of normal width but prelaminar nerve fibres are apparently distorted by an extension of the choroid and Bruch's membrane.

Optic pit

An optic pit appears as a small depression at the rim of the optic disc and is of speculative pathogenesis because a coloboma can be ruled out due to the common temporal location. It is usually asymptomatic and unilateral. Exudative retinal detachment and paracentral arcuate field defects can occur and are most visually threatening when the pit is temporal and there is an exudative detachment of the macula.

Histologically, there is herniation of the retina and a surrounding layer of fibrous tissue into the meninges and adjacent substance of the optic nerve (Figure 6.25). The origin of the subretinal exudate is not understood, but in view of the histological findings may involve leakage from the subarachnoid space.

Optic nerve hypoplasia

Optic nerve hypoplasia is an abnormally small optic nerve head and has been described as one of the three leading causes of blindness in children in the USA.

Morning glory anomaly (MGA)

Morning glory anomaly is a rare sporadic condition characterised by funnel-shaped excavations of both optic discs. Most authors differentiate MGA from an optic disc coloboma.

Clinical presentation

Visual acuity is usually reduced to 6/60. The retina emerging from the excavated optic cup has a constricted appearance and the linear retinal vessels run a straight course from the disc to periphery: the appearances resemble the morning glory flower. Within the recess there may be a mound of glial tissue on the surface of the retrodisplaced nerve head. Periodic movement of the optic disc due to contraction of the smooth muscle within the meninges may be related to light exposure or may be spontaneous.

Morning glory anomaly appears to be an isolated condition unrelated to multisystemic disorders. However, it may be associated with transphenoidal encephelocoele and hypopituitarism – these patients have a wide head, hypertelorism, and a flattened nasal bridge.

Pathogenesis

The pathogenesis is unknown but two common theories have been proposed:

1 Failure of closure of the fetal fissure; it is therefore a variant of an optic nerve coloboma.
2 A primary mesenchymal disorder on the basis of scleral and vascular abnormalities, the presence of adipose and smooth muscle tissue around the scleral canal, and an absence of the lamina cribrosa (Figure 6.26).

Genetics

Unknown as almost all cases are sporadic.

Possible modes of treatment

Treatment is usually conservative, although in up to a third of cases, rhegmatogenous retinal detachment may occur due to a break at the optic disc margin or cup. Subretinal neovascularisation at the disc and macula has been described.

Macroscopic

The anterior part of the optic nerve is enlarged and a cut across the edge will reveal folded retina within dilated meninges. The retina is continuous with a retrodisplaced optic disc (Figure 6.26, left). At the scleral canal, the retina is constricted by a partially pigmented fibrovascular band.

Microscopic

The architecture of the retina and optic nerve is preserved in most cases, but there may be photoreceptor atrophy within the globe due to secondary detachment. The constricting band around the retina is formed by metaplastic retinal pigment epithelium and fibrous tissue (Figure 6.26, right). Smooth muscle bundles can be identified in the meninges.

Whole eye anomalies

Coloboma

A coloboma of the eye is defined as an arrestment in the complete closure of the embryonic fissure of the developing eye resulting in a defect in the inferior nasal quadrant affecting at least one layer of the eye. This condition is commonly sporadic, bilateral, and may occur in the absence of other ocular or systemic abnormalities. Numerous associations with widespread organ abnormalities have been described in the literature. Many of these abnormalities are identified with genetic disorders and numerous teratogenic agents have been implicated. The following text should be considered as a simplified account.

Any structure derived from the optic cup may be subject to a colobomatous malformation.

Coloboma of the iris

This appears clinically either as a notch or a hole of varying size. Paradoxically, this condition cannot be due to a failure of closure of the embryonic fissure because the iris is formed after the fissure is closed and is probably related to abnormalities in the tunica vasculosa lentis. Iris colobomas may be found in isolation or in conjunction with ocular conditions such as microphthalmos. Associations with other colobomas of the ciliary body, choroid, retina, and optic disc have been described. Microscopic examination of the iris notch reveals simple hypoplasia with an absent musculature (Figure 6.27).

Malformation - Optic disc pit

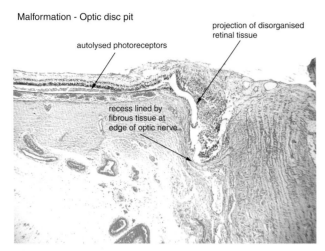

autolysed photoreceptors

projection of disorganised retinal tissue

recess lined by fibrous tissue at edge of optic nerve

Figure 6.25

Malformation - Morning glory anomaly

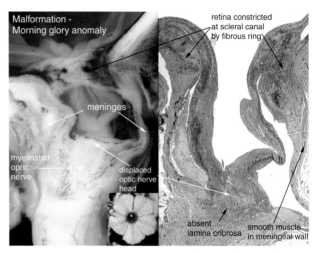

myelinated optic nerve

meninges

displaced optic nerve head

absent lamina cribrosa

retina constricted at scleral canal by fibrous ring

smooth muscle in meningeal wall

Figure 6.26

Malformation - Coloboma of iris

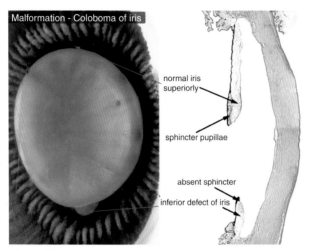

normal iris superiorly

sphincter pupillae

absent sphincter

inferior defect of iris

Figure 6.27

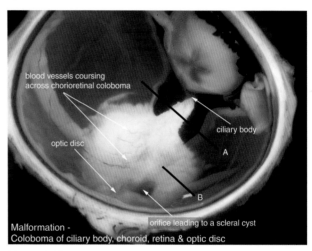

blood vessels coursing across chorioretinal coloboma

optic disc

ciliary body

A

B

orifice leading to a scleral cyst

Malformation - Coloboma of ciliary body, choroid, retina & optic disc

Figure 6.28

Malformation - Coloboma

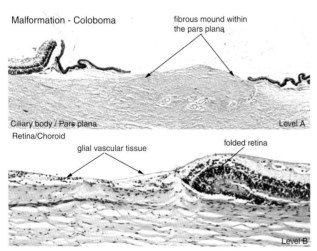

fibrous mound within the pars plana

Ciliary body / Pars plana

Level A

Retina/Choroid

glial vascular tissue

folded retina

Level B

Figure 6.29

Figure 6.25 An optic disc pit is histologically represented by a herniation of retinal tissue into a fibrous sac between the nerve and the edge of the scleral canal. Unfortunately, this specimen shows post mortem autolysis of the photoreceptors.

Figure 6.26 In this example of the morning glory anomaly, the optic nerve head is displaced posteriorly within the optic nerve meninges (left). The retina is dragged through a ring of fibrous tissue formed by metaplastic retinal pigment epithelium at the edge of the scleral canal (right). The globe was enucleated along with a long optic nerve stump because ultrasound examination suggested the presence of a cystic glioma. Although smooth muscle is present within the meninges, clinical evidence of disc movement was not identified in this case. The inset shows a morning glory flower. NB: In an optic nerve staphyloma, uveal tissue lines the scleral herniation.

Figure 6.27 On macroscopic examination (left), an iris coloboma may appear as an inferonasal notch as in this case, or as a peripheral hole. Histologically (right), the malformed sector located inferiorly is much smaller than the normal remaining iris. The angle and outflow system are of normal appearance compared with aniridia (see Figure 6.11).

Figure 6.28 A grossly malformed infant was stillborn and extensive colobomas were identified in both eyes. A horizontal section through the right eye revealed a large inferonasal chorioretinal coloboma extending into the ciliary body. An orifice communicated with a scleral cyst adjacent to the optic nerve. Lines A and B respectively show the histological appearances in Figure 6. 29.

Figure 6.29 The best way to study a coloboma histologically is to take levels transversely across the malformation, shown as A and B in Figure 6.28. A coloboma of the ciliary body is represented by a defect in the pars plana (upper). A chorioretinal coloboma is of interest, because at the edge, the neural retina is folded beneath itself to later fuse with the retinal pigment epithelium. The scleral bed of the coloboma is lined by a membrane which contains glial cells and blood vessels; the latter are easily apparent clinically.

Coloboma of the ciliary body

Colobomas of the ciliary body are often continuous with chorioretinal colobomas (Figure 6.28). The defect in the ciliary body is replaced by a fibrous tissue which projects inwardly towards the lens. This defect often extends posteriorly to include the pars plana (Figure 6.29, upper). Localised absence of zonules may result in a corresponding "coloboma" of the adjacent lens, which appears clinically as a notch.

Coloboma of the choroid and retina

Appears clinically as an inferonasal defect of variable size in the choroid and retina with underlying bare sclera. There is a corresponding superior visual field defect. The coloboma may extend to the ciliary body and optic disc (Figure 6.28). In some cases the bare sclera is lined by a membrane which contains blood vessels (Figure 6.28). Histology across the edge of chorioretinal coloboma demonstrates an infolding of the retina and an extension of glial and vascular tissue across the sclera (Figure 6.29, lower).

Coloboma of the optic disc

Appears as a large bowl-shaped excavation of the optic disc that may extend inferiorly. Exudative retinal detachment is an associated feature.

CHARGE syndrome

There are numerous systemic disorders associated with colobomas, with the most common being: CHARGE syndrome (coloboma of the retina/choroid, heart malformation, atresia choanae, genital hypoplasia, and ear malformation) related to the chorioretinal variant. Genetic abnormalities including deletions in chromosomes 5, 6, and 13 have been documented as well as abnormalities in the *PAX2* (10q24) gene.

Nanophthalmia and microphthalmia

Nanophthalmos

An inherited bilateral condition characterised by very hypermetropic eyes (+10 to +20 D). Each eye has a short axial length (<20 mm), a normal sized lens, and a thickened sclera. This condition is usually autosomal recessive in inheritance although autosomal dominant variants have been described.

Abnormally large collagen bundles and increased glycosaminoglycans result in scleral thickening. Choroidal effusion may occur later in life.

As the lens is normal in size, angle closure glaucoma may result.

Microphthalmos

A disorganised and rudimentary eye is formed when there is arrested development of the optic vesicle. This bilateral condition is commonly associated with many diverse systemic malformations. The degree of visual function varies depending upon the presence of vital ocular structures. An orbital cyst is the most primitive abnormality if there is a failure in invagination of the optic vesicle.

Gross malformations

Gross ocular abnormalities are often in conjunction with severe systemic abnormalities which are incompatible with survival.

Anophthalmia

Anophthalmia is defined as the absence of an eye within the orbit and is extremely rare.

Synophthalmia

Synophthalmia is the fusion of two eyes due to abnormal axial mesenchyme. Such cases are present in elective terminations for gross malformations of the CNS. A true cyclopean eye (one single central eye) is extremely rare.

Chapter 7
Glaucoma

"Glaucoma" is a generic term for a common group of ocular diseases which, if untreated, can result in an irreversible loss of visual function. An inappropriate intraocular pressure linked to damage to the neuronal tissue in the optic nerve head is common to all forms of glaucoma.

Classification

Glaucoma can be divided into five main subgroups:
1 Congenital.
2 Primary open.
3 Primary closed.
4 Secondary open.
5 Secondary closed.

Normal drainage anatomy

Aqueous humour is produced in the ciliary processes by active transport and diffusion. The aqueous leaves the posterior chamber, passes through the pupil into the anterior chamber, and finally drains via the trabecular meshwork (Figures 7.1, 7.2). Drainage is by two mechanisms: conventional drainage through the trabecular meshwork (90%) and unconventional drainage via the uveoscleral outflow (10%).

Knowledge of the normal chamber angle is crucial to an understanding of many pathological processes in the spectrum of glaucoma (Figure 7.3). The iris root is usually at 45 degrees to the inner surface of the trabecular meshwork. A line can be drawn from the posterior end of Schlemm's canal, through the scleral spur, to the periphery of the chamber angle. This is a useful landmark in identifying the normal location of the iris root and appreciating abnormal relationships, for example early angle closure and angle recession. The meriodonal fibres of the ciliary muscle insert into the scleral spur and the oblique layers insert into the uveal layer of the trabecular meshwork.

The outer part of the trabecular meshwork lies within the scleral sulcus (Figure 7.4) and the inner part fuses with the anterior face of the ciliary body. The trabecular meshwork is formed by collagenous beams and plates lined by endothelial cells. In conventional morphology, the trabecular meshwork is divided into three layers. The two innermost layers are the uveal and corneoscleral. The outermost layer is formed by the endothelial cells loosely arranged within mucopolysaccharides and collagen (Figures 7.4, 7.5). The outermost layer is variously termed juxtacanalicular (USA) or cribriform (Europe).

Several functions are ascribed to the trabecular meshwork. The juxtacanalicular layer provides resistance to maintain intraocular pressure and prevents reflux of blood from Schlemm's canal. The endothelial cells lining the trabeculae within the meshwork have a capacity for phagocytosis. This function is necessary due to the breakdown of the tissues of the anterior segment during life (for example the breakdown of tissues in the iris stroma and iris pigment epithelium).

Abnormalities in the outflow system lead to reduced outflow facility and increased intraocular pressure.

Pathological examination of a glaucomatous eye

A cupped disc is a pathological hallmark of longstanding glaucoma. Enucleation, whilst never carried out for uncomplicated primary open angle glaucoma, is sometimes performed in the secondary forms of aqueous outflow obstruction, i.e. tumours, vascular disease, uveitis, and trauma.

Figure 7.1 A section through the anterior segment of a normal eye demonstrating the anatomical features. The yellow colour of the lens is due to gluteraldehyde fixation.

Figure 7.2 A diagram to illustrate the routes of aqueous movement through the posterior chamber into the anterior chamber. Aqueous leaves the trabecular meshwork through the canal of Schlemm and collector channels drain into the episcleral veins. An alternative drainage pathway is into the supraciliary space (uveoscleral outflow).

Figure 7.3 In a paraffin section, the structures surrounding the chamber angle are easily identified. The trabecular meshwork is located on the inner surface of Schlemm's canal. The ciliary muscle fibres insert into the scleral spur and into the uveal layer of the meshwork. The dilator pupillae is seen as a thin red line above the pigmented epithelium of the iris. The chamber angle should reach as far as the imaginary line drawn from the posterior limit of the canal of Schlemm through the scleral spur and ending at the iris root.

Figure 7.4 The morphological distinction between the various layers in the trabecular meshwork is more easily demonstrated diagrammatically. Traction by the ciliary muscle on the scleral spur and the uveal meshwork opens the tissue and facilitates outflow: this is the action of pilocarpine when used to treat open angle glaucoma. The lining endothelium of Schlemm's canal transports aqueous by the formation of giant vacuoles and transcellular channels. The inset shows: (1) the resting stage, (2) an invagination from the inner surface, (3) the transcellular channel, and (4) recovery after the pressure in the canal is equal to that in the juxtacanicular layer. The scleral sulcus represents a groove on the inner peripheral surface of the cornea and contains the outer part of the trabecular meshwork and Schlemm's canal.

Figure 7.5 In a thin plastic section (1 μm) stained with toluidine blue it is possible to see the difference between the uveal layer which fuses with ciliary muscle and the corneoscleral layer which bridges the space between the scleral spur and cornea. The juxtacanalicular layer is inconspicuous. The endothelium which lines Schlemm's canal contains empty spaces (giant vacuoles). The thick line extending from the tip of the scleral spur to the peripheral cornea separates the uveal and the corneoscleral layers.

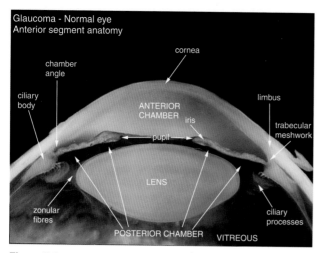

Glaucoma - Normal eye
Anterior segment anatomy

cornea

chamber
angle

ciliary
body

ANTERIOR
CHAMBER

iris

limbus

pupil

trabecular
meshwork

LENS

zonular
fibres

POSTERIOR CHAMBER

ciliary
processes

VITREOUS

Figure 7.1

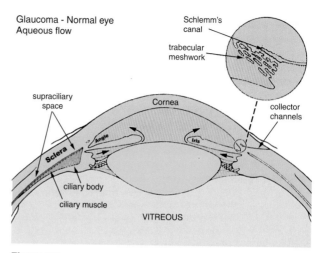

Glaucoma - Normal eye
Aqueous flow

Schlemm's
canal

trabecular
meshwork

supraciliary
space

Cornea

collector
channels

Sclera

Angle

Iris

ciliary body

ciliary muscle

VITREOUS

Figure 7.2

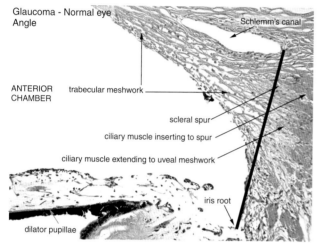

Glaucoma - Normal eye
Angle

Schlemm's canal

ANTERIOR
CHAMBER

trabecular meshwork

scleral spur

ciliary muscle inserting to spur

ciliary muscle extending to uveal meshwork

iris root

dilator pupillae

Figure 7.3

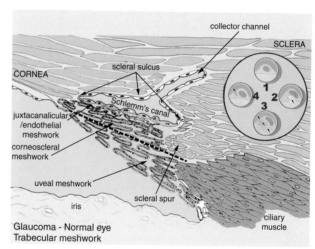

collector channel

SCLERA

CORNEA

scleral sulcus

Schlemm's canal

juxtacanalicular
/endothelial
meshwork

corneoscleral
meshwork

uveal meshwork

scleral spur

iris

ciliary
muscle

Glaucoma - Normal eye
Trabecular meshwork

Figure 7.4

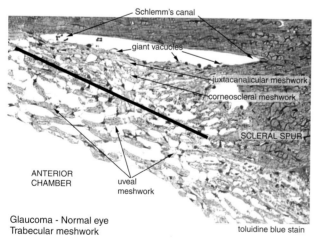

Schlemm's canal

giant vacuoles

juxtacanalicular meshwork

corneoscleral meshwork

SCLERAL SPUR

ANTERIOR
CHAMBER

uveal
meshwork

Glaucoma - Normal eye
Trabecular meshwork

toluidine blue stain

Figure 7.5

Congenital/infantile/juvenile

Congenital glaucoma is defined as a glaucoma that arises in children before the age of 2. The incidence is 1 in 10 000, although there are considerable variations amongst different racial groups. The raised intraocular pressure is due to an increased outflow resistance of an abnormally developed trabecular meshwork.

Clinical presentation
Involvement is usually bilateral with a triad of symptoms:
1 Photophobia.
2 Epiphora.
3 Blepharospasm.

As a result of the raised intraocular pressure, enlargement of the eye (buphthalmos) may occur up to the age of 3, at which stage in life the scleral collagen is more elastic.

Other features include corneal oedema/haze, Haab's striae, and amblyopia.

Gonioscopic examination often shows the iris insertion positioned more anteriorly when compared to a normal infant angle, but appearances can be very variable. A thin membrane initially described by Barkan may be observed straddling the angle. Existence of Barkan's membrane is controversial and histopathological descriptions are scarce.

Pathogenesis
Congenital glaucoma is a result of abnormal development of the trabecular meshwork. However, there is some development and maturation of the trabecular meshwork following birth and this may explain unilateral and arrested cases.

Genetics
There is a difference among races (possibly higher in black races) in the incidence of congenital glaucoma. About 10% of all cases have a strong hereditary component with variable penetrance. Both autosomal dominant and recessive types have been reported.

Possible modes of treatment
Treatment is usually surgical with the most common procedures being goniotomy and trabeculotomy.

Macroscopic and microscopic
Successful treatment of, and the low incidence of, this disease has resulted in a paucity of pathological material and it is only possible to provide a brief outline of the suggested abnormalities:
1 A membrane (Barkan's) lining the inner surface of the uveal layer (Figure 7.6).
2 Hypercellularity of the trabecular meshwork, i.e. a failure of resorption of primitive embryonic tissue located in the chamber angle in early embryonic life (Figure 7.7).
3 Abnormal insertion of the ciliary muscle into the trabecular meshwork occurs due to the absence of an intervening scleral spur (Figure 7.7).

Pathological evidence of treatment
Specimens from enucleated globes with a past history of treated congenital glaucoma often reveal pathology which is so complicated that the primary pathology is obscured.

Primary open angle

Primary open angle glaucoma (POAG) is a chronic, usually bilateral but asymmetric disease that affects 1–2% of the population over the age 40 years. If untreated, it may to lead severe visual loss and blindness.

Clinical presentation
The onset is insidious and the patient is unaware of areas of visual deficit until the disease has progressed to a late stage.

Many clinical and investigative factors are involved in the diagnosis of POAG and are constantly evolving. Traditionally the following criteria are diagnostic: raised intraocular pressure, thinning of the neuroretinal rim (optic disc cupping), and evidence of progression of characteristic visual field loss (enlarged blind spot and arcuate scotoma).

Pathogenesis
The disease is multifactorial and remains poorly understood. An imbalance between intraocular pressure and vascular perfusion of the optic nerve head will lead to sectorial atrophy. Similarly, mechanical pressure on the axons at the neuroretinal rim may interfere with axoplasmic flow and result in retrograde neuronal degeneration.

Genetics
Family history is a risk factor, although the specific genetic abnormality has not been identified in disease affecting elderly individuals.

Topical steroid treatment, in some individuals, will lead to increased intraocular pressure (steroid responders). Individuals with POAG are more likely to be steroid responders and steroid challenges were used in the past to assist in the diagnosis of POAG.

Initially, a gene on chromosome 1 (the trabecular meshwork induced glucocorticosteroid response or TIGR gene) was found in juvenile open angle glaucoma and later in 10% of adults with POAG. This gene is also known as the myocillin (MYOC) gene. Subsequently, other genes have been implicated but, as yet, the precise molecular genetics of POAG are poorly understood and multiple genes are probably involved.

Possible modes of treatment

This is beyond the scope of this text; in brief, standard glaucoma treatment involves lowering the intraocular pressure. Basic principles:

1 *Medical treatment:* includes topical preparations which reduce aqueous production and others that increase aqueous outflow. The latest generation (prostaglandin analogues) increase uveoscleral outflow.
2 *Surgical treatment:* various forms of trabeculectomy with or without antiscarring therapy.
3 *Laser treatment:* includes laser trabeculoplasty or cyclophotocoagulation for end-stage cases.

Microscopic

Unfortunately, the morphological study of trabeculectomy specimens has not provided definitive diagnostic features. Using a variety of sophisticated techniques, the appearance of the outflow system in trabeculectomy specimens showed no significant difference from that of age-matched normal tissue.

Primary angle closure

A form of glaucoma in which there is obstruction to outflow of aqueous by iridotrabecular contact. Factors involved in this condition include:

1 *Race:* especially Eskimos and East Asians.
2 *Gender:* more common in women.
3 *Age:* middle age.
4 *Refractive error:* hypermetropes having smaller globes.
5 *Family history:* positive.
6 *Predisposed anatomy:* eyes with narrow angles or plateau iris (Figure 7.8).

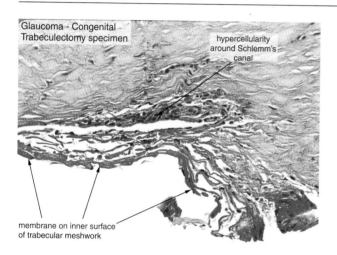

Figure 7.6

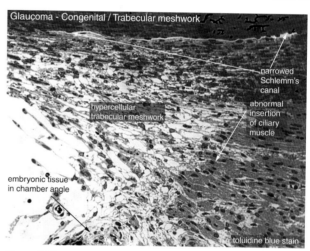

Figure 7.7

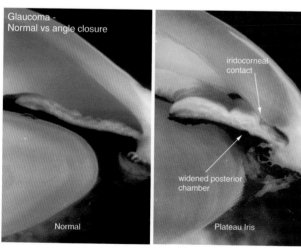

Figure 7.8

Figure 7.6 A trabeculectomy was performed in the treatment of a case of congenital glaucoma. A membrane was identified on the inner surface of the meshwork – this may possibly correspond to the Barkan's membrane, which is sometimes claimed to be observed on gonioscopy.

Figure 7.7 In congenital glaucoma, there is excessive cellular tissue within the trabecular meshwork. Schlemm's canal is narrowed. The ciliary muscle is displaced into the posterior part of the trabecular meshwork. Incomplete resolution of embryonic tissue in the chamber angle appears to be the cause of increased outflow resistance. (Thin plastic section – toluidine blue.)

Figure 7.8 It is extremely rare for a globe to be enucleated for primary closed angle glaucoma, but this chance finding of a plateau iris illustrates the pathogenesis of one type of angle closure (right). A normal angle is included for comparison (left).

Pathogenesis and clinical presentation

The anterior displacement of the peripheral iris is due to several factors:

1 Relative pupil block interrupts aqueous flow from the posterior to anterior chamber. Enlargement of lens with age contributes to the partial pupil block.
2 The pressure behind the peripheral iris rises, causes iris bombé and the angle progressively closes.

Several clinical presentations are possible:

1 *Acute:* a complete iridotrabecular block with rapid loss of vision, ocular pain with nausea, and vomiting. Clinically, there is conjunctival congestion, hazy cornea, raised intraocular pressure (>50 mmHg), anterior chamber flare and cells, and a fixed pupil. Gonioscopy will reveal a peripheral iridocorneal contact.
2 *Intermittent:* periodic iridotrabecular block depending on iris movement. The signs and symptoms during an angle closure attack are similar to those described in acute angle closure glaucoma.
3 *Creeping angle closure:* steadily progressive iridotrabecular contact (progression from 12 to 6 o'clock). The intraocular pressure rise is gradual without acute symptoms.
4 *Chronic:* the end-stage result of creeping closure in which the iridotrabecular contact is complete and permanent (peripheral anterior synechiae). The final intraocular pressure may be very high with an absence of acute symptoms and the field loss and optic disc appearance are similar to POAG.

In most parts of the world, acute and subacute cases represent the commonest forms of angle closure. However, in regions such as India, chronic angle closure is very common without any history of acute attacks.

Genetics

There is a familial as well as a racial tendency, but the molecular genetics have not been identified.

Possible modes of treatment

Treatment is dependent on the stage of disease.

1 *Medical:* initially to control intraocular pressure prior to definitive treatment and also in chronic cases.
2 *Laser iridotomy:* perforation to equalise pressure differentials between the anterior and posterior chambers. The presence of fibrinolysins in the aqueous prevents fibrin deposition so that scar tissue does not form in the iris defect (see below).
3 *Surgical:* lens extraction, iridectomy, goniosynechiolysis, and trabeculectomy.

Pathology

In an untreated globe, a large lens will be evident. The anterior chamber is shallow and the angles closed (Figure 7.9).

The large lens blocks the pupil and initially part of the angle is closed off (Figure 7.10). As the intraocular pressure rises, the remainder of the peripheral iris becomes adherent to the trabecular meshwork (Figure 7.11).

There may be evidence of a laser peripheral iridotomy (Figure 7.12) or surgical iridectomy.

Secondary open

Exfoliation syndrome (ES)

Other names: pseudoexfoliation syndrome (PEX/PXF).

A systemic disorder which is manifest clinically as deposits on the anterior surface of the lens and glaucoma. Deposition is frequently asymmetrical and density increases with the patient's age. The title pseudoexfoliation syndrome was adopted initially to distinguish this condition from true exfoliation (splitting of the anterior lens capsule) which occurs when the lens is exposed to excessive infrared light.

Clinical presentation

Exfoliation syndrome is usually an incidental finding on the lens surface on routine examination – dilatation of the pupil shows a bull's eye pattern of central white deposits surrounded by a clear zone with coarser deposits in the periphery extending to the zonules.

Iris transillumination defects may be evident in the peripupillary region.

There may be an association with primary open angle glaucoma – the surface of the lens should be examined in all types of glaucoma. ES may be associated, less commonly, with angle closure as the deposits weaken the zonules and forward movement of the lens may occur causing pupil block.

Gonioscopy may show heavy pigmentation in the trabecular meshwork.

Pathogenesis

Previously this was considered a primary ocular disease due to release of material from the anterior surface of the lens, hence the term "pseudoexfoliation". In the past two decades it has been shown that material with the same immunohistochemical and ultrastructural characteristics can be found in extraocular tissues (for example orbit, eyelid, lung, kidney, heart, liver, and gallbladder) of affected individuals. Hence, the disorder is systemic with focal deposition in other connective tissues. The ocular pathology is due to precipitation from the aqueous as the substance circulates through the anterior segment.

Genetics

Certain races have a higher incidence (for example Scandinavians).

Possible modes of treatment

Treatment is required only if glaucoma is present and with similar principles to those described in POAG. Intraocular pressures tend to be higher and glaucoma progression is frequently more rapid than with POAG. Laser trabeculoplasty is reported to have a greater effect on lowering intraocular pressure, although the response is temporary.

Cataract surgery is associated with more complications due to poor pupil dilatation and a higher incidence of zonular dehiscence.

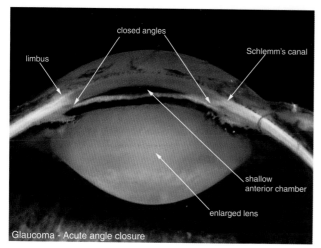

Figure 7.9

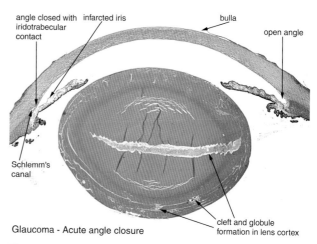

Figure 7.10

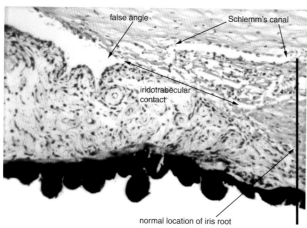

Figure 7.11

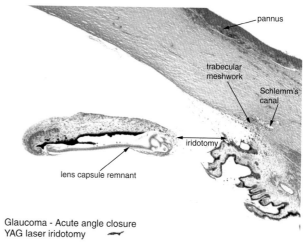

Glaucoma - Acute angle closure
YAG laser iridotomy

Figure 7.12

Figure 7.9 This enucleated globe is used to illustrate an enlarged lens with pupil block and angle closure. The cornea is opaque secondary to corneal oedema and the surface is irregular due to bulla formation. NB: Enucleation is not the current treatment for acute angle closure in our institution – this is an archival case!

Figure 7.10 A low-power micrograph of the anterior segment in angle closure glaucoma demonstrates the effects of an enlarged lens and pupil block which has closed off one angle. The lens substance contains clefts and globules which are forming in the cortex and the nucleus. The result of corneal oedema is the separation of the epithelium with bulla formation. An acute rise in intraocular pressure leads to infarction of the iris stroma and the dilator pupillae – hence the irregular pupil seen clinically.

Figure 7.11 A false angle is formed when the iris stroma comes in contact with the trabecular meshwork in the case of early angle closure. The abnormal iris displacement is evident when this figure is compared with Figure 7.3. When the same line is drawn from the posterior limit of Schlemm's canal through the scleral spur, it is evident that the true angle is completely occluded.

Figure 7.12 A patient developed acute raised intraocular pressure from angle closure glaucoma which did not improve with YAG laser iridotomy. Extracapsular lens extraction was carried out which was later complicated by postaphakic corneal decompensation (bullous keratopathy). Unfortunately, the patient reported late in the development of the disease and had irreversible loss of vision: an enucleation was performed for comfort.

Macroscopic

In an enucleated globe, exfoliation substance appears as fluffy white material on the surfaces of the zonular fibres (Figures 7.13, 7.14).

For a globe to be enucleated, it is likely that the disease will be manifest as longstanding glaucoma and its associated complications (for example trabeculectomy, central retinal vein occlusion, or complicated cataract surgery).

Microscopic

In an H&E preparation, the irregular clumps of exfoliation substance have a pink amorphous appearance (Figure 7.15). Staining with PAS is not strong but is positive (Figure 7.15, inset).

In the iris, the site of deposition is on both surfaces and within the walls of blood vessels (Figure 7.16). The pigmented epithelium has a characteristic "saw-toothed" appearance, although in the peripupillary region it is often atrophic. It is thought that this atrophy is secondary to contact abrasion with the exfoliative material on the lens surface (Figure 7.17).

In the trabecular meshwork, the material is located on the inner surface of the uveal layer, in the outer part of the corneoscleral layer and is concentrated in the juxtacanalicular layer (Figure 7.18). Pigment deposition is seen in the trabecular meshwork; the melanin granules are liberated by rubbing of iris pigmented epithelium on the irregular anterior lens surface.

Immunohistochemistry

Immunohistochemistry and immunolabelling have identified a remarkable number of constituents mainly of basement membrane type (for example laminin, fibrillin, elastin, amyloid-P component, fibronectin, and vitronectin).

Special investigations/stains

The ultrastructural appearance of exfoliation substance is characteristic and consists of fine fibrillogranular material.

Pigment dispersion syndrome (PDS)/ pigmentary glaucoma (PG)

In some individuals, there is a predisposition to dispersion of iris pigment from the iris pigmented epithelium (pigment dispersion syndrome – PDS). This typically occurs in 30 year olds and the quantity of pigment released decreases with age. Phagocytosis of melanosomes by the trabecular endothelial cells may lead to obstruction of aqueous outflow and glaucoma (pigmentary glaucoma – PG) in approximately one third of cases and usually within 15 years of presentation.

Clinical presentation

Gender In PDS, the male to female ratio is equal whereas in PG, the male to female ratio is 3 : 1.

Pigment dispersion syndrome The following signs are found:
1 Krukenberg spindle – deposits of melanin pigmentation in a vortex pattern on the posterior surface of the cornea reflecting aqueous circulation.
2 Iris transillumination defects – radially arranged in the midperipheral region. The iris is described as posterior bowing with a deep anterior chamber.
3 Darkly staining trabecular meshwork – from melanin deposition.

Pigmentary glaucoma The signs in PG are similar to PDS but, in addition, these signs include a raised intraocular pressure and glaucomatous nerve damage.

Figure 7.13 Exfoliation substance can be identified in the anterior segment of an enucleated globe (for choroidal melanoma) by the presence of white fluffy material within the zonular fibres and on the anterior surface of the lens. There is a pericentral circular clear zone on the lens surface due to abrasion by the iris. Note the patchy pigmentation of the trabecular meshwork.

Figure 7.14 Previous extracapsular cataract surgery was attempted in this eye with the complication of zonular dialysis, which necessitated intracapsular cataract surgery, and the eye was left aphakic. It is possible to identify exfoliation substance on the posterior surface of the iris. The iris pigment epithelium is deficient in the peripupillary region, most probably secondary to previous contact abrasion with the exfoliation substance on the anterior surface of the lens. A peripheral iridectomy suggests the presence of a previous trabeculectomy.

Figure 7.15 Exfoliation substance appears as pink amorphous material on the surface of the ciliary processes and zonular fibres. Clumps of the material are present on the anterior surface of the iris. On the posterior surface, the material causes "saw-toothed" distortions of the peripheral iris pigment epithelium (H&E). The inset (PAS stain) shows the linear deposits of exfoliation substance on a zonular fibre.

Figure 7.16 In addition to deposition on the anterior and posterior surfaces of the iris, exfoliation substance can be identified in the walls of the small iris vessels. Contact with the anterior lens surface and the exfoliation substance results in the disruption of continuity of the pigmented epithelium, which otherwise has a "saw-toothed" appearance.

Figure 7.17 The deposits of exfoliation substance on the anterior surface of the lens adopt a "tree-like" configuration. The material stains weakly with the PAS stain and contains melanin pigment derived from the iris pigment epithelium.

Figure 7.18 Aqueous outflow is impeded by deposits of exfoliation substance on the inner surface of the meshwork and in the region of Schlemm's canal. The canal of Schlemm is replaced by fibrovascular tissue.

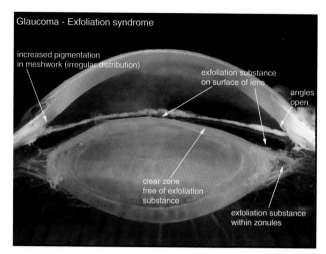

Figure 7.13

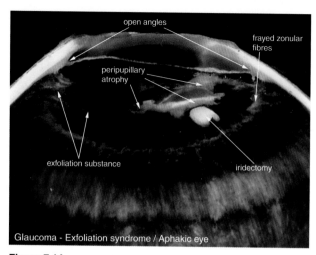

Figure 7.14

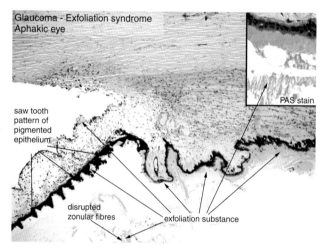

Figure 7.15

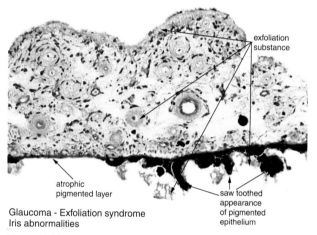

Figure 7.16

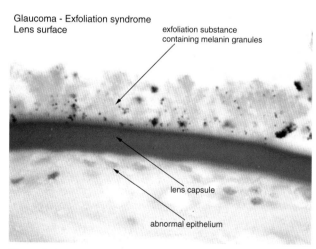

Figure 7.17

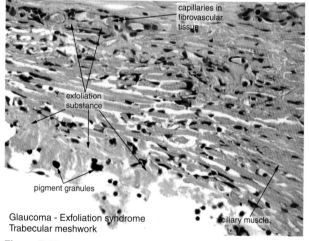

Figure 7.18

Pathogenesis

The mechanical theory suggests that in individuals with pigment dispersion there is a posterior bowing of the iris resulting in a zonule–iris rub. Reverse pupil block occurs in these eyes and may be responsible for this posterior bowing. Aqueous is pumped into the anterior chamber, the pupil acts as a one-way valve and this creates the posterior movement of the peripheral iris.

Genetics

Primarily a Caucasian condition.

Possible modes of treatment

Treatment is similar to POAG if the intraocular pressure is raised. As in ES, intraocular pressure may respond temporarily to laser trabeculoplasty. Some authors propose peripheral iridotomy as a treatment for pigment dispersion syndrome to reverse the posterior bowing of the iris.

Macroscopic and microscopic

The disease is most commonly studied in trabeculectomies.

Melanin pigment granules are phagocytosed by trabecular endothelial cells, which become swollen and eventually disintegrate (Figure 7.19).

Lens-related glaucoma

Degenerative lens disease or lens abnormalities can result in several forms of glaucoma:

1 A hypermature swollen cataract may lead to pupil block and secondary unilateral angle closure glaucoma (phacomorphic glaucoma). The pathology is similar to that described for primary angle closure glaucoma.

2 Liquefaction of the lens cortex may lead to the release of particulate material into the anterior chamber which blocks the trabecular meshwork (lens particle glaucoma). As an alternative, a macrophagic response to liquefied lens matter fills the anterior chamber with swollen mononuclear cells which obstruct the outflow system (phacolytic glaucoma).

This section will describe phacolytic glaucoma.

Clinical presentation

A patient with a hypermature cataract is at risk of glaucoma secondary to the release of liquefied cortical material through an intact or ruptured lens capsule. The rise in pressure is acute and the deep anterior chamber contains floating white particles that may coalesce to form a pseudohypopyon.

Possible modes of treatment

After stabilisation of the intraocular pressure, surgical removal of the cataract and an anterior chamber washout is required.

Macroscopic

Although rare in developed countries, some neglected cases provide the opportunity to study phacolytic glaucoma. The sclerotic nucleus, within a capsular bag, which may or may not contain liquefied cortical material, can be identified easily (Figures 7.20, 7.21).

Microscopic

Macrophages containing lens matter can be found in an aqueous tap in phacolytic glaucoma (Figure 7.22). The original liquefied cortex may not be apparent in an H&E section (Figure 7.23). The macrophages accumulate on the anterior surface of the iris and in the inner layer of the trabecular meshwork blocking the intertrabecular spaces (Figures 7.24–7.26).

The macrophages label with appropriate markers (for example CD68).

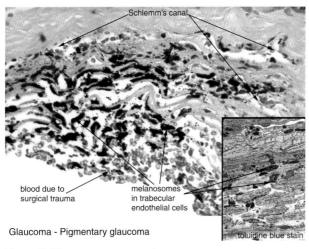

Glaucoma - Pigmentary glaucoma

Figure 7.19

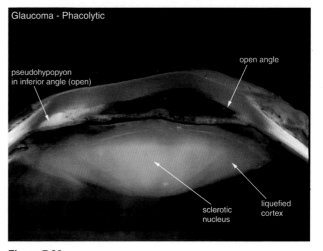

Figure 7.20

Figure 7.19 Melanin pigment granules are phagocytosed by trabecular endothelial cells and intracytoplasmic accumulation, if excessive, reduces the facility of outflow and a trabeculectomy may be required. The surgical procedure causes distortion of the trabeculae and may be complicated by haemorrhage, as in this case. The inset is taken from a plastic embedded semi-thin section to show detail of the melanosomes within the endothelial cells.

Figure 7.20 One form of lens degeneration is manifest as a persistent sclerotic nucleus within a liquefied cortex. The proteinaceous material, in liquid form, has leaked through the capsule and was in sufficient quantity to accumulate in the anterior chamber inferiorly to form a pseudohypopyon.

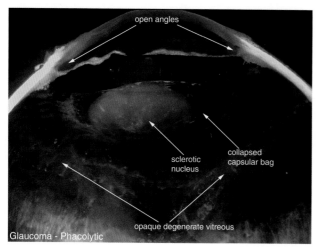

open angles

sclerotic nucleus

collapsed capsular bag

opaque degenerate vitreous

Glaucoma - Phacolytic

Figure 7.21

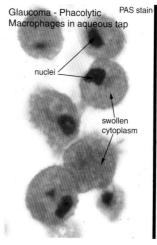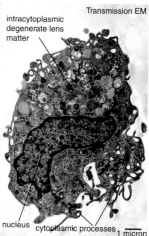

Glaucoma - Phacolytic Macrophages in aqueous tap

PAS stain

Transmission EM

intracytoplasmic degenerate lens matter

nuclei

swollen cytoplasm

nucleus

cytoplasmic processes

1 micron

Figure 7.22

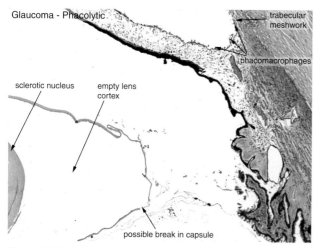

Glaucoma - Phacolytic

trabecular meshwork

phacomacrophages

sclerotic nucleus

empty lens cortex

possible break in capsule

Figure 7.23

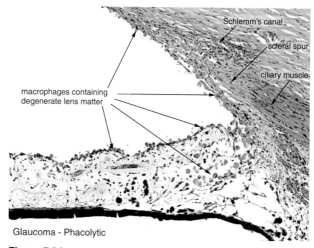

Schlemm's canal

scleral spur

ciliary muscle

macrophages containing degenerate lens matter

Glaucoma - Phacolytic

Figure 7.24

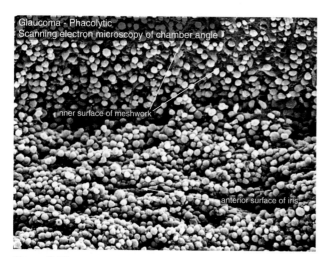

Glaucoma - Phacolytic
Scanning electron microscopy of chamber angle

inner surface of meshwork

anterior surface of iris

Figure 7.25

Figure 7.21 In this example of phacolytic glaucoma, a sclerotic nucleus lies within a collapsed capsular bag following the escape of liquefied cortical lens matter. The liquefied material presumably has escaped into the anterior chamber and passed through the outflow system.

Figure 7.22 In phacolytic glaucoma, an aqueous tap will identify swollen macrophages containing degenerate lens matter staining pink with the PAS stain (left). At the ultrastructural level (right), the granular vesicular structures within the cytoplasm are identical in appearance to the cytoplasmic and cell membrane fragments seen in disintegrating lens fibres in a cataract.

Figure 7.23 A low power view of the anterior segment of a case of phacolytic glaucoma reveals collapse of the capsule around a persistent sclerotic nucleus. Phacomacrophages are identified with difficulty at this level of magnification.

Figure 7.24 Pink staining, round macrophages are present in the iris stroma on the anterior surface of the iris and the inner surface of the trabecular meshwork where they are inconspicuous.

Figure 7.25 Scanning electron microscopy shows the true extent of phacomacrophage accumulation in the chamber angle in phacolytic glaucoma. It is difficult to identify the intertrabecular spaces as the cells are plugging every available opening.

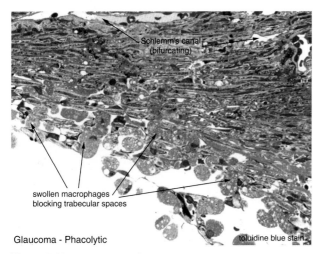

Glaucoma - Phacolytic

swollen macrophages blocking trabecular spaces

Schlemm's canal (bifurcating)

toluidine blue stain

Figure 7.26

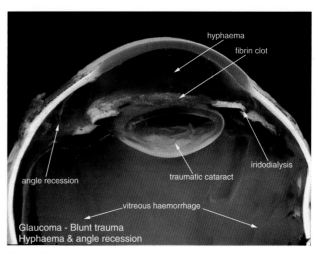

Glaucoma - Blunt trauma
Hyphaema & angle recession

hyphaema

fibrin clot

angle recession

traumatic cataract

iridodialysis

vitreous haemorrhage

Figure 7.27

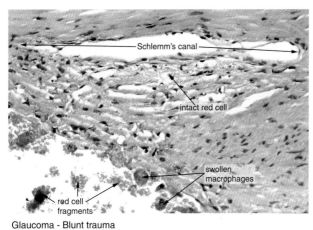

Schlemm's canal

intact red cell

swollen macrophages

red cell fragments

Glaucoma - Blunt trauma
Hyphaema

Figure 7.28

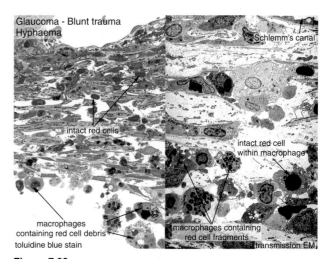

Glaucoma - Blunt trauma
Hyphaema

Schlemm's canal

intact red cells

intact red cell within macrophage

macrophages containing red cell debris
toluidine blue stain

macrophages containing red cell fragments

transmission EM

Figure 7.29

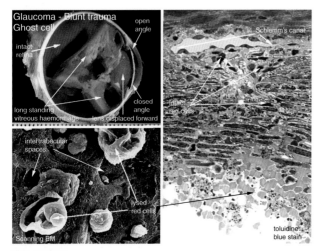

Glaucoma - Blunt trauma
Ghost cell

open angle

intact retina

long standing vitreous haemorrhage

closed angle

lens displaced forward

Schlemm's canal

intact red cells

intertrabecular spaces

lysed red cells

Scanning EM

toluidine blue stain

Figure 7.30

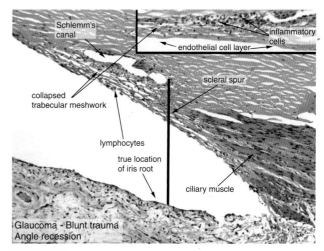

Schlemm's canal

inflammatory cells

endothelial cell layer

collapsed trabecular meshwork

scleral spur

lymphocytes

true location of iris root

ciliary muscle

Glaucoma - Blunt trauma
Angle recession

Figure 7.31

Post-traumatic glaucoma

Blunt and penetrating trauma can produce a variety of injuries that lead to acute or chronic glaucoma, but the following are the most common:

1 Bleeding (hyphaema) can result from a tear in the peripheral iris (iridodialysis) or separation of the ciliary body from sclera (cyclodialysis).
2 A tear into the anterior face of the ciliary body leads to separation and retraction of the ciliary muscle and leaves a large recess (angle recession). Figure 7.27 illustrates both 1 and 2.
3 An epithelial downgrowth via a corneal or limbal wound can form a membrane on the inner surface of the trabecular meshwork.

Angle recession and epithelial downgrowth are secondary glaucomas which are difficult to treat.

Hyphaema

Exposure of the trabecular meshwork to blood products in excess leads to obstruction of aqueous outflow. The acute effects are mechanical and occur because macrophages and lysed red cells are unable to penetrate the intertrabecular spaces (Figures 7.28, 7.29). The trabecular endothelial cells phagocytose the red cell residues and the resultant accumulation of iron from haem breakdown (siderosis) is toxic. The endothelial cells degenerate and eventually fibrous replacement contributes to outflow obstruction.

Ghost cell glaucoma

If the anterior vitreous face remains intact, a vitreous haemorrhage is incarcerated and red cells are lysed progressively for many weeks. A spontaneous or traumatic rupture of the vitreous face releases lysed red cells into the anterior chamber and these rigid swollen (ghost) cells are unable to pass through the trabecular interspaces, resulting in an acute rise in intraocular pressure (Figure 7.30). A vitrectomy in addition to an anterior chamber washout is required for treatment.

Angle recession

The inner uveal layer of the trabecular meshwork is supported by the oblique and circular layers of the ciliary muscle. At this potential point of weakness, shockwave movement from blunt trauma on the iris root can result in the formation of a split in the ciliary body (Figure 7.31). The consequence is a posterior displacement of the iris root and collapse of the trabecular meshwork. The migration of corneal endothelial cells across the inner surface of the trabecular meshwork and the subsequent formation of a secondary Descemet's membrane play a part in traumatic outflow obstruction. In early trauma, there may be infiltration by lymphocytes, particularly if there is an anterior uveitis, and this may explain an acute rise in intraocular pressure.

Figure 7.26 A thin plastic section (toluidine blue stain) provides better detail of the extent of infiltration by macrophages into the uveal and corneoscleral layers of the meshwork. The cells are large and have a foamy vesiculated cytoplasm and an eccentric nucleus.

Figure 7.27 In this specimen, blunt trauma caused anteroposterior compression of the corneoscleral envelope. On one side, the iris root has separated from the ciliary body (iridodialysis). On the other side, there is a complete tear in the face of the ciliary body (angle recession). The anterior chamber is completely filled with blood. There is also blood in the vitreous and the lens is cataractous.

Figure 7.28 In prolonged hyphaema, the inner surface of the meshwork is lined by the breakdown products of blood and macrophages. The intertrabecular spaces of the uveal layer are blocked. There is little penetration into the corneoscleral layer, where the intertrabecular spaces are patent.

Figure 7.29 Two mechanisms can lead to obstruction of the outflow system after prolonged haemorrhage. Large macrophages filled with red cell debris are unable to pass through the intratrabecular spaces: intact red cells are malleable and pass easily through the trabecular meshwork (left – plastic section, toluidine blue stain). Transmission electron microscopy shows that the macrophages containing the red cell debris are confined to the corneoscleral layer (right).

Figure 7.30 A longstanding haemorrhage in the vitreous adopts a yellow appearance ("ochre membrane" – upper left) and an abrupt release of lysed red cells causes an acute obstruction to aqueous outflow (ghost cell glaucoma). The toluidine blue stained section (right) shows a thick layer of lysed red cells on the inner surface of the trabecular meshwork. These inflexible swollen cells (scanning EM, bottom left) are too large to pass through the intertrabecular spaces.

Figure 7.31 Recognition of a recessed angle is aided by the identification of Schlemm's canal and the scleral spur. A vertical line drawn through these two structures should end at the iris root. In this example, there is a tear into the anterior face of the ciliary body. The trabecular meshwork is collapsed. The inset shows a later stage of trabecular collapse when the compressed tissue is lined by an endothelial layer (derived from corneal endothelial cells) and a thin secondary Descemet's membrane.

Epithelial downgrowth

Any form of perforating trauma through the cornea or limbus, whether surgical or civil, may be complicated by epithelial migration especially if the wound edges are not accurately opposed (Figure 7.32). Cells resembling corneal or conjunctival epithelium migrate easily over the posterior corneal surface, trabecular meshwork, iris stroma, and onto the vitreous face (Figure 7.33).

Neoplastic

Melanomas of the iris can infiltrate the trabecular meshwork leading to a secondary glaucoma (Figure 7.34; see Figure 11.5). Infiltration can proceed as far as Schlemm's canal and the collector channels before the onset of glaucoma. When glaucoma occurs secondary to an iris melanoma, enucleation is the sole option – filtering surgery enhances extraocular spread of the tumour.

A ciliary body melanoma can also invade the angle and spread in the anterior chamber, but glaucoma is much more likely to be due to lens displacement and pupil block with secondary angle closure (see Figures 11.9, 11.10).

A retinoblastoma may become necrotic and release a shower of viable tumour cells and tumour debris causing a pseudohypopyon, simulating an acute inflammatory process: the intraocular pressure may be raised.

Miscellaneous

Silicone oil

Silicone oil used in retinal detachment surgery can emulsify and escape as tiny globules into the upper part of the anterior chamber. The globules are rapidly ingested by macrophages, which become trapped in the intertrabecular spaces of the meshwork (Figure 7.35). The trabecular endothelial cells are also able to phagocytose very small globules. Breakdown of anterior uveal tissue with the release of melanosomes occurs in complicated end-stage globes after failed detachment surgery. This explains the presence of melanosomes in endothelial cells and macrophages (Figure 7.35). The intraocular complications of emulsification of silicone oil are described in Chapter 10.

Inflammatory (open angle): trabeculitis

Non-granulomatous inflammation in the iris secondary to chronic keratitis is complicated by lymphocytic infiltration in the trabecular meshwork (Figures 7.36, 7.37). The use of topical steroids to control the inflammation is advantageous, but paradoxically it can increase outflow resistance in individuals who are steroid responders (see "Primary open angle" section, p. 138).

A specific clinical entity with trabeculitis is seen in Fuchs' heterochromic iridocyclitis in which there is a unilateral, intermittent, low-grade iritis of unknown aetiology, associated with glaucoma, cataract, keratic precipitates, and iris heterochromia. The pathology is non-specific in both the iris and trabecular meshwork.

Figure 7.32 After a routine cataract extraction, there was a prolonged dehiscence in the corneal wound and this provided an opportunity for the corneal epithelium to migrate into the anterior chamber. The epithelium extends across the angle onto the iris surface. The absence of goblet cells in the epithelial downgrowth indicates a corneal epithelial origin as opposed to a conjunctival orgin.

Figure 7.33 In this example, the epithelial downgrowth lines the iris and the anterior vitreous face in an aphakic eye.

Figure 7.34 A low power micrograph showing ring spread of a poorly cohesive iris melanoma. In this example, the tumour lines the inner surface of the meshwork and has spread onto the posterior surface of the cornea and the anterior surface of the iris. The inset shows the macroscopic appearance of ring spread in an iris melanoma.

Figure 7.35 Silicone oil globules in the trabecular meshwork are seen as empty spaces in a paraffin section (left). The location of oil droplets within the macrophages and endothelial cells is better demonstrated in an electron micrograph (right). This figure is taken from an eye in which there were many secondary complications following retinal detachment surgery including breakdown of iris pigment epithelium. This explains the presence of numerous melanin granules within the macrophages.

Figure 7.36 An inconspicuous lymphocytic infiltrate in the outflow system may obstruct aqueous drainage and lead to secondary open angle glaucoma. A detail of the cells in the trabecular meshwork is shown in Figure 7.37.

Figure 7.37 The small size of the lymphocytes permits easier infiltration of the trabecular meshwork. This explains the greater density of lymphocytes in the corneoscleral and juxtacanalicular layers. Compare this with a macrophagic infiltration (see Figures 7.26, 7.28).

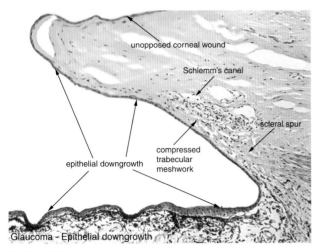

unopposed corneal wound

Schlemm's canal

scleral spur

compressed trabecular meshwork

epithelial downgrowth

epithelial downgrowth

Glaucoma - Epithelial downgrowth

Figure 7.32

Glaucoma - Epithelial downgrowth

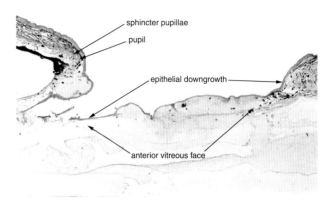

sphincter pupillae

pupil

epithelial downgrowth

anterior vitreous face

Figure 7.33

Glaucoma - Secondary neoplastic
Ring spread of an amelanotic iris melanoma

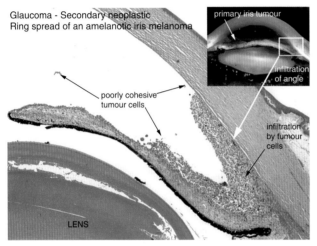

primary iris tumour

infiltration of angle

poorly cohesive tumour cells

infiltration by tumour cells

LENS

Figure 7.34

Glaucoma -
Emulsified silicone oil

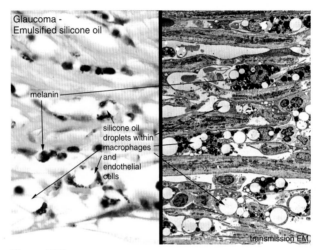

melanin

silicone oil droplets within macrophages and endothelial cells

transmission EM

Figure 7.35

Glaucoma - Trabeculitis

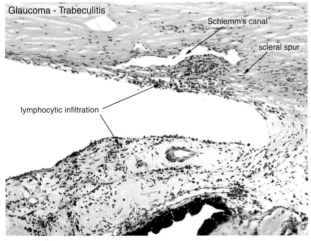

Schlemm's canal

scleral spur

lymphocytic infiltration

Figure 7.36

Glaucoma - Trabeculitis

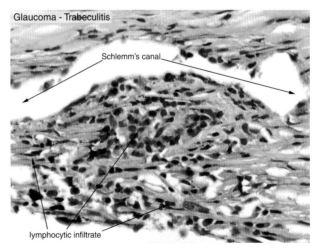

Schlemm's canal

lymphocytic infiltrate

Figure 7.37

Secondary closed

Neovascular

Neovascular glaucoma is commonly seen in enucleation specimens.

Clinical presentation
Early
1 The development of neovascularisation first occurs in the angle and this can be seen by gonioscopy; later new vessels are seen on the anterior iris surface.
2 The initial pressure rise is due to a neovascular membrane on the inner surface of the trabecular meshwork.

Late
1 Contraction of the fibrovascular tissue in the angle leads to iridotrabecular and iridocorneal contact. Gonioscopy reveals closed angles.
2 Fibrovascular proliferation on the iris surface rotates the pupil margin forward so that the pigmented epithelium is visible (ectropion uveae).
3 There may be evidence of glaucomatous decompensation in the cornea (see "Tissue effects" below).
4 A primary cause for ischaemia must always be sought (for example for central retinal vein occlusion or diabetes).

Pathogenesis
Any process which leads to the release of vascular endothelial growth factor (VEGF) into the aqueous could potentially cause neovascularisation of the iris. The sub-categories of possible sources of VEGF are:
1 Ischaemic tissue: for example central retinal vein occlusion, diabetic retinopathy, and prolonged retinal detachment.
2 Neoplasia: for example intraocular melanomas or retinoblastomas.
3 Inflammation: prolonged uveitis of any cause.

Possible modes of treatment
This depends on the primary disease, but the following options are available:
1 Removal of cause: for example panretinal photocoagulation of an ischaemic retina.
2 Medical treatment for inflammation and glaucoma.
3 Ciliary body ablation.
4 Surgical treatment by drainage procedures with or without setons.
5 Enucleation of the painful blind eye for comfort.

Macroscopic
In an enucleation specimen the following changes may be identified (Figure 7.38):
• bullous keratopathy
• peripheral corneal pannus
• ectropion uveae
• cataract
• retinal changes relevant to vascular disease or tumour.

Microscopic
It is important to appreciate that the neovascular membrane consists of small capillaries and fibroblasts. At the earliest stage, the capillaries and fibroblasts are identified on the iris surface and on the inner surface of the trabecular meshwork (Figure 7.39). Fibroblasts proliferate in the chamber angle and subsequently contract to pull the peripheral iris towards the meshwork (Figure 7.40).

The angle eventually closes and the peripheral iris comes into contact with the cornea (Figure 7.41). Contraction of the fibrovascular membrane on the iris surface results in flattening. NB: Any loss of normal iris folds or the presence of ectropion uveae should alert the examiner to the possibility of neovascularisation.

In some cases, the corneal endothelium migrates across the surface of the neovascular membrane (Figure 7.42).

Pathological evidence of treatment
Evidence of surgery or laser as described above, especially pan-retinal photocoagulation (see Figure 10.48).

Tumour

Mechanical displacement of the iris and lens by tumours of the ciliary body, choroid and retina can lead to a pupil block (see Figures 11.9, 11.10, 11.33, 11.43).

Uveitis/inflammation

In inflammation of the anterior uvea, release of a sticky fibrinous exudate promotes the formation of peripheral anterior and central posterior synechiae with resultant secondary angle closure glaucoma. With prolonged inflammation, neovascularisation may also contribute to a rise in intraocular pressure (see above).

Trauma

With civil or surgical trauma involving decompression and perforation of the cornea or limbus, hypotonia and reactionary fibrosis result in anterior synechia formation.

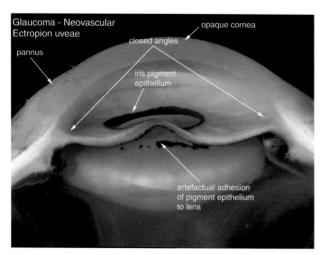

Figure 7.38

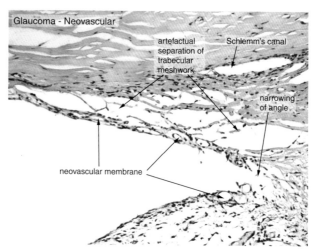

Figure 7.39

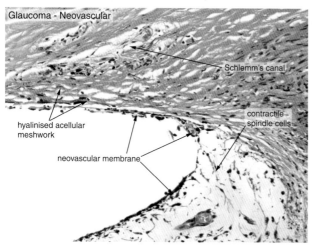

Figure 7.40

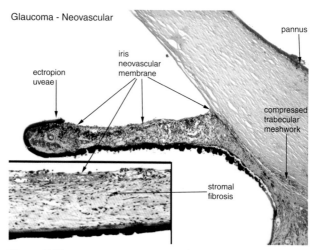

Figure 7.41

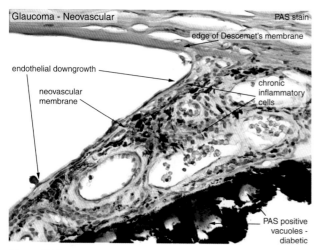

Figure 7.42

Figure 7.38 The macroscopic appearance of the anterior segment in neovascular glaucoma. The iris surface is smooth and the angles are closed. The pigment epithelium of the iris is retracted around the pupil (ectropion uveae). Pigmentation on the lens surface is artefactual but, *in vivo*, occurs in inflammation in the anterior segment.

Figure 7.39 In early neovascular glaucoma, the aqueous outflow is obstructed by a layer of fibrovascular tissue on the inner surface of the meshwork. Similar capillaries are present on the iris surface. This example shows the early stages of secondary angle closure.

Figure 7.40 As the disease progresses, the fibroblastic proliferation and contraction in the chamber angle pulls the peripheral iris forwards. The capillaries are not conspicuous in this example which emphasises the importance of the fibroblast component in angle closure.

Figure 7.41 In late neovascular glaucoma, there is a layer of fibrovascular tissue between the iris stroma and the cornea, the angle is closed, and an ectropion uveae is easily identified. On the iris surface, the neovascular membrane contains capillaries and fibroblasts (inset). The spindle-shaped fibroblasts are responsible for the tissue contraction and pupillary distortion. Note that the iris stromal surface is smooth.

Figure 7.42 In this example of the false angle in neovascular glaucoma, a layer of endothelial cells has migrated across the neovascular membrane (endothelial downgrowth). The presence of PAS-positive lakes within the iris pigment epithelium is a diagnostic feature of diabetes (PAS stain).

Treatment of glaucoma and its complications

Trabeculectomy

Pathological experience is limited to specimens in which surgical treatment of glaucoma has failed. Many procedures were devised to produce a controlled fistula and, of these, a trabeculectomy has proved to be the most commonly employed. The original recommendation was to remove a small block of tissue from the inner sclera, trabecular meshwork, and inner cornea. Currently, a more anterior approach with excision of a small block from the cornea and the anterior part of the trabecular meshwork is favoured. Drainage of aqueous is via the sub-Tenon's space.

Unsuccessful control of intraocular pressure by a fistulising procedure is usually due to fibrosis and scar tissue formation: antimetabolites (5-flurouracil and mitomycin-C) are used to minimise this complication. Iris prolapse is rare, but bleb complications such as leakage and infection are not uncommon (Figures 7.43, 7.44).

Argon laser trabeculoplasty (ALT)

The original intention of ALT was to create a fistula through the trabecular meshwork into Schlemm's canal, but the effects resulting from this pressure lowering were short lived due to fibrosis. Current ALT therapy uses considerably less power and the intention is to stimulate the trabecular endothelial cells. Pathological studies are rare, but in failed cases evidence of ALT is seen in the trabecular meshwork as loss of endothelial cells and fusion of trabecular beams (Figure 7.45).

Transcleral ciliary body ablation – cryotherapy and diode

Destruction of the ciliary processes by transcleral laser or cryotherapy in order to decrease aqueous production appears as areas of ciliary body depigmentation in end-stage glaucomatous eyes (Figure 7.46). In successful ablation, the ciliary processes are fragmented and fibrous tissue containing pigment-laden cells is present in the scar (Figure 7.47).

Tissue effects

While it is convenient to describe the tissue effects of glaucoma under two headings, acute (implying primary angle closure) and chronic (implying primary open angle glaucoma), there is often a considerable overlap between cause and effect.

Table 7.1 summarises the histopathological features in acute and chronic glaucoma.

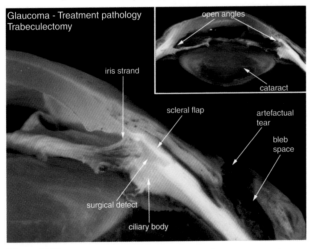

Figure 7.43

Figure 7.43 When the globe is sectioned in the correct plane, it is possible to identify the defect made during a trabeculectomy procedure. The inner limbal defect is located anterior to the ciliary body. In this example iris strands project into the defect. A bleb was present and was artefactually torn. The inset is a lower power view of the anterior segment.

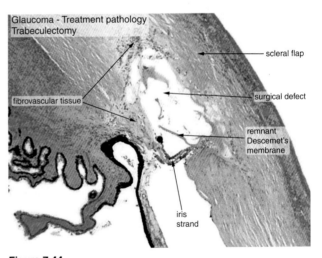

Figure 7.44

Figure 7.44 This figure illustrates some of the potential causes of failure in a trabeculectomy. Fibrovascular scar tissue has drawn the iris over the surgical defect and there is fibrovascular proliferation in the wall of the defect, which contains a strip of Descemet's membrane. The flap is fibrotic and a bleb did not form in this case.

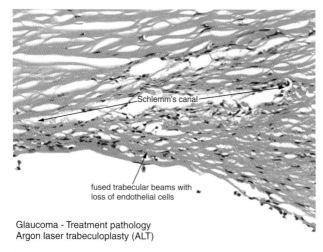

Schlemm's canal

fused trabecular beams with
loss of endothelial cells

Glaucoma - Treatment pathology
Argon laser trabeculoplasty (ALT)

Figure 7.45

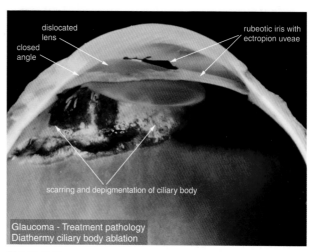

dislocated
lens

closed
angle

rubeotic iris with
ectropion uveae

scarring and depigmentation of ciliary body

Glaucoma - Treatment pathology
Diathermy ciliary body ablation

Figure 7.46

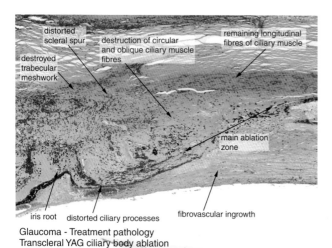

distorted
scleral spur

destruction of circular
and oblique ciliary muscle
fibres

remaining longitudinal
fibres of ciliary muscle

destroyed
trabecular
meshwork

main ablation
zone

iris root   distorted ciliary processes   fibrovascular ingrowth

Glaucoma - Treatment pathology
Transcleral YAG ciliary body ablation

Figure 7.47

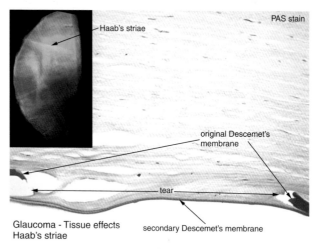

PAS stain

Haab's striae

original Descemet's
membrane

tear

Glaucoma - Tissue effects
Haab's striae

secondary Descemet's membrane

Figure 7.48

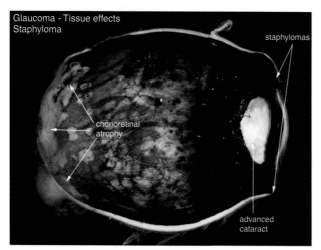

Glaucoma - Tissue effects
Staphyloma

staphylomas

chorioretinal
atrophy

advanced
cataract

Figure 7.49

Figure 7.45 In this example of failure of an argon laser trabeculoplasty (ALT), there is a loss of trabecular endothelial cells and collapse of the meshwork with fusion of the beams.

Figure 7.46 The regions of diathermy ablation can be identified by areas of depigmentation.

Figure 7.47 Transcleral ablation of the ciliary body can be excessively destructive as in this example in which a YAG laser was used. The epicentre of the ablation zone was positioned too far posteriorly. However, sufficient laser energy was applied to destroy the inner layers of the ciliary muscle and the ciliary processes. An exuberant fibrovascular reaction extended across the retina.

Figure 7.48 The inset shows a hemisection of a corneal disc of a patient with a previous history of infantile glaucoma. Slit lamp microscopy shows these fine horizontal lines as tears in Descemet's membrane (Haab's striae). Microscopy of the tears confirms the defect in the original Descemet's membrane. The bare stroma is re-covered by endothelial sliding and there is subsequent formation of a secondary Descemet's membrane. The endothelium is sparse at this end stage and poorly demonstrated in a PAS section.

Figure 7.49 Elongation of the globe and chorioretinal atrophy are features of axial myopia. However, the presence of staphylomas in the region of the ciliary body (intercalary) in this case of secondary angle closure glaucoma indicates longstanding raised intraocular pressure.

Table 7.1 Summary of the histopathological features in acute and chronic (long term) glaucoma.

	Acute	Chronic
Cornea	*Epithelial oedema with or without bulla formation* (see Figure 4.7): prolonged high pressure may lead to loss of endothelium and stromal oedema	*Degenerative keratopathy:* may result if there is sufficiently high pressure (see Figures 4.8, 4.9, 4.11). This may be secondary to endothelial decompensation
		Haab's striae: a sustained rise in intraocular pressure in the neonatal or infantile eye can stretch the cornea to such an extent that linear tears occur in Descemet's membrane. The endothelium covers the bare stromal surface by sliding to form a secondary Descemet's membrane (Figure 7.48). Clinically the tears are horizontal (Figure 7.48, inset)
Sclera	–	*Staphylomas:* occur in the region of scleral canals for vessels and nerves (Figure 7.49)
		Buphthalmos: generalised stretching and thinning of the corneoscleral envelope, which is more elastic in infancy (Figure 7.50)
Iris	*Infarction:* reflex vascular spasm leads to sectorial infarction of the iris stroma and musculature. Clinically this is seen as a sluggish and irregular pupil. Histologically the infarct appears as an acellular sector with loss of muscle and atrophy of the iris pigment epithelium (Figure 7.51)	–
Lens	*Localised epithelial infarction (Glaukomflecken):* focal necrosis of lens epithelial cells (rare pathologically) is seen as white flecks in the anterior cortex	
Retina	Macular and retinal oedema	*Inner retinal atrophy and gliosis:* retrograde atrophy of the ganglion cell layer is due to interruption of nerve fibres at the disc. Consequently, there is a marked reduction in the thickness of the inner retina and preservation of the outer retina (Figure 7.52)
Optic disc	*Papilloedema:* if the intraocular pressure rises rapidly, compression of the nerve head obstructs axoplasmic flow and widespread swelling of the prelaminar nerve fibre layer occurs (Figure 7.53)	*Optic disc cupping:* its distinctive clinical appearance is due to loss of prelaminar axonal tissue (Figures 7.54–7.57). Two main causes are implicated: (1) Mechanical pressure on the prelaminar tissue interferes with axoplasmic flow. The bowing of the lamina cribrosa distorts axons as they pass through the pores in the lamina cribrosa (2) Vascular: it is assumed that in the ageing eye there is diminished blood flow to the optic nerve head. The raised intraocular pressure may interfere with the blood flow from prelaminar capillaries which are supplied by the circle of Zinn
Choroid	Congested	Atrophic

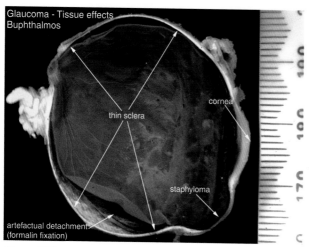

Glaucoma - Tissue effects
Buphthalmos

thin sclera

cornea

staphyloma

artefactual detachment
(formalin fixation)

Figure 7.50

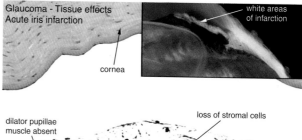

Glaucoma - Tissue effects
Acute iris infarction

white areas
of infarction

cornea

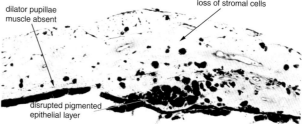

dilator pupillae
muscle absent

loss of stromal cells

disrupted pigmented
epithelial layer

Figure 7.51

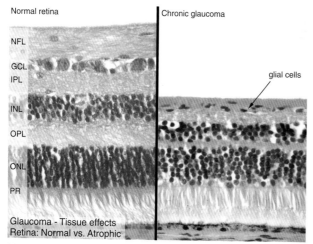

Normal retina

Chronic glaucoma

NFL

GCL
IPL

glial cells

INL

OPL

ONL

PR

Glaucoma - Tissue effects
Retina: Normal vs. Atrophic

Figure 7.52

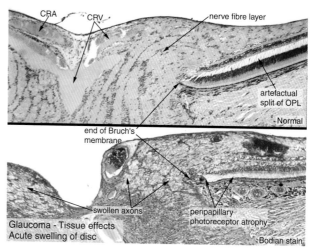

CRA CRV

nerve fibre layer

artefactual
split of OPL

Normal

end of Bruch's
membrane

swollen axons

peripapillary
photoreceptor atrophy

Glaucoma - Tissue effects
Acute swelling of disc

Bodian stain

Figure 7.53

Figure 7.50 The patient had a history of a congenital cataract which was treated with lensectomy surgery in infancy. Glaucoma developed later as a complication. This is an extreme example of buphthalmos – the globe measures nearly 40 mm in diameter. Despite the generalised enlargement of the globe, a co-existing localised staphyloma has occurred.

Figure 7.51 In an infarcted sector of the iris, the stroma is acellular. Macrophages containing melanin derived from necrotic stromal melanocytes are scattered throughout the tissue. The hallmark feature of iris infarction is the loss of the dilator pupillae muscle. The pigment epithelium is disrupted or atrophic. Macroscopically (inset) the infarcted area is white.

Figure 7.52 The extent of inner retinal atrophy in longstanding glaucoma (right) is best demonstrated by comparison with normal retinal tissue (left) from a corresponding region. The thickness of the outer nuclear layer and the distribution of rods and cones in the photoreceptor layer are essentially the

same. The striking abnormality is the absence of recognisable inner retinal layers with glial cell proliferation in the atrophic neural tissue. NFL = nerve fibre layer, GCL = ganglion cell layer, IPL = inner plexiform layer, INL = inner nuclear layer (bipolar cells), OPL = outer plexiform layer, ONL = outer nuclear layer (photoreceptor nuclei), PR = photoreceptors.

Figure 7.53 Upper: normal nerve head; lower: acute glaucoma. An acute glaucoma developed in a patient with a necrotic ciliary body melanoma and the outflow system was blocked by macrophages containing melanin granules. A rapid elevation in intraocular pressure results in optic disc swelling – this is histologically seen as swelling of the nerve fibre layer from an interruption of anterograde axoplasmic flow in the prelaminar part of the optic nerve. The Bodian stain reveals distension of axons and the swollen nerve fibre layer displaces the peripapillary photoreceptor layer. The branches of the central retinal artery (CRA) and vein (CRV) are patent. OPL = outer plexiform layer.

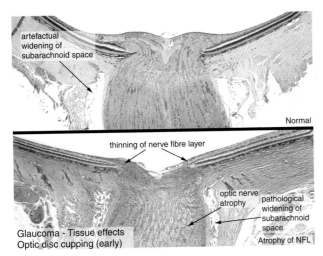

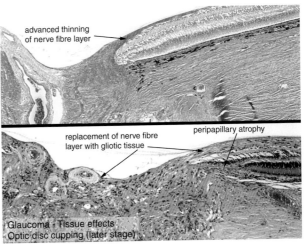

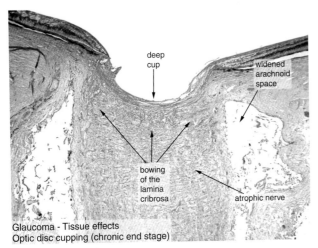

Figure 7.54

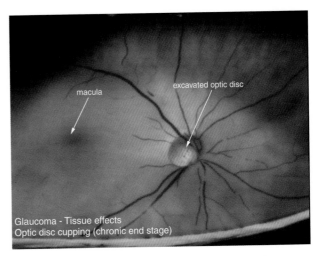

Figure 7.55

Figure 7.56

Figure 7.57

Figure 7.54 The lower figure shows early glaucomatous atrophy of the nerve fibre layer (NFL) by comparison with the normal tissue above. The optic nerve itself is atrophic because of the dropout of axonal tissue and there is enlargement of the subarachnoid space.

Figure 7.55 In the later stages of chronic glaucoma, the nerve fibre layer is extremely thin (upper). Ultimately the optic cup is filled with disorganised gliotic tissue and axonal tissue is absent in the prelaminar portion of the optic nerve (lower).

Figure 7.56 At the end stage of chronic glaucoma, the prelaminar neural tissue is absent and the lamina cribrosa is bowed. The optic nerve is atrophic and the arachnoid space is enlarged.

Figure 7.57 A pathologist's view of advanced optic disc cupping. The macula is easily identified by the presence of luteal pigment and its location within the vascular arcades.

Chapter 8
Inflammation

Basics

This account is confined to the histopathological manifestation of inflammatory disease and the reader should refer to those texts which describe the immunopathology of ocular disorders, for example Forrester J, Dick A, McMenamin P, Lee WR (2002) *The Eye: Basic Sciences in Practice*, second edition. Saunders, London.

Constituents of the inflammatory response

Identification of different types of inflammatory cells is based on their relative size, cytoplasmic inclusions, and nuclear characteristics.

Polymorphonuclear leucocytes (PMNLs)

PMNLs are present in circulating blood and when attracted by the appropriate chemoattractants, they pass through the endothelium of venules and capillaries (Figure 8.1). The PMNL is unique is that its nucleus is *multilobed* and the cytoplasm possesses granules that do not stain in an H&E section but are faint blue in a Giemsa stain. The granules contain proteases, lipases, and lysins. The pale staining of the granules is the reason why this cell is classified as a *neutrophil*. The PMNL is the first response to bacterial infection and is often destroyed by the enzymes and toxins released from ingested bacteria (Figure 8.2).

Eosinophils/eosinophilic polymorphonuclear leucocytes

Eosinophils are the same size as neutrophils but possess bilobed nuclei. In Giemsa stained sections, the cytoplasm contains granular red bodies, hence the terminology (Figure 8.3; see Figure 3.4). The granules contain tissue damaging proteins (eosinophil major basic protein and eosinophil cationic protein). These cells are commonly seen in allergic disease and helminthic infections.

Mast cells

Mast cells resident within tissue are the first to respond to exposure to an allergen. The cell is characterised by an oval eccentric nucleus and a granular cytoplasm in which the granules contain heparin and histamine (Figure 8.4) and stain intensely blue (basophilic) with the Giemsa stain. The equivalent cell in circulating blood is classified as a *basophil*. These cells are three to four times larger than a lymphocyte.

Lymphocytes

Lymphocytes are key elements in the control of immune responses to an antigenic challenge. These are divided into T and B cells. T cells are further subdivided into T-killer, T-helper and T-suppressor cells, each of which has different functions, which are described in detail in immunological texts. B cells have the role in antibody production (see "Plasma cells" below). In a routine histopathological section, the nucleus of a lymphocyte is surrounded by very scanty cytoplasm (Figures 8.4, 8.5). Immunohisto-chemistry has allowed the easy recognition of the different lymphocyte subsets of T and B cells which is useful in the understanding of the complex interactive mechanisms in a chronic inflammatory process.

Plasma cells

A plasma cell is an activated B cell that has the role of producing antibodies (Figure 8.6). It is recognised by an eccentric clockface/cartwheel nucleus and abundant cytoplasm that contains a clear area in the centre (Hof: German for courtyard – this is where antibodies are synthesised).

Figure 8.1 In a hypopyon, PMNLs predominate. Note the multilobed nuclei and the pink cytoplasm in an H&E stain which differs from the appearance seen in a haematological specimen. The inset illustrates margination of polymorphs through the walls of a blood vessel during the acute stages of inflammation. Compare the size of the PMNL with that of a red blood cell (approximately 2 : 1).

Figure 8.2 If the bacterial attack is overwhelming, the organisms, in this case streptococci, destroy the polymorphonuclear leucocytes (PMNLs) which appear as fragmented pink staining bodies (Gram stain).

Figure 8.3 In vernal conjunctivitis, eosinophilic PMNLs are prominent and easily recognised by the presence of fine red intracytoplasmic granules and bilobed nuclei.

Figure 8.4 In the iris stroma, mast cells are much larger than lymphocytes and possess an oval nucleus (compare with an eosinophil, see Figure 8.3). The cytoplasm is pink in an H&E paraffin section and it is not possible to identify intracytoplasmic granules. These are better shown by a metachromatic stain such as toluidine blue (see inset).

Figure 8.5 In a thin section, it is possible to see better nuclear detail within sheets of lymphocytes. These cells are about the same size as the red cells in the lumen of adjacent vessels. The cytoplasm is scanty by comparison with that of a plasma cell.

Figure 8.6 The nuclei of plasma cells are the same size as lymphocytes; the difference is that plasma cells have abundant cytoplasm and oval clear areas are present next to the nuclei. This example is taken from a lacrimal gland. Plasma cells between the acini serve to secrete immunoglobulins into the tears.

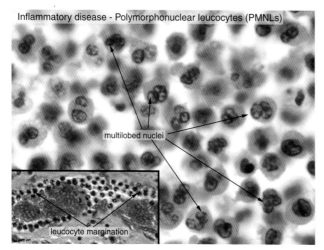

Inflammatory disease - Polymorphonuclear leucocytes (PMNLs)

multilobed nuclei

leucocyte margination

Figure 8.1

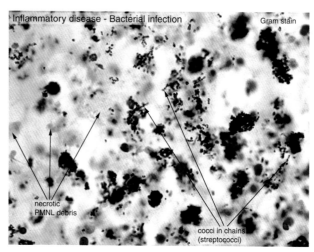

Inflammatory disease - Bacterial infection

Gram stain

necrotic PMNL debris

cocci in chains (streptococci)

Figure 8.2

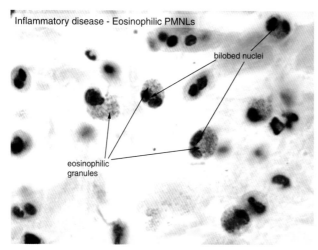

Inflammatory disease - Eosinophilic PMNLs

bilobed nuclei

eosinophilic granules

Figure 8.3

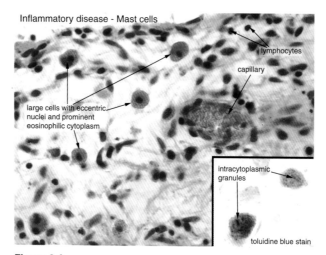

Inflammatory disease - Mast cells

lymphocytes

capillary

large cells with eccentric nuclei and prominent eosinophilic cytoplasm

intracytoplasmic granules

toluidine blue stain

Figure 8.4

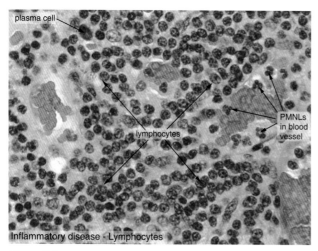

plasma cell

lymphocytes

PMNLs in blood vessel

Inflammatory disease - Lymphocytes

Figure 8.5

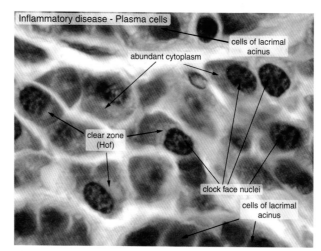

Inflammatory disease - Plasma cells

cells of lacrimal acinus

abundant cytoplasm

clear zone (Hof)

clock face nuclei

cells of lacrimal acinus

Figure 8.6

Macrophages

These cells circulate in the bloodstream and are attracted to locations where phagocytic activity is required. These cells are larger than lymphocytes, plasma cells, and PMNLs (Figure 8.7). Most commonly macrophages are identified by intracytoplasmic phagocytosed debris or microorganisms. Many examples will be found in the section on secondary open angle glaucoma in Chapter 7.

Fibroblasts

These are spindle shaped and their function is to repair damaged tissue by synthesising collagen. The nuclei are relatively large and irregular in shape and the nuclear chromatin is irregularly distributed (Figure 8.8). The cytoplasm of the cell is elongated and it is often difficult to trace the limits since the entire cell often passes out of the plane of section.

Classification of inflammatory reactions

While the identification of different types of inflammatory cells forms a basis for interpretation of patterns in inflammatory disease (for example acute versus chronic), it must be appreciated that the infiltrates almost always contain cells of two or more types.

A convenient broad separation of inflammatory processes is as follows:

1 *Pyogenic reactions:* essentially a polymorphonuclear infiltration in response to pyogenic bacteria such as staphylococci/streptococci and fungi.
2 *Granulomatous reactions:* a chronic inflammatory condition in which the hallmark is the presence of foci of macrophages. These foci are surrounded by chronic inflammatory cells, mainly lymphocytes and plasma cells (and occasionally eosinophils in certain disorders).

In certain conditions the macrophages mature to form epithelial and multinucleate giant cells. The commonest examples of a granulomatous reaction are tuberculosis, sarcodosis, and sympathetic ophthalmitis.
3 *Non-granulomatous reactions:* characterised by lymphocytic and plasma cell infiltrates with only minimal macrophagic involvement. This is often a feature of autoimmune diseases such as collections of lymphocytes (lymphorrhages) in extraocular muscle in thyroid eye disease and diffusely in the uveal stroma in many forms of uveitis.

Endophthalmitis/panophthalmitis

Any inflammatory process that involves some or all the tissues within the eye is referred to as an *endophthalmitis*. If the scleral and episcleral tissues are also involved, the term *panophthalmitis* is employed.

Pyogenic reactions

Endophthalmitis may be classified into the following categories:

1 Exogenous – for example postoperative and traumatic.
2 Endogenous – for example blood borne.

Most commonly bacterial infections complicate (1) while fungal infections are more common than bacterial in (2).

Clinical presentation

The history is most important, especially that of recent intraocular surgery (for example cataract or trabeculectomy) or penetrating eye trauma. Ocular discomfort is accompanied with loss of vision.

Endogenous infections are likely to occur in immuno-compromised patients, intravenous drug abusers, and patients with systemic infections leading to septic emboli (for example subacute bacterial endocarditis).

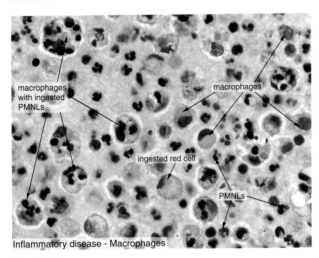

Figure 8.7

Figure 8.7 Macrophages are able to remove necrotic PMNLs after a bacterial infection has been contained. Numerous PMNLs are present within the cytoplasm of enlarged macrophages. A macrophage that has yet to be involved in phagocytosis has an eccentric nucleus and pink cytoplasm. Note the difference in size between a macrophage and a PMNL.

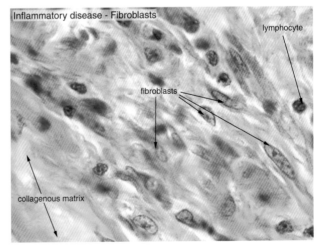

Figure 8.8

Figure 8.8 Fibroblasts are best identified by an elongated nucleus which is much larger than that of a lymphocyte. The cytoplasm of spindle-shaped fibroblasts is indistinct and often extends beyond the plane of section. The cells secrete a collagenous matrix.

Clinical evidence of inflammation:

1 *Anterior (usually exogenous):*
  - a unilateral painful red eye
  - corneal clouding
  - anterior chamber flare and cells that may form a hypopyon.
2 *Posterior (exogenous):*
  - vitritis: cloudy vitreous with or without opacities.
3 *Posterior (endogenous):*
  - Roth's spot – a pale spot within an area of retinal haemorrhage (see below)
  - vascular sheathing
  - vitreous abscess.

Causative organisms are described in detail in the section on microbiology under "Stains for microscopy" in Chapter 1.

Late-stage (saccular) postoperative endophthalmitis

This condition merits consideration due to the popularity of extracapsular cataract surgery. The commonest causative organism is *Proprionibacterium acnes*, an anaerobic Gram positive rod. This disease is characterised by recurrent attacks of anterior uveitis even after several months after surgery. The organism infects the residual cellular tissue left within the capsular bag. The inflammation subsides with topical steroids, but reappears upon cessation with anterior chamber activity (cells and flare) and hypopyon. Treatment requires intravitreal antibiotics, posterior capsulectomy, and vitrectomy (see below).

Pathogenesis

Tissue destruction is the result of toxins released from bacteria or fungi and by lytic enzymes released by necrotic PMNLs. The most serious acute effects are lysis of the retina and generalised vasculitis, which lead to infarction of tissues in the anterior segment. The repair processes which follow, such as fibrosis in the anterior chamber, interfere with aqueous circulation and lead to glaucoma. Traction bands in the vitreous detach the retina and distort the ciliary body so that hypotonia may result.

Possible modes of treatment

The importance of prompt recognition of acute endophthalmitis can not be overemphasised. The management requires an urgent vitreous (+/– anterior chamber) tap for microbiological identification followed by intraocular administration of broad spectrum antibiotic/antifungal agents.

Macroscopic and microscopic

Vitreous biopsy +/– anterior chamber tap A vitreous biopsy in the majority of exogenous cases will contain Gram positive cocci (Figure 8.2). In endogenous infections, fungal elements are more commonly identified (Figure 8.9).

Capsulectomy and vitrectomy In late stage chronic postoperative endophthalmitis (*Proprionibacterium acnes*) the histology shows phagocytosed organisms within macrophages – the pathogens are able to proliferate within the cells (Figure 8.10). With the accumulation of organisms, the macrophages increase in size to eventually rupture with the release of organisms and the inflammatory reaction is intensified. Microbiological diagnosis of *P. acnes* requires prolonged culture (at least 2 weeks) in anaerobic conditions. The bacteriologist should be given prior warning of the possibility of this diagnosis.

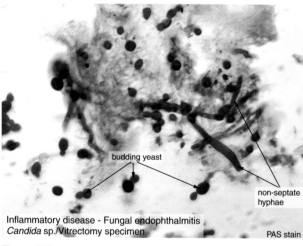

Inflammatory disease - Fungal endophthalmitis
Candida sp./Vitrectomy specimen
PAS stain

Figure 8.9

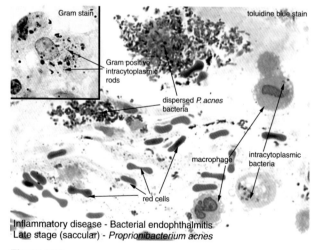

Inflammatory disease - Bacterial endophthalmitis
Late stage (saccular) - *Proprionibacterium acnes*

Figure 8.10

Figure 8.9 A vitreous biopsy was performed in a case of endogenous infection, in this case an intravenous drug abuser. The PAS stain is most commonly used to identify fungal elements. *Candida* sp. are characterised by the presence of budding yeasts and non-septate hyphae.

Figure 8.10 In this example of saccular endophthalmitis, Gram positive rods (*Proprionibacterium acnes*) are seen within the cytoplasm of macrophages (inset). The larger figure is taken from a plastic section stained with toluidine blue to show organisms within the cytoplasm of intact macrophages. The organisms are able to proliferate within macrophages, which increase in size to eventually rupture with release of large clumps of bacteria. This results in cyclical exacerbation of inflammation.

Evisceration Evisceration of ocular contents is preferred by some clinicians for acute uncontrollable infection. The motivation is to reduce the risk of the spread of infection along the optic nerve meninges. Such specimens contain fragments of intraocular tissues and pus. The histopathological abnormalities will be the same as that described in enucleation specimens.

Enucleation An enucleation will be performed for the late stages of infection.

1 *Postsurgical and trauma-related endophthalmitis (exogenous):* purulent material within the vitreous cavity or extrusion through a wound makes the diagnosis of endophthalmitis obvious. The presence of a lens implant is an indication of previous cataract surgery (Figures 8.11, 8.12). If lens tissue is not identified, the possibility of non-surgical trauma should be considered because the lens is often extruded through a scleral or corneal wound in sudden decompression. In a pathological specimen, purulent material is dense white or creamy-yellow in colour: the surrounding vitreous is less opaque (Figure 8.13).

The retina is often necrotic, and the uveal tract may be thickened due to hypotonic exudation (Figure 8.13) or to lymphocytic infiltration (Figure 8.14). Perforation of the cornea may be evident (Figure 8.11).

2 *Blood-borne infection (endogenous):* normal ocular tissues can be recognised in many cases, although there may be varying stages of necrosis. Initially a small septic embolus appears as a white nodule surrounded by a thin layer of haemorrhage (Roth's spot – Figure 8.15). Later, the inflammatory process extends into the vitreous (Figure 8.16). An abscess in the vitreous releases inflammatory mediators which disrupt the integrity of the blood–ocular barrier. Leakage of proteinaceous exudate causes retinal detachment. Retinal ischaemia stimulates the formation of preretinal fibrovascular membranes. Rupture of the anterior vitreous face and damage to the iris vessels is followed by exudation into the anterior compartment (Figures 8.17, 8.18).

Special investigations/stains

See Chapter 1 for specific stains for microorganisms.

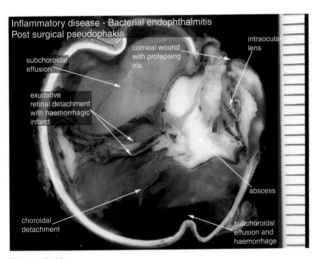

Figure 8.11

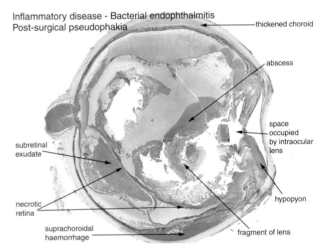

Figure 8.12

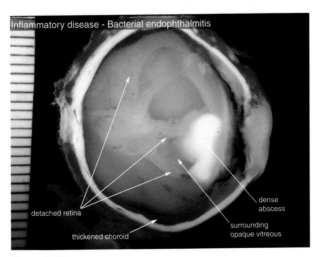

Figure 8.13

Figure 8.11 This is an example of endophthalmitis (*Streptococcus* sp.) following complicated cataract surgery. A lens implant can be identified and there is a dehiscence at the superior limbus. The anterior chamber contains pus and the infection has spread into the cornea. The retina is detached by exudate and the collapsed vitreous is filled with purulent material. Secondary vasculitis has resulted in haemorrhagic infarction of the retina. The exudative detachment of the choroid is due to hypotonia.

Figure 8.12 In this case, cataract surgery was complicated by a dropped lens nucleus. An endophthalmitis (*Staphylococcus* sp.) developed around the lens fragment. The retina and anterior segment are infarcted. The presence of suprachoroidal exudation and haemorrhage confirms the subsequent hypotonia.

Figure 8.13 A vitreous abscess is sometimes localised and this dense white appearance differs from the secondary vitreous opacification. The uveal tract is the "lymph node" of the eye and the choroidal thickening is due to lymphocytic infiltration – see Figure 8.14.

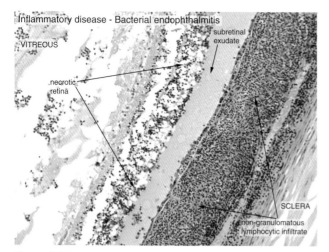

Inflammatory disease - Bacterial endophthalmitis

Figure 8.14

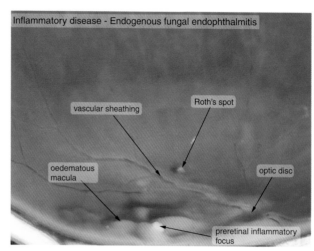

Inflammatory disease - Endogenous fungal endophthalmitis

Figure 8.15

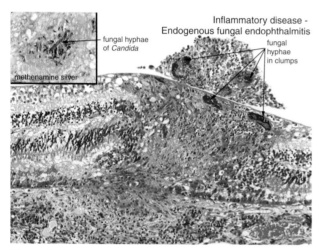

Inflammatory disease - Endogenous fungal endophthalmitis

Figure 8.16

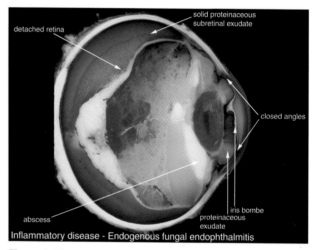

Inflammatory disease - Endogenous fungal endophthalmitis

Figure 8.17

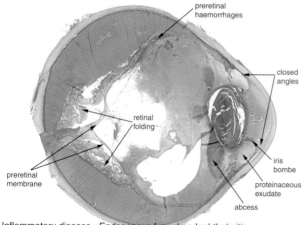

Inflammatory disease - Endogenous fungal endophthalmitis

Figure 8.18

Figure 8.14 In an infarcted retina due to an occlusive vasculitis, the tissue has disintegrated into basophilic fragments. The choroid contains a dense lymphocytic infiltrate.

Figure 8.15 The globe was removed at autopsy in this case of disseminated *Candida* infection in a drug addict. The features of early septic embolism are small white areas surrounded by a ring of haemorrhage (Roth's spots) and sheathing of the retinal vessels. The chorioretinal infection also spreads into the vitreous forming a preretinal inflammatory focus. In autopsy tissue, the retina swells particularly in the region of the macula.

Figure 8.16 This section is at the level of the preretinal nodule shown in Figure 8.15. The choroid and retina have been destroyed by the invading fungi and the inflammatory process. Fungi are not easily seen in an H&E section and the inset shows one of the special stains used to demonstrate fungal elements (methenamine-silver).

Figure 8.17 At the end stage of fungal infection, there is extensive disorganisation of the ocular tissues. Fungal abscesses are present in the anterior vitreous and there is exudation behind the iris with posterior synechiae formation. An iris bombé has resulted. The thickened white appearance of the retina is deceptive, the thickened tissue consists of folded retina behind a preretinal membrane which is the source of bleeding into the posterior vitreous (see Figure 8.18).

Figure 8.18 A section through the globe shown in Figure 8.17 illustrates the pathogenesis of disorganisation due to fungal infection. Damage to the endothelium of the blood vessels results in a massive leakage of proteinaceous fluid into all the ocular compartments. Subretinal exudation has contributed to the detachment but the traction by a preretinal fibrovascular membrane explains the folding of the retina. Friable blood vessels within the preretinal membrane have ruptured and bleeding into the vitreous has occurred. This case illustrates two possible causes of retinal detachment – exudative and tractional.

Granulomatous reactions

In the introduction, the basic cellular constituents (lymphocytes, plasma cells, and macrophages) of a granulomatous reaction were simplified. It is important to appreciate that the various patterns described in the following section vary quite markedly but, in some conditions, the patterns can provide a specific diagnosis.

Infective

Tuberculosis

Infection in tuberculosis (along with sarcoidosis and syphilis) can present in any form of ocular granulomatous inflammatory disease, particularly anterior uveitis and chorioretinitis.

Ocular infections due to mycobacteria (*Mycobacterium tuberculosis* and *Mycobacterium avium-intracellulare*) are more common in individuals in whom the cell mediated immunity response is suppressed. The organisms are occasionally present in large numbers when examined by Ziehl–Neelsen stain (Figure 8.19).

In patients with an intact immune system, the histopathological pattern can vary between caseating and non-caseating granulomas. In both, Langhans' multinucleate giant cells are characteristic (Figure 8.20). Caseation represents intensive necrosis in the infiltrating inflammatory cells (Figures 8.21, 8.22).

Leprosy

Infection by *Mycobacterium leprae* remains endemic in the tropics and subtropics. The ocular manifestations are variable. Involvement of nerves leads to paralytic lagophthalmos and is an indirect cause of exposure keratitis. Damage to autonomic nerve fibres leads to a mild iridocyclitis, and this is the most common manifestation of ocular leprosy. Anterior chamber cells and flare with sparse keratic precipitates are the usual features.

Infections vary depending on the immune status: tuberculoid leprosy (active cell mediated response) or lepromatous leprosy (poor response). In the tuberculoid form, the histopathological patterns are similar to those described in tuberculosis with non-caseating granulomas and scanty organisms. An infiltrate containing macrophages, lymphocytes, and overwhelming numbers of organisms is characteristic of lepromatous leprosy.

Syphilis

Like tuberculosis, syphilis has the potential to present in any form of ocular inflammatory disease. Pathological experience of this condition will be either in the form of a penetrating keratoplasty specimen or a globe, but is rare. Infection is by the spirochaete *Treponema pallidum*. It may be congenital or acquired. The latter is essentially a sexually transmitted disease but may also be acquired via blood transfusions and direct contact with a surface lesion. Although potentially treatable with antibiotics, the incidence of syphilitic infection is rising due to prophylactic and treatment complacency.

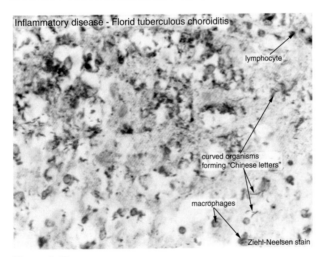

Figure 8.19

Figure 8.19 In an eye removed at the autopsy of an immunosuppressed patient, nodules were identified in the choroid. Histological examination revealed massive accumulations of slender tubercle bacilli. The organisms are curved and are red in colour with the Ziehl–Neelsen stain, and form patterns described previously but incorrectly as "Chinese letters".

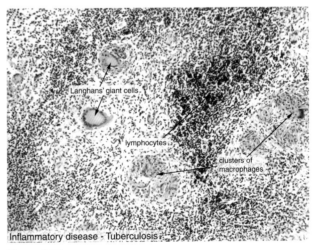

Figure 8.20

Figure 8.20 The histological pattern in tuberculosis varies according to the status of the cell-mediated immune response. In this example, there is no evidence of caseation but the clusters of macrophages contain Langhans' giant cells. In this type of reaction, very few tubercle bacilli will be identified.

Clinical manifestations of ocular syphilis will depend on the stage of disease:

1 *Primary:* chancre of the eyelid or conjunctiva.
2 *Secondary:* iridocyclitis, neuroretinitis, and chorioretinitis.
3 *Tertiary:*
  - Cornea: interstitial keratitis with the appearance of ghost vessels. The majority of cases are congenital (see Chapter 4).
  - Uveal tract: the inflammation may be granulomatous or non-granulomatous.
  - Visible dilated capillaries on the iris surface (roseola) are a characteristic feature. A chorioretinitis may be present which eventually resolves and takes the form of a pigmentary retinopathy.
  - Retina: vasculitis with retinal exudation which may be bilateral, multifocal, or diffuse. Retinal oedema with cotton wool spots may also be present.
  - Optic nerve: optic disc oedema with haemorrhage and exudate.

Non-infective

Sympathetic ophthalmitis

A rare bilateral autoimmune granulomatous choroiditis resulting from trauma to one eye. If untreated, the condition leads to bilateral blindness.

Clinical presentation

A history of a penetrating trauma to one eye (surgical and non-surgical) is essential.

By definition, this condition is bilateral, although it may be variable in severity and symmetry.

The clinical signs vary from a localised uveitis to a panuveitis with features including:

1 *Anterior chamber:* mutton-fat keratic precipitates.
2 *Choroid:* diffuse thickening with white nodules (Dalen–Fuchs spots) representing focal elevated sub-retinal infiltrates. A vitritis, which obscures the view of the fundus, may be present.

Pathogenesis

The pathogenesis is poorly understood but it is generally considered to be the sensitisation of the systemic immune system to antigens present in the retina or uveal tissue. It is assumed that the proteins in chorioretinal tissue are sequestered and are exposed by trauma.

This condition is commonly associated with lens-induced uveitis (see below) by the nature of the trauma involved.

In animal models, it is possible to induce a uveitis by sensitising the immune system to retinal and uveal proteins in combination with Freund's adjuvant. Unfortunately, the histological pattern is unlike human sympathetic ophthalmitis.

Possible modes of treatment

Prophylaxis Enucleation of the non-viable injured eye – there have been no published cases of sympathetic ophthalmitis when an injured eye was enucleated within 10 days of injury. As the incidence of sympathetic ophthalmitis is rare and is continuing to decline, it is common in many practices to conserve an injured eye that still maintains some vision.

Treatment With the recognition of sympathetic ophthalmitis, treatment would involve systemic corticorticosteroids and other immunosuppressive agents.

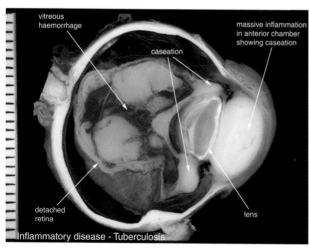

Figure 8.21

Figure 8.21 Some 15 years after treatment for spinal tuberculosis, a male patient developed an episcleral nodule and an anterior uveitis. This progressed to retinal detachment and end-stage disorganisation of the ocular tissues with caseation in the anterior chamber and anterior uvea due to tuberculosis.

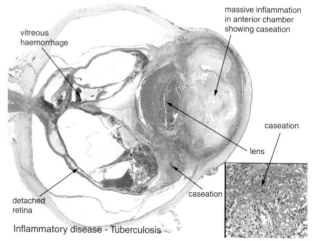

Figure 8.22

Figure 8.22 A histological section showing the globe in Figure 8.21. The inset shows amorphous eosinophilic material (caseation) and fragmentation of inflammatory cells. No more than four tubercle bacilli were identified in this case using the Ziehl–Neelsen stain.

Macroscopic

The only specimen likely to be submitted would be an enucleated eye. With the onset of this disease, in either the injured or non-injured (sympathising) eye, a prominent thickened choroid is evident macroscopically (Figures 8.23, 8.24).

At late stages, hypotonia due to ciliary body shutdown leads to uveal effusion and eventual phthisis.

Microscopic

The granulomatous reaction is confined to the choroid, but in an appropriate plane of section, extension into the scleral canals will be evident (Figure 8.25). The choriocapillaris is usually spared. Multinucleate giant cells are sparse and the accumulations of macrophages are less compact (Figure 8.26) than in sarcoidosis (see below). The macrophages may contain a fine dusting of melanin granules (Figure 8.27). Macrophagic infiltration beneath and within the retinal pigment epithelium (Figure 8.28) is a characteristic feature (Dalen–Fuchs nodule).

Immunohistochemistry/immunopathology

There are no specific markers but conventional immunohistochemistry has revealed T cells (CD3), B cells (CD20), and macrophages (CD68) within the infiltrate.

Sarcoidosis

A chronic multisystem disease of unknown aetiology characterised by the formation of non-caseating granulomas within the eye, conjunctiva, and orbit (see Chapters 3 and 5).

Clinical presentation

The first presentation of the systemic disease is usually within the third to sixth decades, and approximately 80% of cases have ocular involvement.

Any or all parts of the eye may be involved:

1 *Anterior uveitis:* often bilateral, with "mutton-fat" keratic precipitates; formation of anterior and posterior synechiae; secondary open and closed angle glaucoma.
2 *Posterior uveitis:* vitritis, chorioretinitis, neovascularisation, haemorrhage.
3 *Granulomas:* note that granulomas can also occur in conjunctiva, eyelid, orbit, optic nerve, and lacrimal drainage systems.
4 *Vascular:* peripheral retinal periphlebitis, exudates, "candle wax drippings", neovascularisation, and haemorrhage, branch or central retinal vein occlusion.
5 *Optic nerve:* swelling, granuloma, atrophy, and neovascularisation. Field defects may be evident.

It is important to refer the patient for investigation of systemic involvement, especially the lung, liver, skin, and central and peripheral nervous systems.

Basic investigations include a chest X-ray for bilateral hilar lymphadenopathy, serology to detect a raised serum angiotensin converting enzyme (ACE), and a gallium scan. A confirmatory biopsy of a suspicious nodule is preferred, especially with the prospect of committing the patient to long term steroid treatment.

Pathogenesis

Unknown with considerable variation in disease onset and progression.

Genetics

- *Gender:* females > males.
- *Race:* black to white, 10 : 1.

Possible modes of treatment

Treatment is mainly with corticosteroids and other immunosuppressive/antimetabolic therapy.

Figure 8.23 This globe was badly traumatised and enucleation was delayed for a month. Several months later, the patient developed choroiditis in the fellow non-traumatised eye and sympathetic ophthalmitis was diagnosed. In the enucleated globe, the retina was avulsed and the iris was incarcerated into the limbal wound. The thickened choroid is described as having a "marble-like" appearance. In this case, there is an associated lens-induced uveitis and the anterior uvea is thickened by inflammatory cell infiltration.

Figure 8.24 In this low power micrograph from the specimen in Figure 8.23, the choroid and anterior uvea contain a purple granulomatous infiltrate. Lens remnants were found within a fibrous ingrowth and this gave rise to the inflammatory infiltration in the anterior uvea. The avulsed retina forms a nodule surrounded by scar tissue from a fibrous ingrowth from the limbal wound.

Figure 8.25 A granulomatous reaction in sympathetic ophthalmitis is not confined to the choroid but spreads along the scleral canals through which the nerves and arteries penetrate.

Figure 8.26 In sympathetic ophthalmitis, the granulomatous reaction is not compact (compared with sarcoidosis, see below). The macrophages are loosely intermingled with lymphocytes. The multinucleated cells are useful diagnostic features.

Figure 8.27 Within multinucleate giant cells in sympathetic ophthalmitis (left), the nuclei are irregularly distributed unlike the Langhans' giant cells in tuberculosis (see Figure 8.20). Macrophages are identified by their oval nuclei and light dusting of melanosomes in the cytoplasm (right).

Figure 8.28 Clusters of macrophages on the inner surface of Bruch's membrane are the histological equivalent of the white spots (Dalen–Fuchs) as seen clinically in sympathetic ophthalmitis. Note the photoreceptor atrophy.

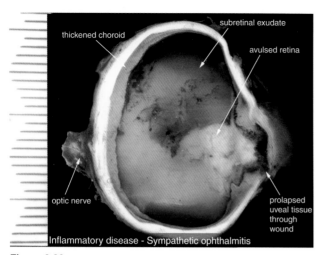

Inflammatory disease - Sympathetic ophthalmitis

Figure 8.23

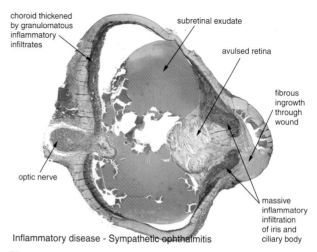

Inflammatory disease - Sympathetic ophthalmitis

Figure 8.24

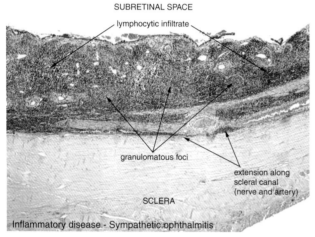

Inflammatory disease - Sympathetic ophthalmitis

Figure 8.25

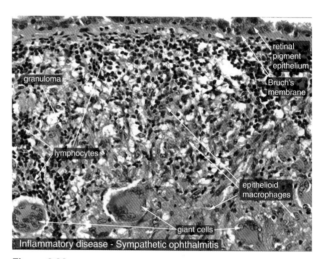

Inflammatory disease - Sympathetic ophthalmitis

Figure 8.26

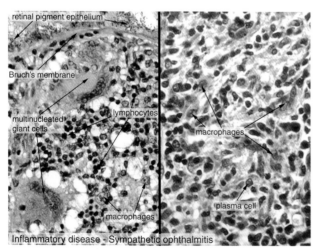

Inflammatory disease - Sympathetic ophthalmitis

Figure 8.27

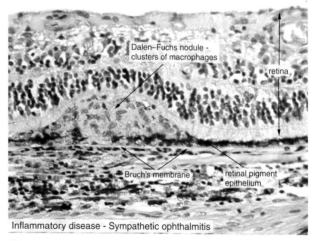

Inflammatory disease - Sympathetic ophthalmitis

Figure 8.28

Macroscopic

The specimen presented would usually be in the form of a diagnostic/confirmatory biopsy, although enucleations may be performed for end-stage secondary complications. In an enucleated eye, perivascular granulomatous nodules (Figure 8.29) and perivascular sheathing are present. The anterior segment may show secondary changes of iritis with angle closure.

With the many new and established investigatory modalities, conjunctival "blind biopsies" are less commonly performed (see Chapter 3), and are usually restricted to areas where small suspicious granulomatous nodules are present.

Complications/secondary effects

1 Secondary glaucoma and cataract from persistent anterior uveitis – open and closed angle.
2 Central and branch retinal vein occlusion due to periphlebitis.

Microscopic

The hallmark pathological feature of sarcoidosis is a non-caseating granuloma with lymphocytes intermingled with epithelioid macrophages. Multinucleate cells are rarely seen.

The granulomas are usually small and can be identified in the retina around blood vessels, in the uveal tract, and in the vitreous (Figures 8.30–8.32). Sarcoid granulomas in the trabecular meshwork are rare (Figure 8.33).

Lens-induced uveitis

Lens-induced uveitis can be divided into the following categories:
1 Phacolytic glaucoma.
2 Phacoanaphylactic endophthalmitis.

The former is not a true uveitis and has been described in Chapter 7. The remainder of this section refers to phacoanaphylaxis.

Phacoanaphylactic endophthalmitis is a severe autoimmune granulomatous reaction against lens matter exposed through a disrupted lens capsule by surgical and non-surgical trauma. Occasionally, "spontaneous" cases are encountered.

Clinical presentation

The patient presents with a unilateral painful red eye. A history of surgical or non-surgical trauma (blunt or penetrating) is significant. The reaction may take several weeks to develop after the initial insult, but the onset may be within 24 hours if there was prior sensitisation to lens matter (for example cataract surgery in the other eye).

Severe granulomatous anterior uveitis appears as "mutton-fat" keratic precipitates, synechiae, and hypopyon. There may be a secondary elevation of intraocular pressure. The posterior segment is relatively unaffected.

Infection and sympathetic endophthalmitis are important differential diagnoses.

Pathogenesis

The aetiology is not well understood. Exposure to certain components of (possibly degenerate) lens proteins sensitises and activates the humoral and cell mediated responses to the remaining exposed lens matter.

Possible modes of treatment

Corticosteroids may be used to decrease the immune response but ultimately surgical removal of residual lens matter is required.

Macroscopic

Opportunities for pathological studies are in the form of an irretrievably damaged globe (Figures 8.34, 8.35) or excised lens tissue.

Trabeculitis and anterior and posterior synechiae may lead to secondary open or closed angle glaucoma.

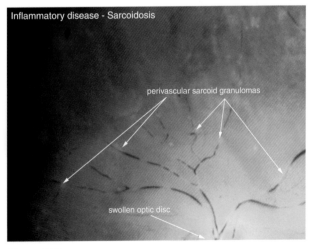

Figure 8.29

Figure 8.29 A patient suffering from sarcoidosis also experienced extreme pain from scleritis. She requested bilateral enucleation. The retina contains small white granulomatous foci located around blood vessels. The optic disc is swollen due to the accumulation of granulomatous foci.

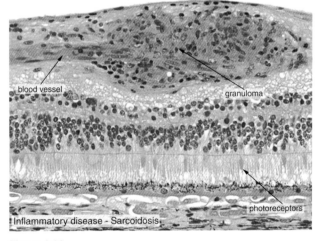

Figure 8.30

Figure 8.30 In retinal sarcoidosis, the granulomatous reaction is compact and consists of macrophages and intermingled lymphocytes. Multinucleate giant cells are rare.

Inflammatory disease - Sarcoidosis

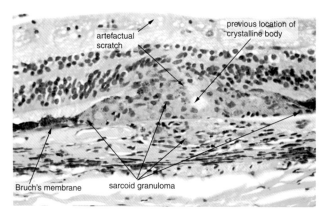

Figure 8.31

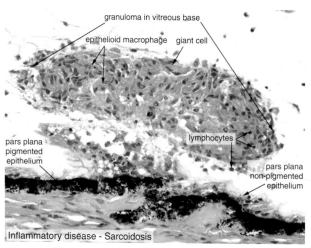

Inflammatory disease - Sarcoidosis

Figure 8.32

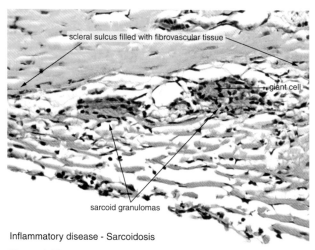

Inflammatory disease - Sarcoidosis

Figure 8.33

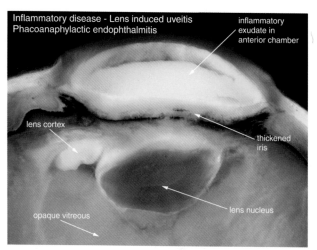

Inflammatory disease - Lens induced uveitis
Phacoanaphylactic endophthalmitis

Figure 8.34

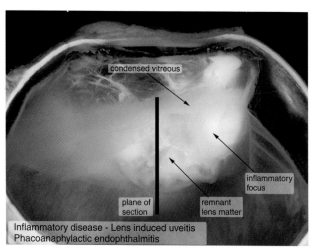

Inflammatory disease - Lens induced uveitis
Phacoanaphylactic endophthalmitis

Figure 8.35

Figure 8.31 In this example of sarcoidosis, the granulomatous reaction involves the retinal pigment epithelium and the underlying choroid. Sometimes granulomas contain crystalline bodies – in this example the microtome knife has sheered off the crystalline body and has left a scratch mark in the retina.

Figure 8.32 Sarcoid granulomas can be found in the vitreous base adjacent to the pars plana. The macrophages with their pink cytoplasm are larger than the lymphocytes, which have heavily stained nuclei.

Figure 8.33 A multinucleate giant cell is present in one of the two small granulomas in the outer part of the trabecular meshwork.

Figure 8.34 An elderly female patient with a morgagnian cataract had accidental blunt trauma to her eye resulting in disruption of the lens and its contents. The brown sclerotic nucleus is surrounded by a yellow inflammatory infiltrate. The iris is thickened by inflammatory cell infiltration and the anterior chamber contains a dense inflammatory exudate.

Figure 8.35 An intracapsular cataract operation was complicated by lens zonule dehiscence, with dislocation of the lens remnants against the ciliary body. An intense inflammatory reaction ensued several days later, with intractable anterior uveitis and raised intraocular pressure. An endophthalmitis was suspected, but was resistant to treatment and the eye was subsequently enucleated. A section was taken in the plane of the black line and is shown in Figure 8.36.

Microscopic

At the earliest stages, focal granulomatous cellular infiltration occurs on the surface of the exposed lens matter (Figure 8.36). There may be evidence of rupture of the lens capsule. A zonal distribution of inflammatory cells is often evident. Neutrophils line the lens matter and are surrounded by macrophages (epithelioid and multinucleate giant cells), lymphocytes, and plasma cells (Figure 8.37). Eosinophils may also be identified – these cells are thought to be a critical component of anaphylaxis, hence the usage of the term "phacoanaphylaxis". The capsule is also eroded by inflammatory cells once the reaction is established (Figure 8.38).

The most vigorous reaction is encountered when the lens matter comes to rest against the ciliary body or is adherent to the iris. The iris often contains a dense lymphoplasmacytoid infiltrate.

Any reaction in the choroid should raise the suspicion of concomitant sympathetic ophthalmitis. Care should be taken to exclude the presence of a bacterial endophthalmitis by using a Gram stain.

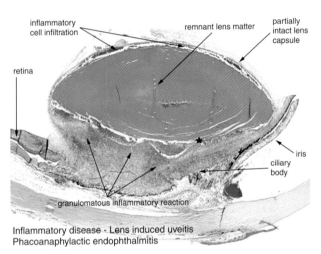

Inflammatory disease - Lens induced uveitis
Phacoanaphylactic endophthalmitis

Figure 8.36

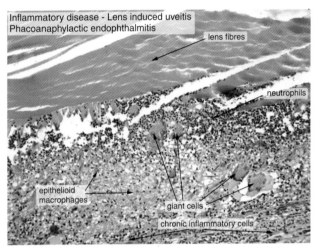

Figure 8.37

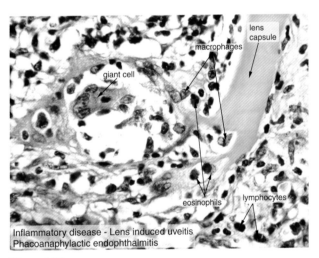

Inflammatory disease - Lens induced uveitis
Phacoanaphylactic endophthalmitis

Figure 8.38

Figure 8.36 A granulomatous mass fuses the exposed lens matter to the iris and ciliary body epithelium. The inflammatory cells have cleaved a space between the capsule and lens matter. The iris stroma contains an inflammatory cell infiltrate. The angle is open and is filled by a hyphaema. The area marked with an asterix is magnified and shown in Figure 8.37.

Figure 8.37 The magnified area (marked with an asterix in Figure 8.36) shows erosion of lens matter by a giant cell granulomatous reaction consisting of epithelioid macrophages, neutrophils, and lymphocytes.

Figure 8.38 As a rarity, the lens capsule is consumed by the giant cell granulomatous process. In this example, the infiltrate contains eosinophils, hence the adoption of the term "phacoanaphylactic endophthalmitis".

Scleritis

Destruction of the corneoscleral envelope by a granulomatous or non-granulomatous inflammatory process is the primary abnormality. The corneal manifestations are described in Chapter 4. A milder form of the disease, episcleritis, should be differentiated from anterior scleritis as the aetiology and management differ.

Scleritis is an idiopathic autoimmune disease either confined to the eye or associated with systemic disease. The most common association is *rheumatoid disease*, but the following conditions should be considered in the differential diagnosis:

- Wegener's granulomatosis
- relapsing polychondritis
- polyarteritis nodosa
- inflammatory bowel disease (Crohn's disease)
- sarcoidosis
- systemic lupus erythematosus
- ankylosing spondylitis
- Reiter's syndrome
- psoriatic arthritis.

Scleritis is subgrouped to the following categories which are very different both clinically and pathologically:

1 *Anterior scleritis:* which may be non-necrotising (diffuse or nodular) or necrotising (with or without inflammation). Scleromalacia perforans is a rare non-inflammatory variant of the latter and is a specific painless necrotising condition in untreated rheumatoid disease (see below).
2 *Posterior scleritis:* located behind the equator of the eye (brawny scleritis).

Clinical presentation

Scleritis is more common in females and is often bilateral. The onset of this condition is gradual and the main symptom is often a severe ocular ache along with visual loss.

1 *Anterior scleritis:* the affected areas may be translucent revealing the underlying purplish choroid. Staphylomas may develop over previously necrotic areas. The cornea may be affected with sclerokeratitis and marginal keratolysis (see Chapter 4). It is common to find a concomitant anterior uveitis. It is important to emphasise that surgical interventions in the anterior segment (for example trabeculectomy, an intraocular procedure, and penetrating keratoplasty) may all be complicated by scleritis.
2 *Posterior scleritis:* the diagnosis presents many more difficulties than anterior scleritis. The patient may be asymptomatic, although pain and visual disturbance are still common. The sclera is usually thickened by inflammation resulting in exudative retinal and choroidal detachments, chorioretinal inflammation, and disc swelling. The severe thickening of the sclera and retro-ocular tissue can produce a proptosis. Ultrasound or CT imaging is required to confirm the thickened sclera.

With the high visual morbidity and mortality in many of the associated systemic conditions, it is common to have a protocol of investigations that would help to differentiate the many possible causes of scleritis.

Pathogenesis

The pathogenesis is commonly thought to be secondary to the formation of antigen–antibody complexes resulting in a vasculitis. In some cases of posterior scleritis, T cells have also been implicated in the inflammatory reaction.

Genetics

Genetics may have relevance depending on any underlying systemic disease.

Possible modes of treatment

Systemic non-steroidal anti-inflammatory medications, corticosteroids, and immunosuppressive therapy may be required. Topical steroids may be used to treat the anterior uveitis. Reinforcement of a weakened sclera may occasionally require patch grafting with sclera or fascia lata.

Macroscopic and microscopic

It is very rare to receive a scleral or corneal biopsy to confirm a scleritis due to the risk of perforation or stimulation of the disease process. Enucleations are performed for intractable symptoms, irretrievable damage after perforation, in misdiagnosis of malignancy, and for cosmesis.

1 *Anterior scleritis:* at a macroscopic level, the necrotic sclera has a creamy yellow appearance (Figure 8.39). On section, the normal white condensed scleral tissue is replaced by partially pigmented granular tissue (Figure 8.40). Corneoscleral collagenolysis with a predominant lymphocytic infiltrate is characteristic; giant cell granulomatous reactions are inconspicuous (Figures 8.41, 8.42). A dense lymphocytic infiltration may replace the normal sclera (Figure 8.43).
2 *Posterior scleritis:* in contrast with the anterior variant, the progress of posterior scleritis is much more chronic and the inflammatory cell infiltration is accompanied by massive reactionary fibrosis (Figure 8.44). When the process is diffuse, the term *brawny scleritis* is appropriate (Figures 8.45, 8.46).

The fibrous reaction can be so extreme that an episcleral mass causes a proptosis (Figures 8.47, 8.48). The mass may also extend into the globe and may simulate an intraocular melanoma (Figure 8.49).

Complications/secondary effects

Severe inflammation can result in scleral thinning with staphyloma formation as well as perforation. Bacterial superinfection may result.

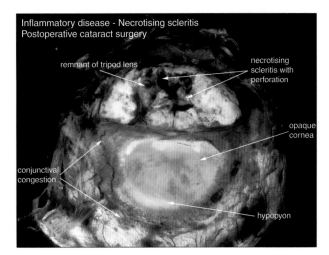

Figure 8.39

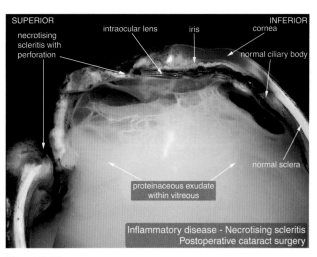

Figure 8.40

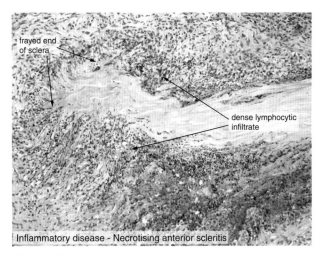

Figure 8.41

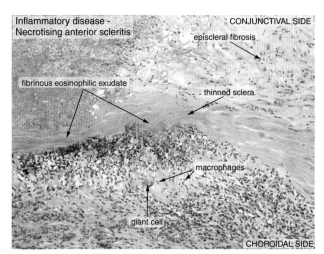

Figure 8.42

Figure 8.39 A massive anterior necrotising scleritis developed after a lens extraction and insertion of a tripod lens into the posterior chamber. The necrotising process extends into the cornea which is opaque due to iridocorneal contact. One haptic of the lens is identified externally.

Figure 8.40 A cut across the anterior segment of the globe shown in Figure 8.39 reveals the intraocular lens and the scleral thinning due to scleritis. The vitreous is filled with a gelatinous exudate.

Figure 8.41 Anterior scleritis is characterised by a dense lymphocytic reaction in the region of the scleral disruption and destruction. It is frequently difficult to demonstrate giant cells and macrophages in such cases.

Figure 8.42 In some cases of scleritis, a granulomatous reaction with epithelioid macrophages and multinucleate giant cells can be demonstrated. Leakage of fibrin into the necrotic sclera gives the tissue a brick-red appearance.

Inflammatory disease - Necrotising scleritis

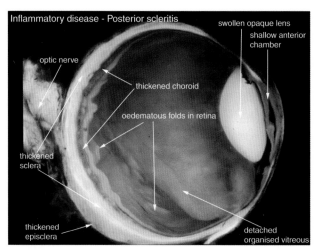

open angle

pupillary membrane

mild disc oedema

necrotising scleritis (scleromalacia perforans)

closed angle

lens removed before sectioning

Figure 8.43

Inflammatory disease - Early posterior scleritis

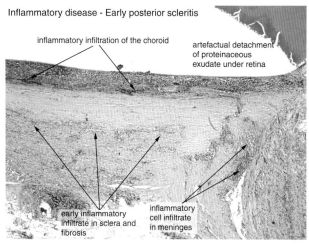

inflammatory infiltration of the choroid

artefactual detachment of proteinaceous exudate under retina

early inflammatory infiltrate in sclera and fibrosis

inflammatory cell infiltrate in meninges

Figure 8.44

Inflammatory disease - Posterior scleritis

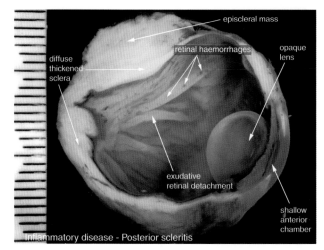

swollen opaque lens

shallow anterior chamber

optic nerve

thickened choroid

oedematous folds in retina

thickened sclera

thickened episclera

detached organised vitreous

Figure 8.45

Inflammatory disease - Posterior scleritis

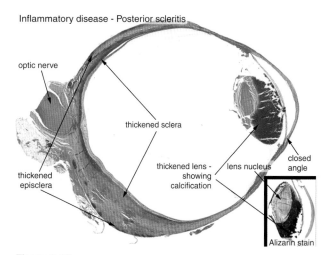

optic nerve

thickened sclera

thickened episclera

thickened lens - showing calcification

lens nucleus

closed angle

Alizarin stain

Figure 8.46

episcleral mass

retinal haemorrhages

opaque lens

diffuse thickened sclera

exudative retinal detachment

shallow anterior chamber

Inflammatory disease - Posterior scleritis

Figure 8.47

Figure 8.43 A patient suffering from rheumatoid arthritis had intractable pain due to extensive anterior necrotising scleritis with imminent perforation. Enucleation was the only option available. Note the dense cellular infiltrate in the pars plana region with severe scleral thinning. Ocular hypotonia has resulted in retinal and optic disc oedema.

Figure 8.44 In the early stage of posterior scleritis, there is a lymphocytic infiltration within the sclera and this is accompanied by a fibrovascular proliferation in the episclera. Lymphocytic infiltration in the choroid interferes with the integrity of the choriocapillaris and retinal pigment epithelium, and the release of proteinaceous fluid detaches the retina. Note the involvement of the meninges.

Figure 8.45 The macroscopic appearance of posterior scleritis. The posterior sclera and episclera are diffusedly thickened. Involvement of the choroid has led to exudation in the retina which is thrown into folds. The vitreous is semiopaque and is detached posteriorly. The cataractous lens is unusually white – see Figure 8.46.

Figure 8.46 A low power photomicrograph of the specimen shown in Figure 8.45 reveals the extent of inflammatory cell infiltration in the choroid, sclera, and episclera. The white macroscopic appearance of the lens is due to calcification. The inset is stained to demonstrate the presence of calcium in the lens (alizarin is a red stain which chelates calcium).

Figure 8.47 A patient presented with a proptosis. In this more advanced case, the fibrous proliferation extends internally into the globe and the secondary complications are exudative detachment and haemorrhage in the retina. Enucleation of such a deformed globe can be difficult, and in this case the surgeon did not excise the anterior part of the optic nerve with the globe.

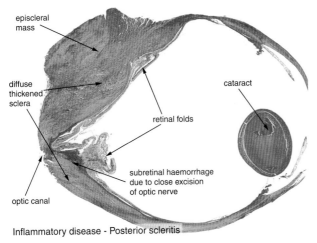

Figure 8.48

episcleral mass

diffuse thickened sclera

cataract

retinal folds

optic canal

subretinal haemorrhage due to close excision of optic nerve

Inflammatory disease - Posterior scleritis

Figure 8.48 A section of the same globe illustrated in Figure 8.47 shows that there is massive inflammation and fibrosis throughout the posterior sclera. The haemorrhage around the optic nerve is a surgical artefact.

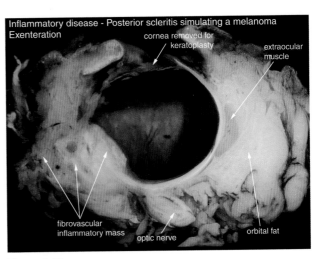

Inflammatory disease - Posterior scleritis simulating a melanoma
Exenteration

cornea removed for keratoplasty

extraocular muscle

fibrovascular inflammatory mass

optic nerve

orbital fat

Figure 8.49

Figure 8.49 The patient presented with a proptosis which appeared to be due to an intraocular mass with extension into the orbit. A diagnosis of an amelanotic melanoma with extraocular extension was made. The possibility of posterior scleritis was excluded as the changes were so localised and the remainder of the ocular tissues appeared normal. An exenteration was performed in view of the possibility of extraocular spread into the orbit.

Vogt–Koyanagi–Harada (VKH) syndrome

A systemic granulomatous condition characterised by bilateral panophthalmitis of unknown aetiology. It is more common in pigmented races and was formerly divided into two different groups according to systemic findings:

1 *Vogt–Koyanagi:*
   • skin: alopecia, poliosis, and vitiligo
   • anterior uveitis.
2 *Harada:*
   • *neurological:* headache, encephalopathy, inner and middle ear symptoms (deafness, tinnitus, and vertigo), cerebrospinal fluid pleocytosis
   • *posterior uveitis:* in conjunction with disc swelling and exudative retinal detachments.

VKH is now commonly thought of as being one condition with a wide spectrum of presentations, although bilateral ocular involvement occurs in every case.

Clinical presentation

Ophthalmic findings will depend on the stage of the disease:

1 *Prodromal stage:* flu-like illness. Eye signs are non-specific with visual disturbance, photophobia, ocular pain, and conjunctivitis.
2 *Uveitic phase:* bilateral uveitis, disc swelling, and exudative retinal detachment.
3 *Chronic phase:* fundus depigmentation, subretinal and optic disc neovascularisation.

Investigations are extensive to exclude other causes. Fluorescein angiography demonstrates multiple retinal pigment epithelium (RPE) window defects.

An important differential diagnosis is sympathetic ophthalmitis and a history of penetrating trauma should be sought.

Pathogenesis

An autoimmune granulomatous reaction against melanocytes, melanin, and retinal pigment epithelium. A viral agent has been suggested although not proven.

Genetics

Females are more commonly affected. There is an association with HLA DR4.

Possible modes of treatment

Principles involve high dose systemic corticosteroids with a long tapering off period. Immunosuppressants may also be used.

Macroscopic and microscopic

The appearances within a globe are indistinguishable from sympathetic ophthalmitis (see above).

Immunohistochemistry

The infiltrating lymphocytes are of T-cell type (suppressor-cytotoxic subsets).

Behçet's syndrome

A systemic vasculitic condition that manifests itself in the eye as a panuveitis. It is most common in Japan and Turkey.

Clinical presentation

Diagnostic criteria is recurrent oral ulceration with any two of the following:

1 Eye lesions: anterior and posterior uveitis.
2 Recurrent genital ulcerations.
3 Skin lesions: for example erythema nodosum.
4 Positive pathergy test.

Pathogenesis and genetics

The aetiology is unknown. The geographical distribution of the disease follows that of the "silk road". Association with HLA-B51 for ocular involvement is recognised.

Possible modes of treatment

Despite treatment, visual prognosis is poor with progression to blindness within 4 years of disease onset.

Macroscopic and microscopic

By the time enucleation is required, secondary pathology obscures the nature of the primary disorder.

Retinal haemorrhage, exudation, and detachment are the result of retinal vasculitis. The uveal tract is thickened by a non-granulomatous lymphocytic infiltrate with a prominent CD4+ T-cell population.

Chorioretinitis

Many infective organisms can lead to chorioretinitis. As a rule of thumb, a viral infection results in a diffuse necrotising retinitis, while parasitic and fungal infections are focal (see section on microbiology under "Stains for microscopy" in Chapter 1).

Viral: herpes simplex virus (HSV), herpes zoster virus (HZV), and cytomegalovirus (CMV)

The clinical patterns of disease in viral infections vary and have become of great importance due to the increase in incidence of AIDS and immunosuppression therapy. Thus it is convenient to consider viral retinitis in terms of the patient's immune status.

Immunocompetent

Acute retinal necrosis (ARN)

In HSV and HZV infections, there is a unilateral necrotising retinitis, initially patchy and subsequently becoming confluent, accompanied by a non-granulomatous choroiditis – this is classified as acute retinal necrosis (ARN). Severe vitritis, vasculitis, and papillitis are important features of this condition. The emphasis for prompt antiviral treatment is to avoid bilateral involvement (BARN).

Macroscopic and microscopic

The likely specimen submitted to the pathologist would be an enucleation for end-stage ARN (Figure 8.50). Microscopic examination reveals total retinal infarction, vitreous exudation, and infiltration by inflammatory cells (Figure 8.51). A retinal biopsy may be taken at the earlier stages of the disease and it is possible to demonstrate intranuclear inclusions formed by proliferating herpes simplex viral particles (Figure 8.52). The ultrastructural characteristics of HSV are identical to those of CMV and consist of a central core surrounded by a capsid (Figure 8.53).

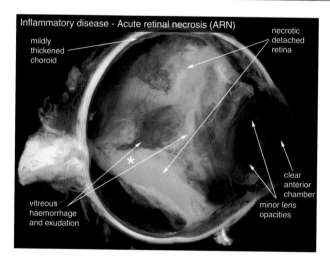

Figure 8.50

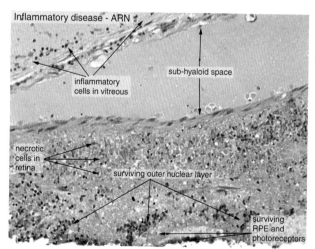

Figure 8.51

Figure 8.50 An immunocompetent patient known to be suffering from acute retinal necrosis (ARN) was treated with systemic acyclovir which protected against infection in the opposite eye. The disease in the affected eye however progressed to a haemorrhagic retinitis with detachment and an enucleation was performed for discomfort. A section through the centre of the eye reveals a normal anterior segment, early lens opacities, and a haemorrhagic exudate in the vitreous. The necrotic retina is grey in colour. The minor thickening of the choroid is due to lymphocytic infiltration. The asterix shows the region shown histologically in Figure 8.51.

Figure 8.51 In the higher power view of the area marked with an asterix in Figure 8.50, there is total destruction of the retinal cells which appear as smudgy pink structures. Some of the cells in the outer nuclear layer have survived (in contrast with progressive outer retinal necrosis). The vitreous is detached by a proteinaceous exudate and the vitreous gel contains an inflammatory cell infiltrate which would be minimal in an immunocompromised patient.

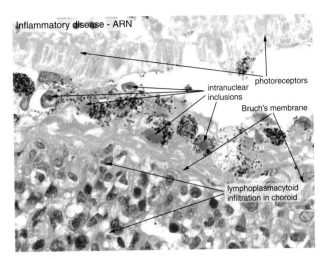

Figure 8.52

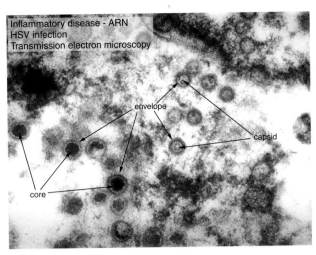

Figure 8.53

Figure 8.52 In the early stages of infection, herpes virus can be identified by intranuclear inclusions within the retinal pigment epithelium cells and macrophages. Compared with cytomegalovirus (CMV) inclusions, the parent cell in a herpetic infection is much smaller and similar in size to a macrophage. Degeneration and fragmentation is present in the photoreceptor layer. The choroid contains a dense lymphoplasmacytoid infiltrate and the choriocapillaris is obliterated.

Figure 8.53 This electron micrograph illustrates the architecture of viral particles within a retinal cell infected with herpes simplex virus (HSV). Note that the viral morphology is identical in HSV and CMV infections. The viral particles vary in appearance because replication requires migration into the cell nucleus for the formation of viral DNA. The envelope is derived from the nuclear membrane.

Herpes zoster ophthalmicus (HZO)

HZO involving the fifth cranial nerve (shingles) can cause a mild neuritis in the ciliary nerves and a non-granulomatous nodular choroiditis (Figure 8.54) which is evident on fundoscopy.

Immunocompromised

The hallmark feature of viral retinitis in the immunocompromised patient (for example when CD4+ T cells are reduced below 50 cells/mm^3 in peripheral blood) is an absence of the inflammatory response, particularly in the vitreous. It is important to note that it is not always possible to reliably differentiate clinically between the infections caused by herpes simplex virus (HSV), herpes zoster virus (HZV), cytomegalovirus (CMV), and toxoplasmosis. Simultaneous infections may also occur. Thus, it is important in biopsies to perform PCR for the entire herpes family to achieve a precise diagnosis, because the treatments can vary.

Cytomegaloviral (CMV) retinitis

Small areas of retinal necrosis increasing in size, with or without haemorrhage, in any region of the retina are characteristic (Figure 8.55). As the infection progresses, the retina becomes thickened and linear perivascular infiltrates extend laterally from the vessel (frosted branch angiitis – Figure 8.56). Untreated, the condition is progressively destructive to the whole retina resulting in blindness with the further complication of retinal detachment.

Destruction of the neurones in the retina by the virus leaves a relatively thin strand of tissue containing inflammatory cells and scattered surviving neurones (Figure 8.57). Extremely large infected cells, diagnostic for CMV infection, may contain obvious viral inclusion bodies within the nuclei (Figure 8.58).

Progressive outer retinal necrosis (PORN)

This is the result of HSV/HZV retinitis in the absence of an active immune response. The lack of vitritis, vasculitis, and papillitis are important differentiating features from ARN.

The condition is characterised by extensive destruction of the outer retina (compared with ARN), which can be located in any region of the fundus. The clinical appearance is characteristic: it begins with a blanching of the fundus which later progresses to extensive destruction of the outer retina. The histological features are similar to ARN, but the destruction of the outer retina predominates. There is also relative sparing of the retina adjacent to retinal vessels.

Human immunodeficiency virus (HIV)

Infection by HIV alters the immune system by selective destruction of the CD4+ helper and inducer cells with an increased incidence of secondary infections apart from those described above. An awareness of the complexities which occur in the management of AIDS patients will be apparent from the following list of ocular opportunistic infections and malignancies (refer to relevant chapters):

- *Toxoplasma gondii* (see below)
- fungal chorioretinitis (*Histoplasma capsulatum*, *Coccidioides immitis*, *Pneumocystis carinii*, *Candida* sp.)
- endogenous bacterial endophthalmitis (*Mycobacterium intracellulare* and *M. avium*)
- molluscum contagiosum
- Kaposi's sarcoma
- lymphomas.

NB: HIV causes a specific microvasculopathy which is manifest in early cases as retinal microinfarcts due to viral parasitisation of vascular endothelial cells.

Inflammatory disease - Herpes zoster ophthalmicus

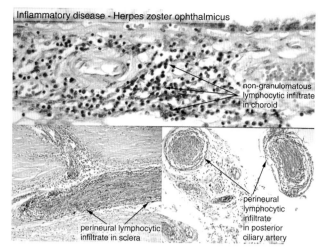

non-granulomatous lymphocytic infiltrate in choroid

perineural lymphocytic infiltrate in posterior ciliary artery

perineural lymphocytic infiltrate in sclera

Figure 8.54

Inflammatory disease - CMV retinitis

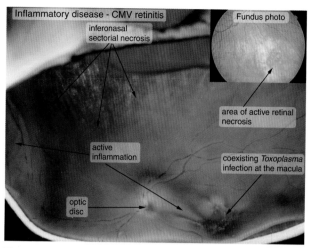

inferonasal sectorial necrosis

Fundus photo

area of active retinal necrosis

active inflammation

coexisting *Toxoplasma* infection at the macula

optic disc

Figure 8.55

Inflammatory disease - CMV retinitis

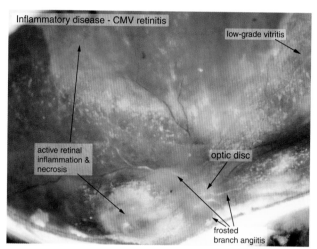

low-grade vitritis

active retinal inflammation & necrosis

optic disc

frosted branch angiitis

Figure 8.56

Inflammatory disease - CMV retinitis

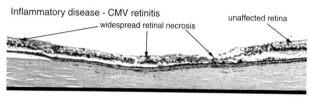

widespread retinal necrosis

unaffected retina

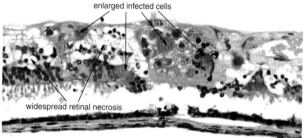

enlarged infected cells

widespread retinal necrosis

Figure 8.57

Inflammatory disease - CMV retinitis

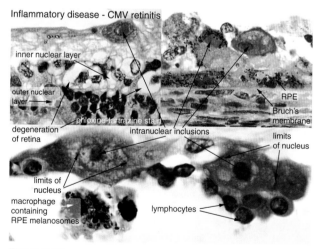

inner nuclear layer

outer nuclear layer

RPE

Bruch's membrane

degeneration of retina

phloxine-tartrazine stain

intranuclear inclusions

limits of nucleus

limits of nucleus

macrophage containing RPE melanosomes

lymphocytes

Figure 8.58

Figure 8.54 The histological features of herpes zoster ophthalmicus include a non-granulomatous lymphocytic infiltrate in the choroid (upper), and in the perineurium of intrascleral nerves (lower left) and posterior ciliary nerves (lower right). Intranuclear viral inclusions are not demonstrated in lymphocytes but are present in the epithelium in shingles.

Figure 8.55 A patient suffering from Hodgkin's disease was immunosuppressed and died as a result of disseminated toxoplasmosis in addition to cytomegaloviraemia. Five weeks prior to his death, an area of active inflammation and necrosis was noted in the inferior nasal quadrant of his right eye consistent with CMV retinitis (inset). In the right eye enucleated at autopsy, a triangular defect in the retina exposed the underlying choroid (marked sectorial necrosis). Thickened white areas in the retina indicate more recent infection. The necrotic focus at the macula was found on histology to be due to toxoplasma chorioretinitis. Note that the vitreous is clear.

Figure 8.56 A middle aged man with a long history of HIV infection lost vision due to massive CMV retinitis. His T-cell CD4+ counts were less than 20 cells/mm³. After death, the globes were removed at autopsy. The affected areas in the retina appear to contain yellow granular material which is becoming confluent. Vascular sheathing away from necrotic areas is evident and the appearance is consistent with frosted branch angiitis as seen clinically.

Figure 8.57 Histology from the necrotic area shown in Figure 8.55 illustrates widespread retinal necrosis with sharp demarcation at the edge of the unaffected retina (upper). At higher magnification, the necrotic retina contains extremely large cells indicative of cytomegaloviral infection (lower) – see Figure 8.58.

Figure 8.58 With a phloxine-tartrazine stain, intranuclear inclusions in CMV are easily demonstrated (upper left). In this example the infected cell is present in the inner retina and only thin strips of cells represent the surviving inner and outer nuclear layers. Extremely large infected cells are present in the debris on the inner surface of the retinal pigment epithelium (RPE) (upper right). The size of the large infected cells (with intranuclear inclusions) should be compared with that of the adjacent lymphocytes (lower).

Parasites

Toxoplasma

Toxoplasma gondii is the commonest protozoal parasite to infect the eye. This organism is neurotrophic and infection is limited to the neural retina and the brain. Whereas it was previously thought that toxoplasma retinochoroiditis was due to reactivation of congenital infections, there is growing evidence for acquired disease.

Clinical presentation

Congenital In this category, acute infection of the mother during pregnancy proceeds to transplacental infection of the fetus. If infection occurs during the first trimester, still-birth usually results. The fetus can survive a later infection but often the triad of convulsions, cerebral calcifications, and chorioretinitis are clinical manifestations after birth. With this potential outcome, mothers who have toxoplasma chorioretinitis during pregnancy may choose to have an elective termination of pregnancy.

Reactivation or acquired infection in adulthood The patient presents with reduced vision and floaters. Examination reveals a moderate to severe vitritis with underlying single or multiple patches of necrotising retinitis. A pre-existing chorioretinal scar is evident in cases of reactivation of infection – "headlight in the fog" appearance. Satellite lesions are common. The parasitisation is usually situated in the inner retina leading to retinal oedema.

The surrounding inflammation may be severe enough to affect other regions producing choroiditis, scleritis, and anterior uveitis of differing severity.

Pathogenesis: life cycle of Toxoplasma gondii

The cat is the definitive host in which the organism undergoes sexual reproduction (Figure 8.59). Oocysts are passed in cat faeces which may be directly ingested by domestic animals. Human infection occurs either from direct ingestion of oocysts in contaminated soil or from uncooked meat of infected animals. The organism can exist in a free form (trophozoites) or an encysted form (bradyzoites). Parasitisation within neural cells provides protection from the immune system. Multiplication within intermediate hosts is by asexual reproduction.

Possible modes of treatment

Infections are usually self limiting and treatment is conservative. The indications for treatment are:
1 Sight threatening: involving macula, papillomacular bundle, and optic disc.
2 Vasculitis: overlying a major retinal vessel.
3 Persistence: more than a month.

4 Severity: severe vitritis leading to significant visual loss.
5 Immunosuppression.
Treatment involves multiple drug combinations:
1 *Folic acid antagonists – sulfadiazine and pyrimethamine:* the *Toxoplasma* organism has an inability to transport folate which is an essential component for DNA synthesis, and antagonists inhibit synthesis in the active trophozoite. Folinic acid supplement is added to prevent patient folate deficiency.
2 *Clindamycin, azithromycin, and atavaquone:* although many of these agents are found to have cysticidal properties *in vitro*, recurrence of infection has been known to occur following treatment.
3 *Corticosteroids:* introduced systemically at a later stage to modulate the inflammation and secondary damage.
4 *Other treatment modalities:* these include argon laser ablation, cryotherapy, and vitrectomy.
The difficulty in management lies in the treatment resistance of the parasite when it is in an encysted form.

Macroscopic

Acute Most cases of acute disease are observed in autopsy material obtained from aborted fetuses or stillborn infants.

Chronic or healed Sites of previous infection may be observed as an unrelated finding in an enucleated eye (Figure 8.60). This has the appearance of an irregular white chorioretinal scar with clumps of pigmentation usually in the periphery.

The associated uveitis may lead to secondary glaucoma.

Microscopic

Acute In the centre of the infected sector in the retina, there is a thickened strip of hypocellular pink-staining tissue. Adjacent to this, there is a more cellular zone containing inflammatory cells. The adjacent recognisable retina is thickened by oedema and contains a scattered infiltrate of inflammatory cells – lymphoplasmacytoid cells and macrophages (Figure 8.61). Bradyzoite cysts are most commonly identified at the edge of the surviving retina: freeform trophozoites are identified less easily (Figure 8.62). The complex morphology of *Toxoplasma gondii* is best appreciated at the ultrastructural level (Figure 8.63).

Chronic A healed scar consists of a thin strip of gliotic retina separated by clumps of retinal pigment epithelium from a fibrotic choroid.

Immunohistochemistry

Labelled antitoxoplasma antibodies identify the organisms (Figure 8.62). PCR may also be used.

Inflammation - Toxoplasmosis
Life cycle

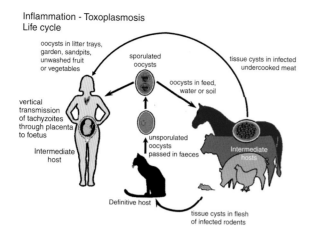

Figure 8.59

Inflammatory disease - Adult toxoplasmosis
Healed chorioretinal scar

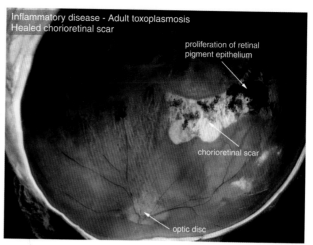

Figure 8.60

Inflammatory disease - Acute toxoplasmosis

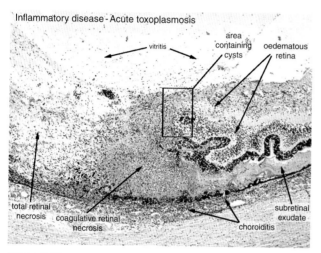

Figure 8.61

Inflammatory disease -
Toxoplasma gondii

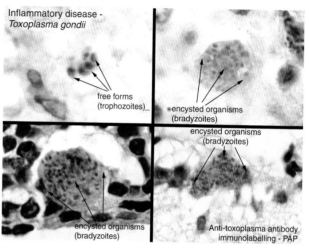

Figure 8.62

Inflammatory disease - *Toxoplasma gondii*
Transmission electron microscopy

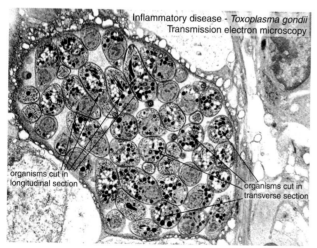

Figure 8.63

Figure 8.59 Diagram to show the lifecycle of *Toxoplasma gondii*. (Courtesy of Dr Fiona Roberts.)

Figure 8.60 This globe was enucleated for angle closure glaucoma secondary to recurrent anterior uveitis. A typical chorioretinal scar is identified in the midperiphery. It was not possible to histologically identify *Toxoplasma* cysts in the retina adjacent to the scar, and this is often the case in healed disease.

Figure 8.61 An eye from a stillborn infant was found to contain an area of acute retinal necrosis associated with dense choroiditis. *Toxoplasma* cysts are found at the edge of the necrotic area outlined by a box. An exudative retinal detachment is evident.

Figure 8.62 Identification of *Toxoplasma* organisms requires the high magnification of an oil immersion lens. Free forms or trophozoites (top left) are identified by a basophilic spot within an elongated eosinophilic tail. Most commonly the organisms are identified within cystic structures containing blue or purple dots (bradyzoites – top right and bottom left). The organisms can also be identified with antitoxoplasma antibody immunolabel (bottom right).

Figure 8.63 Electron microscopy demonstrates the complex structure of *Toxoplasma* organisms within a retinal cyst. The organisms are cut in different planes.

Toxocara

This infection results from a common parasitic intestinal roundworm (*Toxocara canis*) that resides in the dog.

Clinical presentation

Infection by *Toxocara* larvae is systemic and involves both the lung and liver (visceral larva migrans). The ocular manifestations include:

1 A solitary nodule which resembles a small retinoblastoma. The location may be in the posterior pole or in the periphery.
2 Retinal detachment due to an inflammatory reaction in the peripheral retina and resultant vitreous traction.
3 Endophthalmitis.

In the past, the globe of an infected child would be enucleated if the eye was blind and there was a suspicion of a retinoblastoma.

Current diagnosis involves the use of ELISA titres for antitoxocara antibodies in serum or vitreous and may include ultrasonography.

Pathogenesis

Puppies are infected and the organisms are passed in the faeces in a cyst form. Humans are infected by direct ingestion of contaminated food or soil in the case of young children (pica). The cysts dissolve in gastric juice and the larvae (or microfilaria) pass through the intestinal wall into the blood-stream. The organism evades immune recognition by secretion of a surface coat that has the property of changing antigenicity. An inflammatory reaction only occurs when the organism dies.

Possible modes of treatment

The main damage occurs if the organisms are killed. The main therapy therefore is to modulate the inflammatory response in the form of corticosteroids. Antihelminthic therapy (for example thiabendazole) is only indicated in exceptional cases.

Vitrectomy is used for retinal complications such as traction detachment and folds. Surgical removal of a parasitised focus requires retinectomy. Argon photocoagulation is sometimes used if a mobile larva is identified.

Macroscopic

In the past, opportunities to observe *Toxocara* ocular infections came from enucleations for suspected retinoblastomas.

A fibrogranulomatous mass at the posterior pole can resemble a small endophytic retinoblastoma. A misdiagnosis of a retinoblastoma can also occur when a chronic infective focus at the retinal periphery leads to vitritis and the formation of vitreous traction bands (Figure 8.64). The inflammatory foci within the retina stimulate exudation and retinal detachment (Figure 8.65).

Currently a pathologist may be required to examine a retinectomy specimen for the presence of *Toxocara* larvae.

Secondary glaucoma can result from chronic inflammation.

Microscopic

When a *Toxocara* infection simulates a retinoblastoma, a large fibrotic inflammatory mass is located within the retina (Figure 8.66). More commonly, the enucleated eye will contain the following features: necrotic foci in the retinal periphery and detachment of the retina (tractional and exudative). *Toxocara* larvae are multicellular organisms which appear as rows of nuclei within a cuticle. It may not be possible to identify intact larvae within the microabscess but intact organisms may be observed in the adjacent tissue (Figure 8.67).

Special investigations/stains

Serial sections are required to demonstrate the sparsely distributed larvae. *Toxocara* antibody labels are also available.

Non-granulomatous uveitis

Pathological studies have so far failed to unravel the many causes of non-granulomatous uveitis. In clinical practice, these are divided according to anatomical location (anterior, intermediate, and posterior) and usually respond well to immunomodulatory therapy.

Rare infections

The reader should be aware that the above descriptions are restricted to the commoner entities encountered in pathological material in Europe. In other continents, a wider variety of fungal and protozoal parasitic infections commonly occur. The ophthalmologist should be aware of the possibility of exotic diseases as a consequence of international travel.

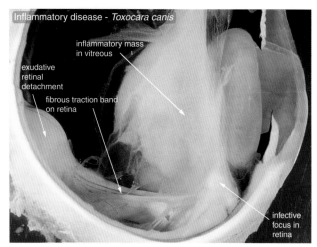

Figure 8.64

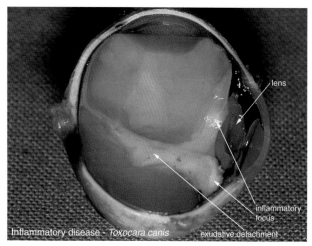

Figure 8.65

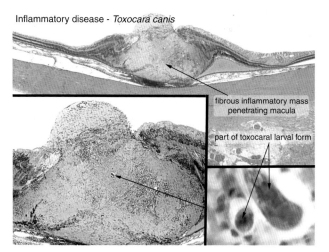

Figure 8.66

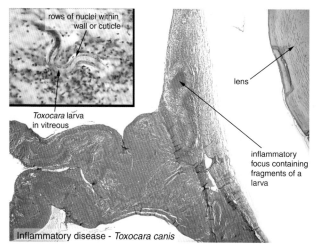

Figure 8.67

Figure 8.64 This eye was enucleated for suspicion of retinoblastoma due to the presence of vitreous opacities. A necrotic focus in the retinal periphery in association with tractional bands suggests the diagnosis of *Toxocara* infection.

Figure 8.65 This archival specimen shows the end stage of a *Toxocara* infection with a complete retinal detachment and the suggestion of infective foci in the retinal periphery. The histology of this case is shown in Figure 8.67.

Figure 8.66 The first time that *Toxocara* was identified in the UK as a cause of a pseudo-retinoblastoma was when Professor Norman Ashton studied this case

by serial section. The same inflammatory fibrous mass is displayed at differing levels of magnification. At the highest magnification, in the centre of this fibrous inflammatory mass, a filarial structure is identified. The oblique section through the pathogen demonstrates the multiple nuclei of a metazoal organism.

Figure 8.67 Histology from the specimen shown in Figure 8.65 reveals the microabscess in the retina after serial sections have been studied. It was only possible to demonstrate fragments of a filarial worm within the abscess, but an intact larva was found in the adjacent vitreous (inset).

Chapter 9
Wound healing and trauma

Accidental and non-accidental trauma is common in ophthalmic practice and is the leading cause of blindness in young adults. Depending on the type of trauma, there may be specific patterns of tissue damage on both clinical and pathological examination.

Healing and repair in ocular tissues

Repair of damage to intraocular tissues often leads to fibrous proliferation within the ocular compartments, fibrous metaplasia in the lens epithelium, and proliferation of glial cells (gliosis) in the retina. The most important basic research on wound healing has been carried out on the cornea and this is described in detail below.

The normal anatomy of the conjunctiva and cornea is described in Chapters 3 and 4 respectively.

Cornea

Epithelium

Normal turnover

In the normal process of "wear and tear", there is a constant turnover of corneal surface epithelium with complete replacement of the surface epithelium every 7 days. The maintenance of the corneal epithelium depends upon a slow centripetal migration from the basal stem cells located in the corneal limbus. As the cells migrate, cell division occurs with increasing epithelial differentiation from the basal layer.

Trauma

Any form of trauma disrupting the surface of the epithelium will prompt an increase in the rate of migration to re-establish the epithelial surface. Studies have shown that complex cell-signalling interactions exist between the damaged corneal epithelium, the limbal stem cells, and the underlying stroma.

The stem cell source of corneal epithelium is located at the limbus. The limbus also acts as a barrier against conjunctival migration onto the cornea. Exhaustion of limbal stem cell supply through trauma (for example alkali burn, see below) may lead to "conjunctivalisation" in which the surface layer has the appearance of conjunctival epithelium.

Stroma

Normal turnover

The normal corneal stroma is less metabolically active compared with the epithelium – the keratocytes maintain stromal lamellar collagen and the glycosaminoglycans in the extracellular matrix. Transparency is achieved via a relative state of dehydration of the stroma which is maintained by an intact overlying epithelium via evaporation and active transport of fluid by the endothelial cells.

Summary of corneal stromal healing

1 Trauma with apoptosis of keratocytes at wound edges. The proposed signalling is via multiple cytokine pathways (for example Fas-ligand and interleukin 1 (IL-1)) from damaged epithelial cells to underlying keratocytes.
2 Replacement of apoptosed keratocytes by proliferation and migration of remaining adjacent keratocytes.
3 Metaplasia of stromal keratocytes to myofibroblasts, which in turn restore collagen, glycosaminoglycans, and other matrix constituents. Note that collagen in the normal cornea is principally type I with lesser amounts of types III, V, and VI. Replacement collagen, however, is primarily type III.
4 Myofibroblasts also produce hepatocyte growth factor (HGF), keratinocyte growth factors (KGFs), and other cytokines. HGF promotes epithelial hyperplasia.
5 Cross linking of collagen reinstates the mechanical strength of the cornea but only rarely is complete transparency restored.

NB: Bowman's layer of the corneal stroma is formed in embryogenesis – any disruption or loss of this tissue is an indication of previous corneal damage, including surgery, for example in the case of photorefractive keratectomy (PRK) or penetrating keratoplasty.

Matrix metalloproteinases (MMPs)

MMPs are a group of degradative enzymes that play a very significant role in the healing responses in the corneoscleral envelope. Overactivity of these enzymes is also of great importance in disorders such as rheumatoid eye disease and is responsible for severe collagenolysis. The characteristics of these enzymes are as follows:

1 Degradation of at least one component of the extracellular matrix.
2 Each member of the group possesses significant amino acid homology.
3 Optimal activity at neutral pH.
4 Zinc is a co-factor; calcium ions are required for stability. Hence the terminology "metalloproteinase".
5 They are secreted in an inactive state and activation is achieved by cleavage of a small amino peptide.
6 Tissue inhibitors of metalloproteinases (TIMPs) exist within the corneal tissues.

A complex interplay of cytokines and matrix metalloproteinases is present with the main MMPs being:

1 *Collagenases* (for example MMP-1, type I collagenase): cleave collagen types I, II, and III and is sourced mainly from keratocytes. PMNLs also have a similar enzyme (MMP-8).

2 *Gelatinase:* acts on basement membranes and denatured collagen (gelatin, collagen types IV, V, and VII). There are two main subtypes of gelatinases:
   (a) Gelatinase A (MMP-2) is produced by keratocytes and is available in large amounts in inactivated form in the cornea.
   (b) Gelatinase B (MMP-9) is produced in the corneal epithelium and also in monocytes, stromal keratocytes, and PMNLs acting against gelatin and collagen types IV and V. An inhibitor is produced by the corneal epithelium, and is thought to be involved in the resynthesis of basement membrane in repair.

3 *Stromelysin* (for example MMP-3, type IV collagenase): has broad proteolytic activity (for example fibronectin, proteoglycans, laminin, and type IV collagen of basement membrane).

4 *Membrane-type MMPs:* differ by an additional transmembrane domain and a cytoplasmic tail which anchors the enzyme to the extracellular side of the cell membrane.

Abnormalities of MMP activity have been implicated in many ocular and systemic diseases. The main ocular disorders are corneal wound healing, pterygium, keratoconus, and glaucoma. Current research is directed toward modification of MMP activity in relation to altering the outcome of the disease processes.

This area of knowledge is rapidly evolving and the interested reader should pursue the latest journals on new developments. The main reference used here was: Wong TL *et al.* (2002) Matrix metalloproteinases in disease and repair processes of the anterior segment. Surv Ophthalmol 47:239–56.

Endothelium

Normal turnover
The human corneal endothelium has a very limited capacity to divide. Throughout life there is a gradual decline in the total population and depletion is compensated by widening of adjacent endothelial cells.

Trauma
Endothelial cells are delicate and any trauma of sufficient energy (including intraocular surgery) is capable of destroying substantial areas of the monolayer, which are compensated by the spreading of adjacent cells. As these cells have a limited covering capacity, once a declining limit is reached, corneal decompensation ensues from overhydration of the stroma with resultant opacification (see Chapter 4).

Relevance to laser refractive surgery and differences between photorefractive keratectomy (PRK) and laser-assisted *in situ* keratomileusis (LASIK)

Keratocyte apoptosis has been shown to occur in the wound interfaces of both PRK and LASIK procedures. It has been theorised that the resultant epithelial hyperplasia (stage 4 of "Summary of corneal stromal healing" above) could be a factor in the regression of refraction being more significant in PRK (being closer to the epithelium) as compared with LASIK, especially in deep stromal ablations. Experimentally, the epithelial hyperplasia in PRK is lessened with transepithelial PRK (without initial scrape) which may disrupt the amount of cytokine induced apoptosis. There is currently much investigation of agents which may decrease the initial apoptotic response.

Trauma

Mechanical

Most types of mechanical trauma are civil.

Terminology

There has been a confusing array of terminologies to describe mechanical injury to the eye (Table 9.1).

Blunt trauma

Closed globe injury
Severe compression of the corneoscleral envelope and elastic rebound leads to disruption of the intraocular contents.

Conjunctival epithelium
Subconjunctival haemorrhages are located within the stroma.

Corneal epithelium
A corneal abrasion usually heals within days. Recurrent erosions are due to epithelial instability and may be followed by separation of the entire epithelium after minor trauma. Treatment is usually conservative with topical lubrication, although further intervention in the form of debridement or anterior stromal puncture may be required.

Anterior segment damage

This can be subdivided into the following types:

1 *Iris sphincter/root tear (iridodialysis):* may result in hyphaema if a major blood vessel is torn (Figure 9.3, left). Most clinical cases are micro- or macrohyphaemas (with a visible fluid level) which clear spontaneously. A massive bleed, however, can fill the entire anterior chamber ("8-ball" hyphaema: Figure 9.3, right). There is a high risk of rebleeding after surgical evacuation of the anterior chamber. Fibrosis does not occur in the iris after a tear or a surgical wound because the aqueous contains fibrinolysins.

2 *Angle recession:* refers to a tear forming a cleft in the anterior face of the ciliary body. This predisposes to secondary open angle glaucoma (see Chapter 7).

3 *Iridocyclodialysis:* partial or total separation of the iris and ciliary body from the sclera (Figure 9.4). This has a poor prognosis with a tendency to hypotony and phthisis due to ciliary body shutdown and a reduction in aqueous inflow.

Inflammation – traumatic iridocyclitis

Anterior uveitis is due to release of inflammatory mediators.

Lens subluxation/dislocation

Disruption of the zonular fibres may result in displacement of the lens into the anterior chamber (Figure 9.5) or into the vitreous.

Blunt trauma of sufficient force may also rupture the lens capsule and create a lens induced uveitis secondary to sensitisation of the immune system by lens antigens.

Vitreous haemorrhage

Traumatic rupture/tear of retinal vessels results in bleeding into the vitreous.

Ghost cell glaucoma occurs at a much later stage due to movement of lysed red cells from the vitreous into the anterior chamber and angle (see Chapter 7).

Table 9.1 Summary of the different definitions used to classify mechanical trauma (modified from Kuhn F *et al.* (1996) A standardized classification of ocular trauma Ophthalmology 103:240–3).

Term	Definition
Eyewall	Scleral and corneal envelope
Laceration	Single laceration of the eyewall, usually cause by a sharp object (Figure 9.1)
Blunt trauma	
Closed globe injury	The eyewall is intact, but the intraocular contents are disorganised
Rupture	Full-thickness split in the eyewall, caused by a blunt object, the impact results in a massive but momentary increase in the intraocular pressure
Open globe trauma	
Penetrating injury	Full-thickness wound of the eyewall, usually caused by a sharp object. The wound occurs at the impact site by an outside–in mechanism (Figure 9.1)
Intraocular foreign body injury	Retained foreign objects(s) causing entrance lacerations
Perforating injury	Two full-thickness lacerations (entrance and exit) of the eyewall, usually caused by a sharp object or missile (Figure 9.2)

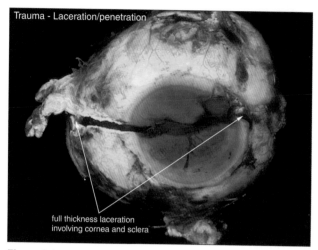

Trauma - Laceration/penetration

full thickness laceration
involving cornea and sclera

Figure 9.1

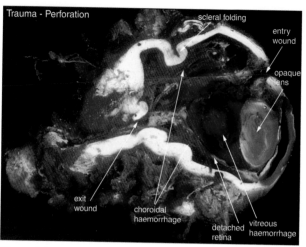

Trauma - Perforation

scleral folding

entry
wound

opaque
lens

exit
wound

choroidal
haemorrhage

detached
retina

vitreous
haemorrhage

Figure 9.2

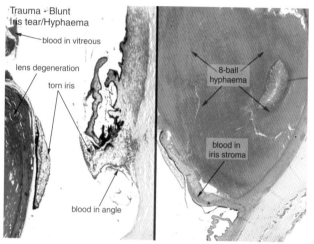

Trauma - Blunt
Iris tear/Hyphaema

blood in vitreous

lens degeneration

torn iris

8-ball
hyphaema

blood in
iris stroma

blood in angle

Figure 9.3

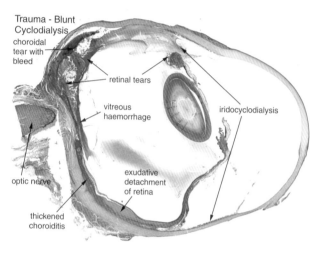

Trauma - Blunt
Cyclodialysis

choroidal
tear with
bleed

retinal tears

vitreous
haemorrhage

iridocyclodialysis

optic nerve

exudative
detachment
of retina

thickened
choroiditis

Figure 9.4

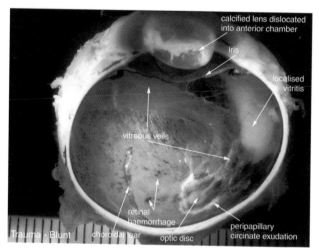

calcified lens dislocated
into anterior chamber

iris

localised
vitritis

vitreous veils

retinal
haemorrhage

Trauma - Blunt

choroidal tear

optic disc

peripapillary
circinate exudation

Figure 9.5

Figure 9.1 The anterior part of the globe was divided horizontally by a fragment of nylon cord while the patient was using a strimmer. This is an example of a lacerating penetration injury of the globe.

Figure 9.2 This patient was stabbed with a knife which resulted in a perforating injury of the eye. This specimen illustrates the extensive ocular disorganisation which occurs after severe trauma.

Figure 9.3 In this example of a torn iris, bleeding occurs from the edge of the tear (left). A massive bleed which fills the anterior chamber after an iris tear is termed clinically as an "eight-ball" or "black-ball" hyphaema (right).

Figure 9.4 A low power view of an enucleated globe following severe blunt trauma. This has resulted in an extensive iridocyclodialysis and retinal tears which are the sources of intraocular haemorrhage. Inflammation in the uveal tract is common in trauma and this can lead to an exudative retinal detachment. The section passes through the edge of the optic nerve and the disc is not included.

Figure 9.5 Important consequences of blunt trauma are dislocation of the lens and choroidal rupture. In this example, the lens has dislocated into the anterior chamber: the white streaks in the lens matter indicate calcification. The vitreous is partially detached and is condensed. There is a circinate exudate around the optic disc and a curved choroidal tear is temporal to the macula.

Retina

Commotio retinae describes localised retinal oedema (Figure 9.6) which appears clinically as pale grey swollen areas. Spot haemorrhages are occasionally observed. The condition resolves spontaneously and is only seen by the pathologist in conjunction with more severe injuries.

Retinal tear/dialysis results from oscillations of the vitreous following blunt trauma. The location of the tear occurs where the vitreous is strongly adherent (vitreous base, peripapillary, macula, and over vessels). Rhegmatogenous retinal detachment is the resultant complication. In severe trauma, these tears can extend beyond 90 degrees to form a giant retinal tear (Figure 9.7).

Post-traumatic pseudoretinitis pigmentosa appears as a *unilateral* pigmentary retinopathy following severe blunt trauma. The aetiology is unknown but is thought to be the result of photoreceptor damage. The clinical and pathological features (Figure 9.8) are indistinguishable from hereditary retinitis pigmentosa (which is a *bilateral* condition – see Chapter 10).

Choroidal tear

Blunt trauma of sufficient force can cause semicircular tears in the choroid around the optic disc and this exposes the underlying sclera. The retinal pigment epithelium (RPE) proliferates at the edge of the defect (Figure 9.5). A rupture in Bruch's membrane predisposes to subretinal neovascularisation.

Optic nerve

Traumatic optic neuropathy may result from direct or indirect trauma to the head. Depending on the type of trauma, theories of indirect optic nerve damage range from avulsion of nutrient vessels to direct transmitted energy to the optic canal. The treatment is variable depending on the institution, and controversial ranging from decompression of the optic canal to high dose systemic steroid therapy.

Avulsion of the optic nerve secondary to severe head injury occurs at the level of the optic foramen.

Miscellaneous

Haemosiderosis bulbi (also found in open globe injuries) occurs after longstanding haemorrhage with breakdown of haemoglobin. Iron salts can be identified in the following tissues: cornea, iris stroma, lens epithelium, ciliary epithelium, and retina. In the retina the metabolic consequences are the most serious due to the toxic effects of iron salts on neurones (Figure 9.9).

Phthisis bulbi occurs from any cause of ciliary body "shut down" resulting in hypotony and a decrease in globe size with shrinkage of the corneoscleral envelope.

Rupture of the corneoscleral envelope

When a blunt impact is extreme, for example by an iron bar, the force is sufficient to burst the corneoscleral envelope.

Most commonly, ruptures occur at the limbus or in the sclera just behind the insertion of the recti muscles where it is thinnest. The sudden hypotony may be followed by massive expulsive choroidal haemorrhage and extrusion of the intraocular contents:

1 *Limbal:* associated with prolapse of anterior uveal tissue and loss of an intact lens or lens matter should the capsule rupture (Figure 9.10).
2 *Scleral:* rupture is complicated by prolapse of uvea, retina, and vitreous (Figure 9.11).

Figure 9.6 At the histological level in commotio retinae, the accumulation of fluid within the substance of the retina creates a folding effect in the outer layers. The inset shows the macroscopic appearance of retinal oedema in a globe after fixation. NFL = nerve fibre layer.

Figure 9.7 After severe blunt trauma, a tear in the retinal periphery may extend 360 degrees. In this case, treatment was not carried out immediately and the detached retina collapsed to form a folded mass on the optic disc. The trauma has also resulted in lens subluxation and a tear in the iris. This specimen was photographed after both calottes were removed, hence the background of the container is seen in the vitreous space.

Figure 9.8 The retina may not be detached after blunt trauma but the outer layers may be damaged and become atrophic and gliotic. The retinal pigment epithelium (RPE) proliferates within the retina, particularly around blood vessels, giving macroscopic (top left) and microscopic (top right and bottom) appearances very similar to retinitis pigmentosa. INL = inner nuclear layer.

Figure 9.9 Prolonged haemorrhage within the globe leads to deposition of iron salts in the retina. In an H&E section (upper), the iron salts appear dark blue and are most striking around the walls of the blood vessels. This abnormality is best demonstrated by the Prussian blue reaction (lower). There is also diffuse staining of the retinal tissue but the subretinal exudate is negative (pink staining on H&E).

Figure 9.10 This patient was hit in the eye by a golf club. A rupture is situated at the limbus and is partially blocked by iris tissue, which prevents lens extrusion. The retina is detached by a gelatinous exudate and is prolapsed towards the limbal wound. A similar exudate is present in the anterior chamber and a recent haemorrhage is located in the posterior chamber. The scleral thickening suggests prolonged hypotony prior to enucleation.

Figure 9.11 For comparison with Figure 9.10, this figure shows a rupture in the sclera just behind the insertion of the medial rectus muscle, which emphasises the importance of careful surgical exploration of this area where the sclera is thinnest. The patient was an elderly gentleman who, in an inebriated state, fell onto a wooden clothes horse! The lens and anterior segment tissues are intact, although there is haemorrhage into the ciliary body. The haemorrhagic vitreous is detached from the disc and has prolapsed into the wound. The retina is detached by a choroidal haemorrhage and a subretinal haemorrhagic exudate.

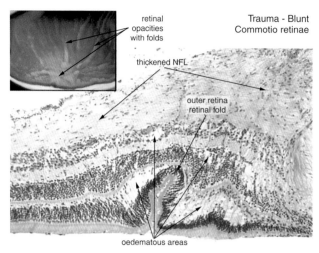

retinal opacities with folds

Trauma - Blunt
Commotio retinae

thickened NFL

outer retina
retinal fold

oedematous areas

Figure 9.6

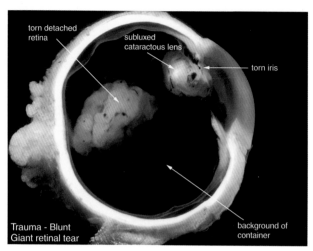

torn detached retina

subluxed cataractous lens

torn iris

Trauma - Blunt
Giant retinal tear

background of container

Figure 9.7

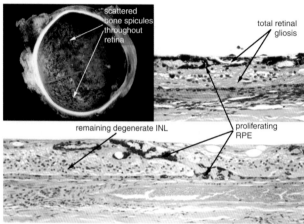

scattered bone spicules throughout retina

total retinal gliosis

remaining degenerate INL

proliferating RPE

Trauma - Blunt / Pseudoretinitis pigmentosa

Figure 9.8

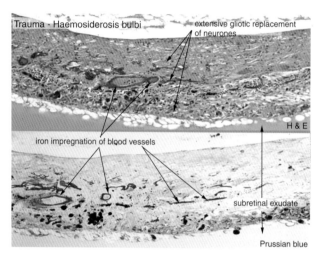

Trauma - Haemosiderosis bulbi

extensive gliotic replacement of neurones

H & E

iron impregnation of blood vessels

subretinal exudate

Prussian blue

Figure 9.9

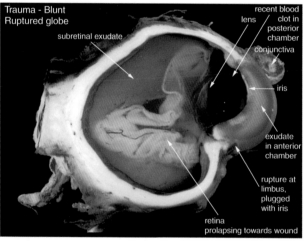

Trauma - Blunt
Ruptured globe

subretinal exudate

recent blood clot in posterior chamber

lens

conjunctiva

iris

exudate in anterior chamber

rupture at limbus, plugged with iris

retina prolapsing towards wound

Figure 9.10

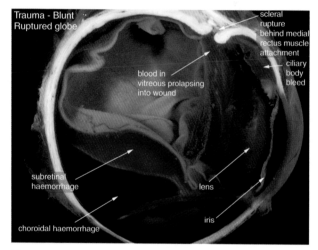

Trauma - Blunt
Ruptured globe

scleral rupture behind medial rectus muscle attachment

ciliary body bleed

blood in vitreous prolapsing into wound

subretinal haemorrhage

lens

choroidal haemorrhage

iris

Figure 9.11

Penetrating injury

A penetrating injury involves entry into a structure without traversing the entire substance. Hence, a penetrating injury of the cornea does not involve the entire thickness, whereas in a penetrating injury of the globe either the cornea or the sclera is perforated (Figure 9.12). In the remainder of this section, penetrating or perforating trauma is discussed in relation to the globe.

Perforating injury

Perforation differs from penetration, in that there are both entry and exit wounds in the globe (see Figure 9.2).

Secondary complications

Epithelial ingrowth
Failure to close a penetrating wound of the cornea allows epithelial migration into the interspace (Figure 9.13). When epithelium grows into a perforating wound of the cornea, the cells migrate across the chamber angle and secondary open angle glaucoma is the result (see Chapter 7).

Fibrous ingrowth
The cells in the corneoscleral envelope react to traumatic laceration by proliferation to form dense scar tissue within the globe (Figures 9.14, 9.15).

Disorganisation of intraocular contents
These include tears in the uveal tract, laceration of the lens capsule, retinal wounds, vitreous detachment, and intraocular haemorrhage (Figure 9.16).

Lens induced uveitis
Trauma to the lens is one of the commoner causes of autoimmunity to lens matter (see Chapter 8).

Sympathetic ophthalmitis
Unilateral trauma involving a corneoscleral wound with uveal prolapse is associated with bilateral granulomatous choroiditis (see Chapter 8).

Intraocular foreign body (IOFB)

By definition, an IOFB can only occur following penetrating injury of the globe, but the foreign body may not be located in the line of trajectory due to a ricochet (Figure 9.17).

Organic
The most commonly encountered organic IOFB is wood. Penetration of the globe by sharp splinters introduces microorganisms into the eye such as fungi and bacteria leading to intractable endophthalmitis. This scenario is regarded as a surgical emergency. In the absence of secondary pyogenic infection, a wood particle becomes surrounded by a giant cell granulomatous reaction (Figure 9.18).

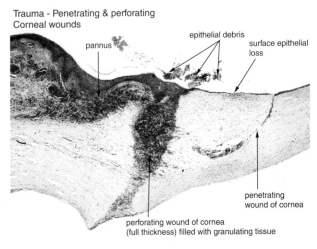

Figure 9.12

Figure 9.12 An assault with a broken glass bottle can cause multiple wounds to the eye – in this case examples of both penetrating and perforating wounds to the cornea are illustrated. The edges of the penetrating wound are not in apposition and the space is filled by fibrovascular tissue and inflammatory cells derived from the adjacent pannus. Note that a perforating wound of the cornea is also a penetrating wound of the globe.

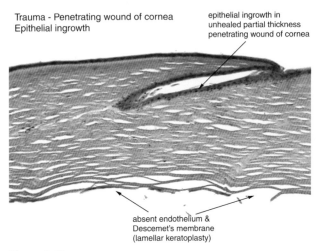

Figure 9.13

Figure 9.13 In general, a penetrating wound heals by fibrosis (see Figure 4.94), but occasionally, there is a failure of apposition and epithelium grows into the defect. This is a lamellar keratoplasty specimen which does not include the posterior corneal layers.

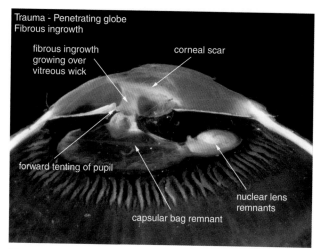

Trauma - Penetrating globe
Fibrous ingrowth

fibrous ingrowth growing over vitreous wick

corneal scar

forward tenting of pupil

capsular bag remnant

nuclear lens remnants

Figure 9.14

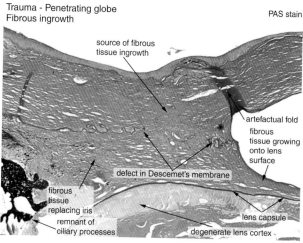

Trauma - Penetrating globe
Fibrous ingrowth

PAS stain

source of fibrous tissue ingrowth

artefactual fold

fibrous tissue growing onto lens surface

defect in Descemet's membrane

fibrous tissue replacing iris

remnant of ciliary processes

lens capsule

degenerate lens cortex

Figure 9.15

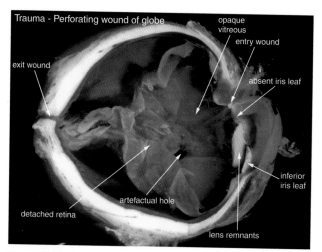

Trauma - Perforating wound of globe

opaque vitreous

entry wound

exit wound

absent iris leaf

inferior iris leaf

detached retina

artefactual hole

lens remnants

Figure 9.16

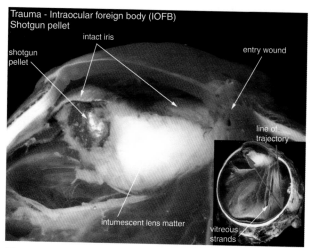

Trauma - Intraocular foreign body (IOFB)
Shotgun pellet

intact iris

shotgun pellet

entry wound

line of trajectory

intumescent lens matter

vitreous strands

Figure 9.17

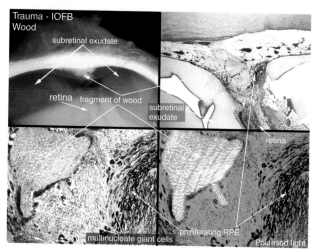

Trauma - IOFB
Wood

subretinal exudate

retina   fragment of wood

subretinal exudate

retina

proliferating RPE

multinucleate giant cells

Polarised light

Figure 9.18

Figure 9.14 A patient developed secondary angle closure glaucoma some years after a penetrating injury resulting in a corneal wound, a lens perforation, and a disrupted anterior vitreous face. A vitreous wick has provided a scaffold for a fibrous ingrowth.

Figure 9.15 A broad peripheral corneal wound can be identified in a PAS stained section which illustrates the edges of Descemet's membrane. A fibrous ingrowth lines the surface of a degenerate lens. The iris was lost during trauma and the defect is now replaced with fibrous tissue.

Figure 9.16 A man was stabbed in the eye with a fine chisel. The entry and exit wounds are in line but the site of retinal perforation is obscured by a retinal detachment. The inferior iris leaf is present, but the superior leaf is absent. This section is taken through the pupil and optic nerve (PO block) of the globe, but in making the second cut an artefactual hole was made in the retina.

Figure 9.17 The momentum of a small metallic particle is markedly reduced by a ricochet within the globe. This shotgun pellet came to rest behind the iris and damaged the lens, which over the next few days became swollen and opaque. The proposed trajectory route is shown in the inset.

Figure 9.18 A young boy was hit in his only seeing eye by a homemade arrow. The arrow was extracted but a small fragment of wood was left behind which induced a giant cell reaction and fibrosis in the choroid. The retinal pigment epithelium (RPE) became metaplastic and was transformed into a fibrous tissue scar which tacked down the retina. Once the retinal defect had been sealed, the retinal detachment converted from a rhegmatogenous to an exudative type (upper left). The tiny wood fragment is surrounded by inflammatory and fibrous tissue (upper right and lower left). The cellulose in the wood is birefringent in polarised light (bottom right).

Table 9.2 Common inorganic intraocular foreign bodies and reactions.

Material	Reaction
Glass	Minimal reaction. Usually from civil trauma
Plastic	Minimal reaction. Intraocular lenses would be most common
Iron	Ferrous ions (Fe^{2+}) are retinotoxic, leading to siderosis bulbi. Histological effects are similar to those described for haemosiderosis*
Copper Brass (copper/tin)	Copper produces a massive acute sterile inflammatory reaction: acute *chalcosis* (Figure 9.19). Chronic chalcosis is due to slow leakage of Cu^{2+} ions with the formation of opacities in the lens (sunflower cataracts). Peripheral corneal stromal copper staining (Kayser–Fleischer ring) may also be found in Wilson's disease, which is a systemic disturbance in copper metabolism
Lead	Usually from a retained airgun pellet injury associated with gross disorganisation of the globe (Figure 9.20). Diffusion of lead salts is minimal. Massive intraocular fibrosis is a non-specific response to a perforating injury of the globe (Figure 9.21)

* The term siderosis also describes deposition of iron salts from an intraocular foreign body and should not be confused with haemosiderosis (Figure 9.9) which is secondary to retained blood (see above).

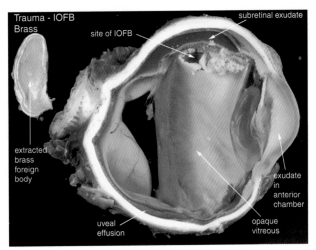

Figure 9.19

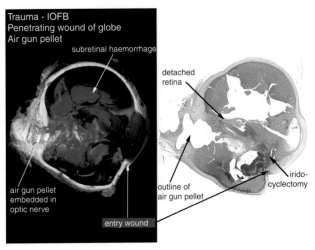

Figure 9.20

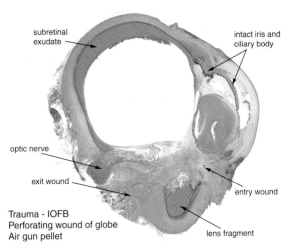

Figure 9.21

Figure 9.19 Brass may contain different concentrations of copper in the copper/tin alloy. In certain concentrations of copper, the response to a brass foreign body leads to a sterile purulent exudate. In this example, pus surrounds the site from which the foreign body was removed (located adjacent to the globe). The vitreous is completely opaque due to inflammatory cell infiltration and the secondary effects are exudative retinal detachment and an exudate in the anterior chamber.

Figure 9.20 An airgun pellet injury is extremely destructive. In this macroscopic and microscopic example, the pellet rotated on entry into the globe and was embedded within the optic nerve. The iris and ciliary body are destroyed at the point of entry and intraocular haemorrhage detached the retina. The lens presumably was lost through the entry wound after decompression at the time of injury.

Figure 9.21 If an airgun is fired at close range, there is sufficient momentum in the pellet to produce a perforating wound of the globe. In this example, the damage to the scleral wall is extensive and surgical closure is incomplete. As a result, massive fibrovascular tissue proliferation leads to distortion and shrinkage of the affected segment of the eye. A fragment of lens matter is displaced and there is histological evidence of an early lens induced inflammation.

Inorganic

The most commonly encountered inorganic IOFBs are metallic, plastic, or glass (Table 9.2).

Surgical pathology

Cataract surgery

Many examples of surgical pathology have been illustrated in other chapters. In the following section the pathological complications of cataract surgery will be discussed.

Historically, cataract surgery developed from the displacement of the lens into the vitreous (couching) and was later followed by surgical lensectomy *in toto* (*intracapsular*) which involved the complete removal of lens matter and capsule. These two procedures had high visual morbidity outcomes due to the required aphakic spectacle correction which distorted and reduced the visual field. The development of plastic intraocular lenses (IOLs) with insertion into the anterior chamber (Figure 9.22) and later into the capsular bag have achieved superior visual outcomes. Currently lens matter is most commonly removed by *extracapsular* cataract extraction (ECCE) with the intention of leaving an intact lens capsule to house a posterior chamber intraocular lens (PCIOL, Figure 9.23). Newer techniques have allowed smaller surgical wounds by means of phacoemulsification of lens matter and insertion of foldable lenses.

Complications

Although complication rates are low, the following are the most important of those recorded.

Endophthalmitis This complication can occur following any form of intraocular surgery. After cataract surgery, the widely quoted incidence of endophthalmitis is approximately 1 in 1000 (Figure 9.24).

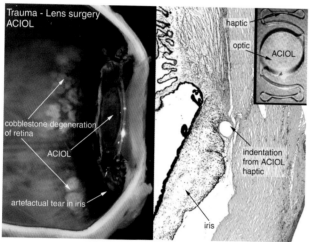

Figure 9.22

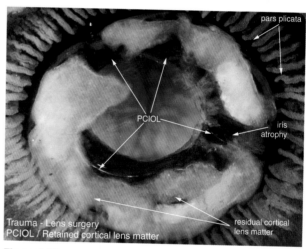

Figure 9.23

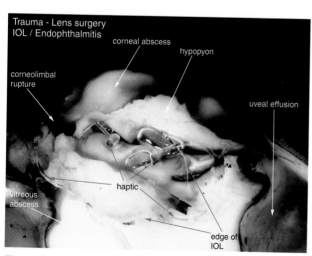

Figure 9.24

Figure 9.22 In an autopsy globe the first cut disturbed an anterior chamber intraocular lens (ACIOL) which led to an artefactual tear in the iris (left). The design of ACIOLs has changed with time and one of the more recent developments is to use thin extensions (haptics) which slot into the anterior chamber angle to fix the lens (right inset). Processing for paraffin histology dissolves the plastic to leave an empty space (right).

Figure 9.23 For technical reasons, it may not always be possible to completely remove lens matter during an extracapsular cataract procedure. In this autopsy case, there was rupture of the posterior capsule with vitreous prolapse into the anterior chamber. Further cortical clean up was difficult and the intraocular lens was inserted into the sulcus.

Figure 9.24 Within a few days after intraocular lens (IOL) implantation, a fulminating endophthalmitis occurred and *Streptococcus pneumoniae* was identified. Despite administration of broad spectrum intraocular antibiotics, the infection was not contained and an enucleation was carried out. The ocular compartments were filled with pus and the intraocular lens was displaced during the initial cut but was still identifiable.

Retained lens matter Evidence of inadequate lens matter clearance is easily identified macroscopically (Figure 9.23). The term "doughnut cataract" describes the residual lens matter at the cortical rim. Histology reveals degenerate lens matter which may be totally or partially enclosed by a residual capsule (Figure 9.25). If the equatorial lens epithelium is not removed, fibrous metaplasia occurs and opaque membranes grow across the posterior capsule (posterior capsular opacity (PCO); Figure 9.26). Photodisruption by a YAG laser is used to treat this condition.

Cystoid macular oedema/edema (CMO/CME) The visual results following cataract surgery are sometimes disappointing due to the development of oedema and cyst formation in the macula (CMO): the aetiology is uncertain. Three theories have been proposed: (1) vitreomacular traction; (2) diffusion of inflammatory mediators (prostaglandins) from the anterior segment; and (3) damage to the integrity of the blood–retinal barrier. CMO is identified by fluorescein angiography which reveals a petaloid pattern of fluid accumulation around the fovea. In the majority of cases, fluid is resorbed and only a small percentage (1%) of cases progress to chronic visual impairment. Studies of acute pathology are rare, but occasionally specimens are received and these show cyst formation in the outer plexiform layer with expansion to involve all the layers (Figure 9.27).

Chemical

The chemicals most commonly involved in eye injuries are acids and alkalis. A useful review article is Wagoner MD (1997) Chemical injuries of the eye: current concepts in pathophysiology and therapy. Surv Ophthalmol 41:275–313.

Acid

Examples: sulphuric (H_2SO_4), hydrofluoric (HF), acetic (CH_3COOH), and hydrochloric (HCl) acids.

Acids damage the ocular surface by denaturation of proteins in the epithelium leading to cell death. Protein precipitation creates a barrier which usually limits further diffusion into the eye. It is for this reason that the resultant damage from an acid burn is superficial scarring. A pathological specimen would most commonly be encountered in the form of a host corneal disc following a penetrating keratoplasty for visual rehabilitation. The pathology at the end stage is non-specific with epithelial instability, stromal fibrosis, and vascularisation. Very concentrated acids, however, may diffuse into the eye with effects similar to alkalis (see below).

Alkali

Examples: ammonia (NH_3), sodium hydroxide (NaOH, Lye), potassium hydroxide (KOH), magnesium hydroxide ($Mg[OH]_2$), and lime ($Ca[OH]_2$).

In comparison with acids, alkalis create more damage to the ocular tissues by saponification of fatty acids within the cell membranes by the hydroxyl (OH^-) ion, resulting in cell wall disruption. Alkali diffusion into the eye is progressive and may damage the cells in the cornea, trabecular meshwork, iris, lens, ciliary body, retina, and optic nerve.

In addition to the primary insult, the secondary effects of alkali burns are destructive to the eye for the following reasons:

1 Destruction of conjunctival cells leads to fibrosis in the fornices and lid distortion (symblepharon).
2 A loss of corneal limbal stem cells reduces the capacity for re-epithelialisation of the corneal surface with migration of surviving conjunctival cells onto the corneal surface.
3 The damage is often made more extensive due to an exaggerated inflammatory and healing response. Stromal melting and thinning from extensive liberation of metalloproteinases from both keratocytes and neutrophils can occur.
4 Fibrosis in the anterior segment tissues is followed by complicated sequelae which include glaucoma and cataract formation.

Severe cases of alkali burns are more likely to reach the pathologist at the end stage of the disease (Figure 9.28).

Physical

Thermal

The damage is mainly superficial to the cornea and episclera. Tissue destruction and subsequent reactions from accidental thermal burns are similar to chemical injuries and result in tissue lysis and scarring.

Thermotherapy using heated applicators or needles has also been employed to form scars in order to promote adhesions between the retina and choroid in retinal detachment treatment. In addition, ciliary body thermoablation has been applied in end-stage glaucoma. Currently lasers such as argon and diode (see below) have replaced direct heat application techniques.

Radiation

The electromagnetic spectrum is categorised according to wavelength, which has varying effects on the ocular tissues by nature of its penetrative ability and amount of energy delivered. Radiation from any source will suppress cell division by its effect on nuclear DNA with chromosome fracture. In addition, the release of free radicals such as superoxides also results in cell damage. Therefore, the ocular tissues which are constantly proliferating (for example corneal epithelium and lens epithelium) are at risk while cells with a low turnover (for example retinal neurones, RPE, corneal endothelium) are radioresistant.

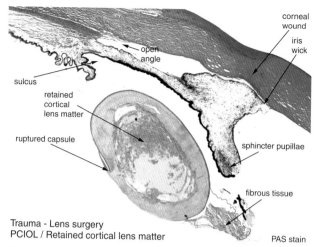

Trauma - Lens surgery
PCIOL / Retained cortical lens matter

PAS stain

Figure 9.25

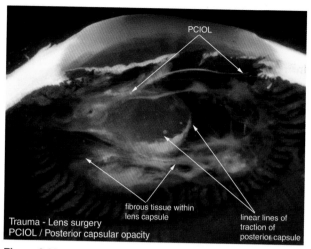

Trauma - Lens surgery
PCIOL / Posterior capsular opacity

Figure 9.26

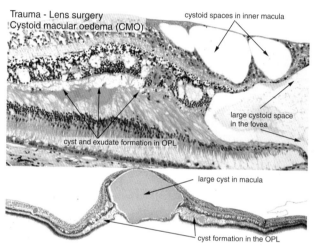

Trauma - Lens surgery
Cystoid macular oedema (CMO)

Figure 9.27

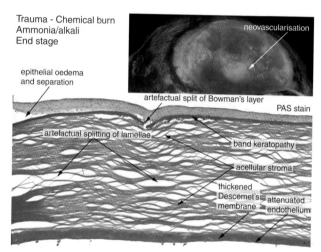

Trauma - Chemical burn
Ammonia/alkali
End stage

PAS stain

Figure 9.28

Figure 9.25 This is an example of failure to remove all the cortical lens matter during cataract surgery. The lens capsule does not completely surround the lens matter, which suggests a capsular rupture during the procedure. Similarly, the presence of iris tissue adjacent to the corneal wound implies an incarceration of the iris at a deeper level of the cornea.

Figure 9.26 This eye was removed at post mortem in 1982 with a presumed history of an extracapsular cataract extraction. The posterior chamber intraocular lens (PCIOL) is surrounded by a capsular bag in which there are dense fibrous strands. The membranes are the result of proliferation of lens epithelial cells undergoing fibrous metaplasia. Contraction of such fibrous tissue may displace the intraocular lens and create traction lines on the posterior capsule. In current practice, such posterior capsular opacities would be disrupted by means of a YAG laser.

Figure 9.27 In advanced cystoid macular oedema, small cysts are present in the outer plexiform layer (OPL) initially and these expand to form larger central cysts (upper and lower). In this and the other cases on file, it has been impossible to demonstrate vitreomacular traction, which is one of the proposed mechanisms for this condition. Similarly, there is an absence of inflammatory cell infiltration, which has also been implicated.

Figure 9.28 Enucleation following an alkali burn takes place usually many years after the injury when secondary complications supervene. In this example, an ammonia burn occurred during childhood and enucleation was carried out in adult life for pain and secondary glaucoma. The cornea is vascularised and scarred (inset). In the histological example (lower), there is calcification of Bowman's layer (band keratopathy), an acellular stroma, and an attenuated endothelium behind a thickened Descemet's membrane. These end-stage findings are non-specific.

Microwave

This has the longest wavelength and is cataractogenic.

Infrared

Unprotected workers in industries depending on the intense heat in processing are at risk: glass blowers, foundry workers, and iron smelters. Splits in the anterior lens capsule (true exfoliation) and degenerative changes in the lens cortex are identified clinically and pathologically.

Ultraviolet

This is absorbed in the corneal epithelium, and excessive exposure (for example from arc welding, reflected light from snow/water/sand) can lead to epithelial necrosis and separation. These cases heal spontaneously and thus would not be presented to a pathologist.

Visible light

If sufficiently intense, visible light can damage the retina. An example of this type of injury would be "sun staring", which destroys the photoreceptors of the macula. A therapeutic form of this type of energy is the xenon-arc photocoagulator which was used for retinal ablation in diabetic retinopathy; this has now been replaced by lasers.

Laser

Laser stands for **l**ight **a**mplification by **s**timulated **e**mission of **r**adiation. A detailed description of lasers and their applications are outside the scope of this text.

The three principle effects of lasers are dependent upon the amount of energy and wavelength:

1 *Photocoagulation* causes heat destruction of target tissues. Examples include the use of the argon laser (green 457, 488, 514 and 610 nm) for panretinal photocoagulation (PRP; see Chapter 10), trabeculoplasty, and treatment of choroidal neovascular membranes. Other lasers commonly used are the krypton laser and diode laser (the latter works in the infrared range and is used for ciliary body ablation and transpupillary thermotherapy).
2 *Photodisruption:* an example is the YAG laser (infrared, 1064 nm) which produces a high intensity energy which mechanically disrupts tissues. Most commonly this is applied to disrupt membranes which form within the capsule after an intraocular lens implant (YAG capsulotomy).
3 *Photoablation:* the high ultraviolet energy from an excimer laser (ultraviolet, 193 nm) directly vaporises tissues by disrupting the molecular bonds. The excimer laser is used in photorefractive surgery.

Ionising

Therapeutic ionising radiation in ophthalmology is used in the treatment of primary and secondary tumours of the eye and orbit.

- *Beta irradiation* has low penetration and is used for surface tumours of the globe, for example dysplasia, pterygium, and melanocytic tumours of the conjunctiva.
- *Proton beams* can be collimated and therefore accurately focused on intraocular tumours. The most appropriate use is teletherapy for uveal melanomas.

- *X-rays* have higher penetration and are used in the treatment of retinoblastomas, lymphomas, and metastatic tumours.
- *Gamma irradiation* is used in plaque brachytherapy such as ruthenium-109 in treatment essentially for melanomas and for other intraocular tumours where appropriate. Collimated gamma rays (gamma knife) are also used for external radiation in teletherapy for melanomas.

Effects of radiation on normal ocular tissues

Dose-related effect

The severity of damage is proportional to the total dose delivered or the size of fractionated dose in the case of teletherapy, and increases sharply once a threshold is reached (see below). In general, retinal vasculopathy is least likely to develop in eyes receiving doses less than 25 Gy in fractions of 2 Gy or less.

Although many parts of the eye are affected by irradiation, much of the damage is secondary to the primary effects on the vasculature and is, therefore, not pathognomonic. However, accidental irradiation in sufficiently high doses (20 Gy in one dose) may result in acute necrosis of the corneal keratocytes, endothelial cells, and scleral fibrocytes, resulting in necrotising keratitis or scleritis (Figures 9.29, 9.30).

Long term sequelae

The conditions described below are long term sequelae from therapeutic radiotherapy for other conditions.

Eyelid and conjunctiva Skin changes are characterised by atrophy of adnexal glands, endarteritis obliterans, and telangiectasia with collagen necrosis. Following radiation, a mild non-specific conjunctivitis is a common early reaction.

Lacrimal gland Dry eye can follow destruction of lacrimal gland tissue with secondary keratoconjunctivitis sicca. Inadequate lubrication may lead to bacterial infection, corneal ulceration, and perforation. (40 Gy)

Lens As low a dose as 5 Gy can cause a posterior subcapsular cataract (Figure 9.31).

Retinal vasculature Vascular disease secondary to radiation occurs months or years after exposure. This is due to radioresistance in the vascular endothelium which is said to replicate every 3 years. Failure of the retinal vascular endothelium to regenerate means that there is a progressive breakdown of the blood–retinal barrier with leakage of lipid-rich plasma constituents. Pathologically, the retina contains areas of lipid-rich proteinaceous exudates (Figures 9.32–9.34). The most important sequel to this ischaemic retinopathy is secondary neovascular glaucoma. Diabetes may exacerbate the severity of the condition, and is an important differential diagnosis in radiation retinopathy. (50 Gy)

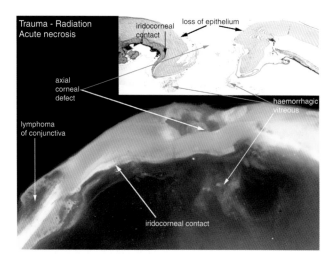

Figure 9.29

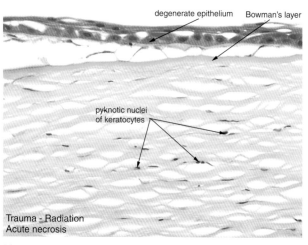

Figure 9.30

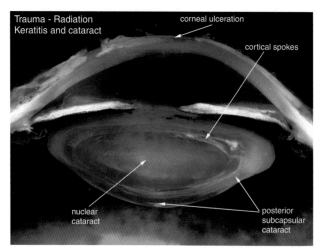

Figure 9.31

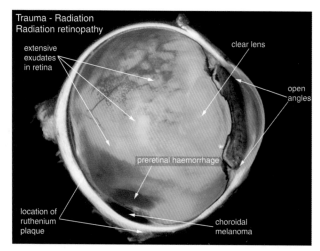

Figure 9.32

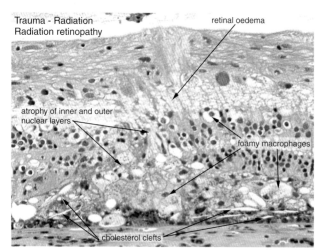

Figure 9.33

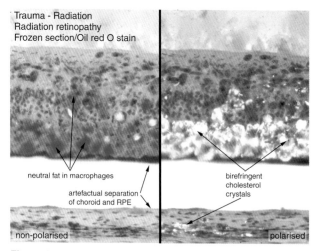

Figure 9.34

Figure 9.29 In treatment of a conjunctival lymphoma, a dose of 20 Gy was delivered unintentionally in one session. This was followed within a few days by an acute corneal perforation with prolapse of the lens and vitreous; the globe was subsequently enucleated. Note the absence of inflammatory infiltration (inset).

Figure 9.30 Histology from the cornea shown in Figure 9.29 reveals pyknosis of the keratocytes and advanced atrophy and degeneration in the corneal epithelium.

Figure 9.31 A radiation cataract and corneal ulceration occurred after deep X-ray therapy for nasopharyngeal carcinoma.

Figure 9.32 An inferior choroidal melanoma was treated with ruthenium (^{106}Ru) plaque brachytherapy. After 3 years, the eye was enucleated due to continuing growth of the tumour. The macroscopic appearance illustrates the extensive lipoidal exudates secondary to radiation vasculopathy.

Figure 9.33 In a paraffin section taken from the specimen shown in Figure 9.32, the lipids were dissolved during routine processing. The presence of an extensive lipid exudate was identified by macrophages and cholesterol clefts in the tissue. The layers of the outer retina have been disrupted by the exudate.

Figure 9.34 Frozen retinal tissue (case shown in Figure 9.32) was embedded in gelatin and sectioned in order to preserve the lipids in the exudate. Using the Oil red O stain, neutral lipids are red in colour and the cholesterol crystals are birefringent in polarised light.

Optic neuropathy Tumouricidal radiotherapy to the orbit results in endarteritis of the ophthalmic artery and its branches with damage to the microvasculature of the optic nerve. The optic atrophy is therefore based on ischaemia rather than radiation induced necrosis of the myelinated nerve fibres. (60 Gy)

Non-accidental injury of infants (NAI)

Other terms: battered baby syndrome (BBS) and shaken baby syndrome (SBS).

Children may be injured by direct force leading to broken bones and organ damage or may suffer chemical or thermal injuries, all of which may be accidental or malicious. A more specific form of abuse occurs when an infant is violently shaken but does not have any further evidence of trauma.

The brain and eye are usually well protected from sudden impacts but are particularly vulnerable to sudden acceleration and deceleration forces giving rise to subdural and retinal haemorrhages, and there is a good correlation between these findings. Repeated translational or torsional forces cause direct trauma to the brain as well as intracranial haemorrhage from the fragile vessels that traverse the subdural and subarachnoid spaces. The main mechanism of brain injury, however, is said to be secondary to hypoxia, caused by stretch (neuraxis) injury at the craniocervical junction with resultant apnoea and hypoxia.

The mechanisms for retinal haemorrhage are uncertain. One theory implicates the oscillation of the lens and vitreous causing tractional tearing to the retinal vessels. Another possibility is that the back pressure from raised intracranial pressure causes retinal haemorrhage by compressing the central retinal vein in the meninges. High morbidity and mortality (up to 33%) are correlated with the presence of retinal haemorrhages.

It is important to note that there are no ocular findings that are pathognomonic of NAI but an ophthalmological examination is often requested in suspect cases in which an infant is admitted in a comatose state or is moribund. Additional evidence of injury to the skeleton or viscera supports the diagnosis of non-accidental injury.

Currently there is much contention regarding the reliability of eye and brain findings alone as evidence in the diagnosis of SBS, as there are cases of accidental death in which retinal haemorrhages occurred following seemingly minor injuries. The reader should be well aware of the medicolegal consequences which can arise in cases of suspected NAI and should refer to the latest publications reflecting the current opinion.

Pathology

It is common for eyes to be enucleated at post mortem for investigation of unexplained neonatal or childhood deaths for exclusion of NAI. On preliminary macroscopic examination, subdural and subarachnoid haemorrhages may be identified in the optic nerves (Figure 9.35). Bleeding in the retina and vitreous may be evident (Figure 9.36). Retinal folds occur in eyes when fixation is delayed or may be due to retinal oedema. Microscopically, haemorrhages may be present in the vitreous or at any level of the retina (Figure 9.37). The Prussian blue stain demonstrates the presence of iron in areas of previous haemorrhage.

Differential diagnosis
Blood dyscrasias and septicaemia should be excluded.

Terson's syndrome
SBS should be distinguished from Terson's syndrome, which is the presence of intraocular haemorrhage secondary to intracranial haemorrhage from many other causes and usually occurs in adults. The popular theory for Terson's syndrome is that excess CSF pressure within the subarachnoid space of the nerve sheath compresses the retrobulbar portion of the optic nerve, and indirectly the retinochoroidal anastomoses and the central retinal vein – the impeded venous drainage results in stasis and haemorrhage.

The shrunken eye (atrophia/phthisis bulbi)

The term "phthisis" is defined as a progressive wasting disease and "phthisical eye" is often written as a clinical diagnosis in the pathology request form to describe a shrunken eye. Trauma is the usual association but many other conditions (for example ocular infection and chronic non-specific inflammation) may be encountered. Hypotonia is the common pathogenic mechanism. The eye is usually enucleated for cosmesis, for relief of pain, or if there is suspicion of an underlying tumour. It should be noted that melanomas are occasionally encountered in phthisical eyes.

There are two separate pathological terms based on the degree of internal disorganisation which are used to describe the shrunken globe:

1 *Atrophia bulbi:* where there is preservation of the choroidal and retinal anatomy.
2 *Phthisis bulbi:* where there is severe internal disorganisation, for example following penetrating trauma of the globe. The remainder of this section describes the phthisical eye.

Pathology

There is usually a long interval between the initial insult and enucleation. The history is often obscure and histopathological examination is often unrewarding in elucidating the primary mechanisms.

Reactive proliferation of three cell types predominates in the phthisical eye:

1 *Fibroblasts:* these cells can form contractile broad sheets within the eye. The source of these cells may be from the corneoscleral envelope, the iris, or the choroidal stroma following penetrating trauma.

2 *Retinal glial cells:* these cells are activated Müller cells and perivascular astrocytes. Any process which destroys neural cells in the retina may be repaired by these proliferating spindle-shaped glial cells.

3 *Epithelium:* these cells are derived from the ciliary body and retinal pigmented epithelium and have the capacity for reactionary proliferation and fibrous metaplasia.

Calcification or ossification can occur within fibrous proliferation in both atrophia and phthisis bulbi. Such specimens would require decalcifying treatment with a weak acid prior to routine histological processing.

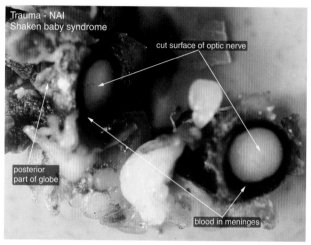

Figure 9.35

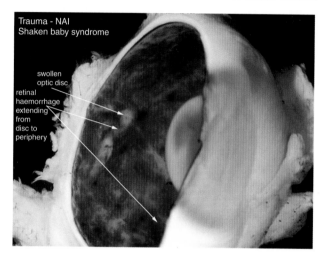

Figure 9.36

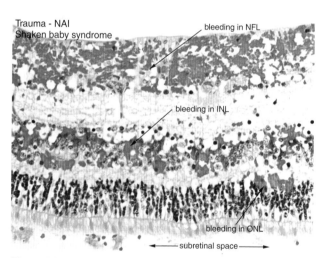

Figure 9.37

Figure 9.35 The routine practice of transecting the optic nerve reveals extensive bleeding into the meninges in the shaken baby syndrome. The optic nerve is normal.

Figure 9.36 The pathologist is most likely to encounter the shaken baby syndrome post mortem when there is often extensive haemorrhage within the retina. In the clinical situation, the haemorrhage may vary in severity. Usually fixation is delayed and the autolysed retina has a corrugated, thickened appearance which would not occur *in vivo*.

Figure 9.37 In the shaken baby syndrome, the distribution of bleeding is throughout the retina but is most extensive in the nerve fibre layer (NFL) and nuclear layers (INL = inner nuclear layer, ONL = outer nuclear layer).

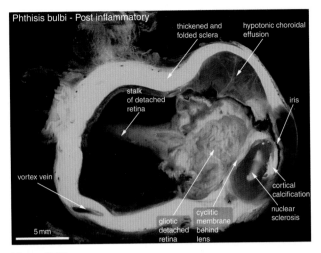

Figure 9.38

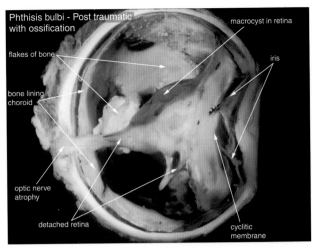

Figure 9.39

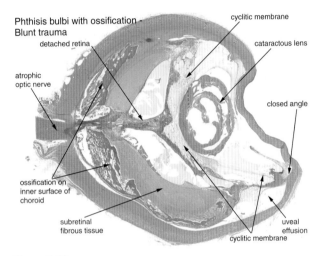

Figure 9.40

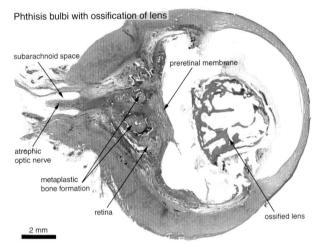

Figure 9.41

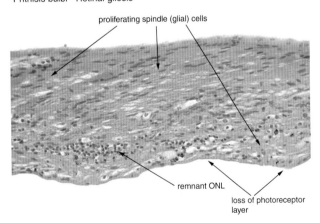

Figure 9.42

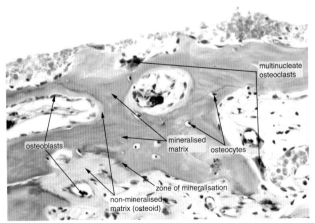

Figure 9.43

Macroscopic

By definition, the dimensions of the globe are reduced (Figure 9.38). There is often advanced distortion of the specimen which is extremely firm on palpation. Calcification and ossification are detectable by X-ray of the specimen but are immediately apparent when the blade meets resistance (Figure 9.39)!

Microscopic

The following descriptions are common findings in a phthisical globe:

1 *Cyclitic membrane:* metaplasia of the ciliary epithelium in response to inflammation or disorganisation leads to the formation of a retrolental fibrous mass or a preretinal membrane (Figure 9.40).
2 *Lens:* interference with lens metabolism promotes degeneration of the lens substance and fibrous meta-

plasia of the lens epithelium. In rare cases, the fibrous tissue is transformed into bone (Figure 9.41).

3 *Retinal gliosis:* irrespective of the nature of trauma to the retina, the end result is loss of neurones and glial cell proliferation (Figure 9.42; see also Figures 10.106, 10.111).
4 *RPE:* the RPE possesses a capacity to undergo fibrous metaplasia to form a collagenous matrix (Figures 9.39–9.41). This is an ideal substrate for calcification and migrating mesenchymal cells (i.e. osteoblasts and osteoclasts) form bone (Figure 9.43).
5 *Choroid:* this is relatively unaffected in phthisis bulbi unless there is evidence of a penetrating trauma in which case fibrous tissue derived from the sclera will proliferate within the choroidal wound.
6 *Optic nerve:* atrophy of the optic nerve corresponds to the extent of retinal degeneration.

Figure 9.38 Postinflammatory hypotonia leads to supraciliary exudation and metaplasia of the ciliary epithelium to form a retrolental "cyclitic" membrane. Retinal detachment follows contraction of the membrane. The lens is often calcified and this may progress to bone formation (see Figures 9.39, 9.40). Shrinkage of the globe leads to thickening and folding of the sclera. The overall dimensions of this specimen were 20 × 17 × 17 mm.

Figure 9.39 The history in this specimen was one of previous penetrating trauma with loss of the lens. This was followed by chronic uveitis and the formation of a cyclitic membrane associated with secondary retinal detachment. Reactive fibrous metaplasia of the retinal pigment epithelium has provided a substrate for calcification and ossification in the choroid and subretinal space. When the globe was divided, a fragment of bone was displaced into the subretinal space.

Figure 9.40 Phthisis bulbi with ossification represents the end stage of a process which is so complicated that the sequence of events may not be determined without an accurate clinical history. This example shows the effects of blunt trauma followed by retinal detachment. A cyclitic membrane arose from the ciliary epithelium to attach to the retina with traction. The membrane has also interfered with lens metabolism and has caused degenerative changes within the lens substance. Reactive metaplasia of the retinal pigment epithelium has progressed from fibrosis to ossification (see Figure 9.43).

Figure 9.41 Disorganisation of ocular tissues in phthisis bulbi is extensive in some specimens. In this post-traumatic example, the retina has collapsed over the scleral canal which suggests that there had been a giant retinal tear. The presence of a thick fibrous membrane on the inner surface of the retina supports this suggestion. Fibrous metaplasia of the lens epithelium proceeds to ossification (cataracta ossea).

Figure 9.42 After trauma with untreated retinal detachment, the neurones of the retina undergo degeneration and few survive. In this example, only the bipolar cell layer is identifiable. The remainder of the retinal substance is replaced by spindle-shaped glial cells. ONL = outer nerve layer.

Figure 9.43 This image is included for interest to show bone formation and remodelling in the process of ossification in a phthisical eye. It is assumed that many of the pigmented cells are derived from retinal pigment epithelium. The matrix, initially formed by osteoblasts, is non-mineralised (osteoid). At the edge of this area is a zone of mineralisation, in which calcium salts are deposited and osteoblasts are buried to become osteocytes. Mineralised bone is resorbed by multinucleate osteoclasts (remodelling in the normal skeleton controls the balance between bone formation and resorption and maintains normal serum calcium and phosphate levels).

Chapter 10
Retina: vascular diseases, degenerations, and dystrophies

Normal anatomy

The function of the retina is to accurately detect light in location and in intensity. In order to recognise the histological appearances of different disease processes that affect the retina, it is important to be aware of the histology of the normal retina in different anatomical locations.

Macula

In a horizontal section above the edge of the optic nerve, the fovea is located 1 mm below an imaginary line drawn through the centre of the optic disc (Figure 10.1). The perimacular area is opaque in a fixed specimen and the fovea and foveola are more easily identified than *in vivo*.

Histologically, the fovea and foveola are seen as a thin layer which consists only of photoreceptors and the nerve fibre layer of Henle. A greatly increased density of ganglion cells thickens the adjacent macula (Figure 10.2). The processes of the photoreceptor cells (Henle's layer) pass obliquely from the foveola to synapse with the bipolar cell processes in the outer plexiform layer. The cone photoreceptors are densely packed at the macula (Figure 10.3).

Periphery

The retinal periphery is that region that extends from the macula and the optic disc to the ora serrata. The retinal thickness decreases progressively towards the periphery, because the density of ganglion cells and bipolar cells is reduced (Figure 10.4). Rod photoreceptors are more numerous than cones (Figure 10.5).

Photoreceptor–RPE interface

To better appreciate the degenerative and dystrophic disorders which will be described subsequently, a basic understanding of the interrelationships between the two layers of the retina (neural and retinal pigment epithelium) is important. The metabolic requirements of the outer retina are provided by the retinal pigment epithelium (RPE). The outer segments contain discs which are formed by lipoproteins. Exposure to photons stimulates an electrochemical reaction in the discs resulting in the generation of a nerve signal. The process of disc replacement in rod renewal depends on the phagocytosis of the tips of the photoreceptors with further breakdown in the cytoplasm of the RPE. New photoreceptor discs are formed in the rod inner segment and this renewal minimises the effects of photic damage. In an electron micrograph, it is possible to identify processes from the RPE extending around tips of the rod outer segments (Figure 10.6). The mechanisms by which the cone outer segments are maintained and renewed are less well understood.

Ora serrata and pars plana

Knowledge of the equatorial and far peripheral retinal pathology is important in interpreting abnormalities as seen by indirect ophthalmoscopy. The retina is limited by the ora serrata which has a scalloped appearance (Figure 10.7).

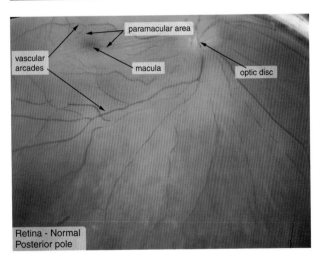

Figure 10.1

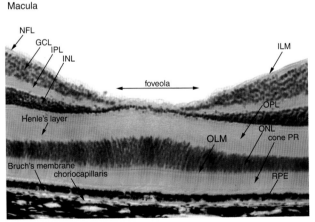

Figure 10.2

Figure 10.1 The fundus in an enucleated globe varies in appearance according to the fixative used. Gluteraldehyde provides an appearance closer to the *in vivo* state; formalin fixation makes the entire retina opaque. In this gluteraldehyde-fixed specimen, the macula is red and the paramacular area is opaque. The vascular arcades contain less blood than would be present in the living eye.

Figure 10.2 The histological architecture of the fovea and macula is distinctive. In the central foveola, the layers are restricted to photoreceptors and Henle's layer. The other retinal layers are present in the adjacent macula. ILM = inner limiting membrane, NFL = nerve fibre layer, GCL = ganglion cell layer, IPL = inner plexiform layer, INL = inner nuclear layer (bipolar cells), OPL = outer plexiform layer (also features Henle's layer in the macula), ONL = outer nuclear layer (photoreceptor nuclei), OLM = outer limiting membrane, PR = photoreceptors (cones only in the macula), RPE = retinal pigment epithelium with the underlying Bruch's membrane (BrM) and choriocapillaris.

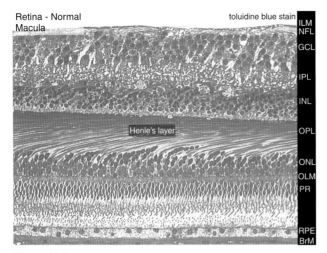

Retina - Normal
Macula

toluidine blue stain

ILM
NFL
GCL
IPL
INL
OPL
ONL
OLM
PR
RPE
BrM

Henle's layer

Figure 10.3

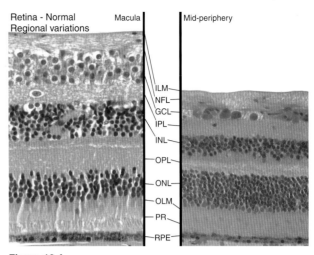

Retina - Normal
Regional variations

Macula

Mid-periphery

ILM
NFL
GCL
IPL
INL
OPL
ONL
OLM
PR
RPE

Figure 10.4

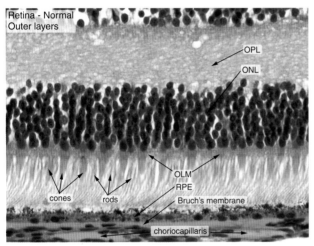

Retina - Normal
Outer layers

OPL
ONL
OLM
RPE
Bruch's membrane
cones   rods
choriocapillaris

Figure 10.5

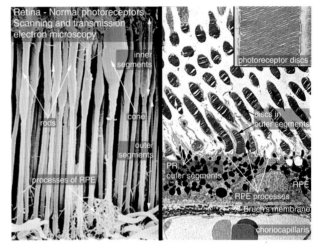

Retina - Normal photoreceptors
Scanning and transmission
electron microscopy

inner
segments
photoreceptor discs
discs in
outer segments
rods   cone
outer
segments
PR
outer segments
processes of RPE
RPE
RPE processes
Bruch's membrane
choriocapillaris

Figure 10.6

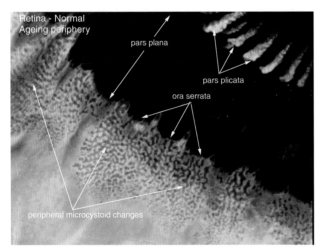

Retina - Normal
Ageing periphery

pars plana
pars plicata
ora serrata
peripheral microcystoid changes

Figure 10.7

Figure 10.3 Detail of the macula is best demonstrated in a plastic section stained with a toluidine blue stain. The oblique arrangement of the nerve fibres in the outer plexiform layer is evident. The cone photoreceptors are densely packed in this region. (Abbreviations as in Figure 10.2.)

Figure 10.4 The macula contains the greatest density of neurones (left). Toward the retinal periphery (right), the density of bipolar cells and ganglion cells declines and the retinal thickness decreases. (Abbreviations as in Figure 10.2.)

Figure 10.5 This is the appearance of the photoreceptors in the mid-periphery in a 24 year old male. The inner segments of the cones appear as thick red tapering ("carrot-shaped") structures while the rods are more uniform ("pencil-shaped") in thickness. The processes of the retinal pigment epithelium interdigitate with the tips of the photoreceptors. (Abbreviations as in Figure 10.2.)

Figure 10.6 Electron microscopy (scanning and transmission) is invaluable in the understanding of interactions between the retinal pigment epithelium (RPE) and the photoreceptors (PRs). Rods and cones have a characteristic three dimensional morphology with distinct separation between the inner and outer segments (left). Transmission electron microscopy of the outer segments (right) reveals the stacks of discs surrounded by a membrane (inset, right).

Figure 10.7 The scalloped interface between the peripheral retina and the pars plana is easily identified in an enucleated eye. The pars plana overlies the ciliary muscle and is limited anteriorly by the ciliary processes which form the pars plicata. The degenerative process shown here, peripheral microcystoid degeneration, is almost always innocuous.

Vasculature

The central retinal artery emerges from the optic disc in several branches. Arterioles are formed at the third branching. The capillaries, which branch off the arterioles, loop down into the outer plexiform layer before joining the retinal venules. These, in turn, drain into retinal veins and merge to form the central retinal vein in the prelaminar part of the optic nerve. A relative narrowing of the vein within the lamina cribrosa is sufficient to maintain pressure in the capillary bed against intraocular pressure. At the microscopic level, the muscular wall of the arteriole is thicker than that of the venule (Figure 10.8). Neither arterioles nor venules possess an internal elastic lamina.

The vascular bed has been examined in classical studies by retinal digest preparations (Figures 10.9, 10.10) in which the neural retina is digested by means of pepsin and trypsin to expose the retinal vasculature.

Vascular disease

Common pathological features in retinal vascular disease

While there are many pathological disorders that result in ischaemic damage to the retina, the manifestations are restricted to the entities outlined in Table 10.1.

Vascular malformations (congenital)

Von Hippel's disease (angiomatosis retinae)

Angiomatosis retinae is part of a spectrum in which vascular hamartomas and vascular neoplasms are present in the retina and within the brain.

Clinical presentation

The most common presenting symptom is visual disturbance, although many cases will be an incidental finding on routine examination or as follow up of an established family history.

Retinal haemangiomas are either solitary or multiple, and can be unilateral or bilateral. The multiple and bilateral cases are more likely to have a hereditary component (autosomal dominant).

These vascular tumours are typically red/orange in colour, with a prominent feeding artery and a draining vein. An exudative retinal detachment may be present.

The tumour has a characteristic clinical appearance but may be investigated further with fluorescein angiogram and ultrasound.

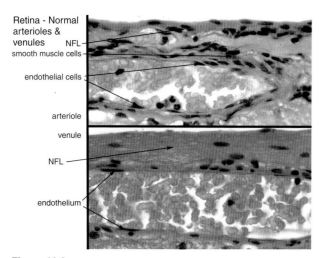

Retina - Normal
arterioles &
venules   NFL
smooth muscle cells
endothelial cells
arteriole
venule
NFL
endothelium

Figure 10.8

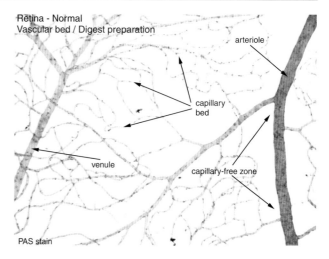

Retina - Normal
Vascular bed / Digest preparation
arteriole
capillary bed
venule
capillary-free zone
PAS stain

Figure 10.9

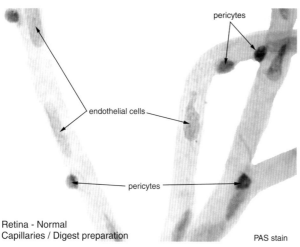

pericytes
endothelial cells
pericytes

Retina - Normal
Capillaries / Digest preparation
PAS stain

Figure 10.10

Figure 10.8 The retinal arterioles and venules are present in the nerve fibre layer (NFL) and ganglion cell layer. The arterioles have a thicker layer of myocytes than the venules. Both are lined by endothelial cells.

Figure 10.9 When the retina is removed from the globe and immersed in pepsin-trypsin solutions, the neural elements are digested away to leave the vascular bed, which can be mounted on a glass slide and stained with PAS. Arterioles are identified by a zone that has no capillaries and a greater density of myocytes in the wall. It is possible to trace capillaries from the branching arterioles to the venules.

Figure 10.10 A capillary is a thin-walled tube lined internally by endothelium. Pericytes are incorporated into the basement membrane of the capillary wall and are seen as small, heavily stained nuclei.

Table 10.1 Common pathological features in retinal vascular disease.

Features	Macroscopic	Microscopic	Commonest causes	Pathogenesis
Retinal haemorrhage	Flame, dot and blot haemorrhages in the retina (Figures 10.11, 10.12)	Flame: red cells in nerve fibre layer Dot: red cells within outer retina Blot: red cells in subretinal space (Figure 10.13)	Central/branch retinal vein occlusion (CRVO/BRVO) Diabetes Arterial embolism Ocular ischaemic syndrome Blood dyscrasias	Interruption of blood flow damages vascular endothelium and the vessel wall. When blood flow is reinstated, the damaged vessel ruptures
	Roth's spot: circular red areas with a central white spot (Figure 10.14)	Haemorrhage in all retinal layers adjacent to an occluded arteriole (Figure 10.15) Inflammatory or neoplastic cell foci will be evident	Subacute bacterial endocarditis (SABE) Leukaemia Other causes of microembolism	Embolism from an infective source or a tumour cell bolus
Microinfarcts/cotton wool spots	Fluffy white areas within retina (Figure 10.16)	Swollen nerve fibre layer Distended interrupted axons containing cytoid bodies (Figure 10.17)	Diabetes Hypertension HIV Systemic lupus erythematosus (SLE) Septic embolism Blood dyscrasias CRVO	Represents a focal infarct in the nerve fibre layer (NFL). Axons are interrupted in an area of infarction in the NFL. The surviving axons become swollen upstream from the infarct and the NFL is thickened
Exudates (Figures 10.18–10.21)	Well circumscribed yellow areas in the retina (Figures 10.18, 10.19)	Pink staining lipoproteinaceous exudates in the outer plexiform layer (OPL) with infiltrating macrophages (Figures 10.20, 10.21)	Diabetes Hypertension Radiation Coats' disease	Ischaemic damage to the endothelial cells disrupts the blood–retinal barrier and lipoproteins leak into the neural tissue
Microaneurysm (Figures 10.53–10.56)	Small red dots within the retina	Small bulges in the walls of capillaries. Eventually filled by endothelial cells and finally replaced by fibrosis (hyalinisation)	CRVO (peripheral) Diabetes (central)	Loss of capillary endothelial cells Loss of capillary pericytes
Neovascularisation (Figures 10.43–10.46)	Vascularised membranes or nodules	Arterioles, venules, capillaries, and fibroblasts proliferate within, upon, and beneath the retina The vitreous also provides a scaffold for preretinal proliferations	Diabetes CRVO	Vascular endothelial growth factor (VEGF) is secreted from an ischaemic retina This and other growth factors stimulate endothelial cell proliferation

Systemic findings – patients with von Hippel–Lindau syndrome (VHLS) may have the following extraocular abnormalities:
1 CNS haemangioblastomas.
2 Cysts of kidneys, liver, pancreas, epididymis, and ovaries.
3 Renal cell carcinoma.
4 Phaeochromocytoma of adrenal gland.

Genetics
Whereas solitary unilateral ocular tumours are mostly sporadic, bilateral multiple tumours are likely to be associated with a deletion in a suppressor gene located on chromosome 3p25–26 (VHLS gene) with incomplete penetrance.

Possible modes of treatment
1 Observation for "quiet" tumours.
2 Photocoagulation, brachytherapy, proton beam teletherapy, or endocryotherapy for exudative tumours.
3 Vitrectomy or conventional surgery for retinal detachments with a rhegmatogenous component.

Retina - Vascular disease / Haemorrhage

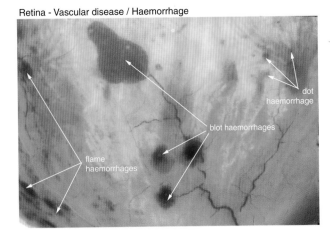

Figure 10.11

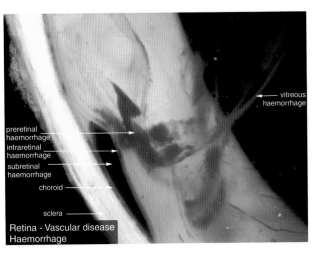

Retina - Vascular disease
Haemorrhage

Figure 10.12

Retina - Vascular disease
Haemorrhage

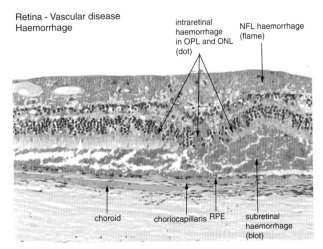

Figure 10.13

Retina - Vascular disease
Roth's spot / Malignant lymphoma

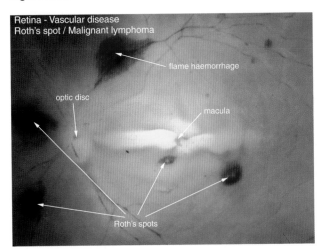

Figure 10.14

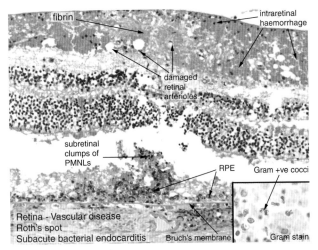

Retina - Vascular disease
Roth's spot
Subacute bacterial endocarditis

Figure 10.15

Figure 10.11 Depending on their location within the retinal layers, haemorrhages have a varying appearance. Flame haemorrhages occur in the nerve fibre layer, dot haemorrhages in the outer plexiform layer, and blot haemorrhages beneath the neural retina.

Figure 10.12 This cross-section through the retina illustrates more extensive haemorrhage extending into the subhyaloid (preretinal) space and vitreous gel. A large subretinal haemorrhage is present which would have a blot appearance clinically.

Figure 10.13 The histological features of haemorrhages in different layers of the retina are illustrated. The corresponding clinical appearances are annotated. (Abbreviations as in Figure 10.2.)

Figure 10.14 In Roth's original description (1907), circular areas of haemorrhage with a white centre were noted in patients suffering from subacute bacterial endocarditis. Currently, this abnormality is seen in patients with blood dyscrasias, in this case a malignant lymphoma with anaemia. This autopsy globe shows autolytic swelling of the macula, and formalin fixation accounts for the white appearance of the retina.

Figure 10.15 A patient died from septicaemia following streptococcal endocarditis. In this microscopic illustration of a Roth's spot, the pale pink area (clinically white) in the centre of the haemorrhage is due to leakage of fibrin consequent upon upstream partial occlusion of the feeder arteriole by a septic embolus. Subsequent ischaemic damage to the vessel wall causes leakage of red cells under pressure covering a wider area. A metastatic abscess is present in the choroids, and the polymorphonuclear leucocytes (PMNLs) in the subretinal space contain Gram positive cocci (inset). RPE = retinal pigment epithelium.

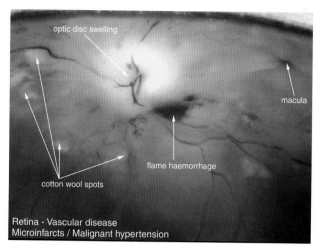

Retina - Vascular disease
Microinfarcts / Malignant hypertension

optic disc swelling
macula
flame haemorrhage
cotton wool spots

Figure 10.16

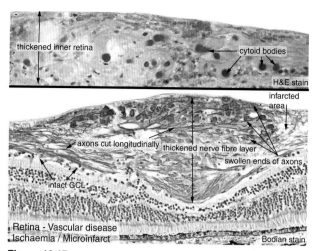

thickened inner retina
cytoid bodies
H&E stain
infarcted area
axons cut longitudinally   thickened nerve fibre layer
swollen ends of axons
intact GCL
Retina - Vascular disease
Ischaemia / Microinfarct
Bodian stain

Figure 10.17

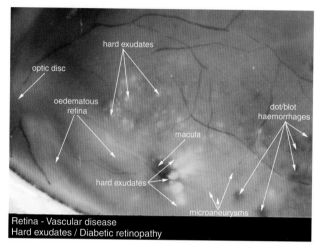

hard exudates
optic disc
oedematous retina
macula
hard exudates
microaneurysms
dot/blot haemorrhages
Retina - Vascular disease
Hard exudates / Diabetic retinopathy

Figure 10.18

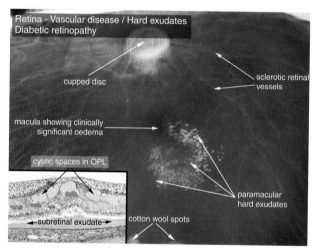

Retina - Vascular disease / Hard exudates
Diabetic retinopathy
cupped disc
sclerotic retinal vessels
macula showing clinically significant oedema
cystic spaces in OPL
paramacular hard exudates
subretinal exudate
cotton wool spots

Figure 10.19

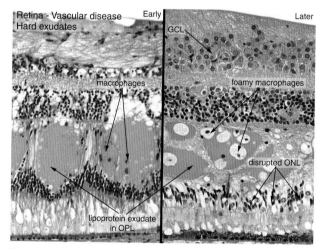

Retina - Vascular disease
Hard exudates
Early
Later
GCL
macrophages
foamy macrophages
disrupted ONL
lipoprotein exudate in OPL

Figure 10.20

Figure 10.16 In an archival autopsy specimen, the features of malignant hypertension are characteristic and include small white retinal swellings (microinfarcts/cotton wool spots) and flame haemorrhages. The optic disc is swollen.

Figure 10.17 In a routine H&E section (upper), a retinal microinfarct is identified by the presence of pink-staining circular or oval structures which are larger than cells (historically these were referred to as "cytoid bodies"). The use of a stain to illustrate the axons (lower) shows that the structures previously described as cytoid bodies are, in fact, the swollen ends of axons at the edge of an infarcted area of retina. As a consequence of localised infarction, the interrupted ends of the axons become sealed. Continuing axoplasmic transport from the parent ganglion cell results in a build up of axoplasm (Bodian stain for axons). GCL = ganglion cell layer.

Figure 10.18 Hard exudates were previously a prominent feature of diabetic retinopathy in enucleated globes. They appear as discrete pale yellow structures of varying size commonly located in the posterior pole. They are usually arranged in a circinate pattern around leaking capillaries, classically around microaneurysms. NB: It is difficult to identify microaneurysms macroscopically in a pathological specimen.

Figure 10.19 This globe was enucleated for failed treatment of secondary neovascular glaucoma in a diabetic patient. An important feature of diabetic retinopathy is macular oedema that is a result of nearby vessel leak often with hard exudate deposition. In this example, there is "clinically significant macular oedema" (CSMO) in which there is retinal exudation with thickening within 500 μm of the fovea. The inset shows histology from a macula in which there are cystic dilatations containing lipoproteinaceous deposits in the outer plexiform layer (OPL) over a proteinaceous exudative detachment.

Figure 10.20 Hard exudates appear initially as homogeneous pink-staining areas within the outer plexiform layer (OPL). At an early stage, macrophages (intrinsic glial cells) migrate into the exudate (left). At a later stage, the macrophages become distended with lipoprotein and disruption of the OPL leads to degeneration of the photoreceptor cells (right). GCL = ganglion cell layer, ONL = outer nuclear layer.

Macroscopic

This disease will probably be observed in enucleated globes in which treatment has failed and the haemangioma may be obscured by the retinal detachment (Figure 10.22).

Microscopic

The tumour mass consists of proliferating endothelial cells forming primitive capillary networks (Figure 10.23).

Coats' disease

An idiopathic condition with the key feature being abnormal retinal telangiectatic vessels with intra- and subretinal leakage of lipoproteinaceous fluid.

Clinical presentation

In a child aged 3–5 years, the classic presentation is that of a leucocoria with reduced vision and strabismus.

Most cases are unilateral (80%).

Depending on the extent of vascular abnormality and, hence, leakage of lipoprotein, the fundus appearance varies from localised yellow subretinal exudates to total exudative retinal detachment. Telangiectatic vessels and microaneurysms may be apparent in the periphery.

Further investigations with ultrasound, fluorescein angiogram, and CT may be necessary to differentiate this condition from other causes of leucocoria (see Chapter 11).

Pathogenesis

The presence of abnormal endothelium in sectors of the retinal vasculature leads to a breakdown of the blood–retinal barrier with resultant exudation.

Genetics

More common in males.

Possible modes of treatment

1 Observation.
2 Photocoagulation or cryotherapy for areas of retina in which leakage can be demonstrated by fluorescein angiography.
3 Vitrectomy and retinal detachment surgery.

Macroscopic

In an enucleated globe, Coats' disease should be suspected if the gelatinous subretinal exudate contains numerous cholesterol crystals and yellow clusters of cells. It may be possible to demonstrate a thickened area of retina which would represent the sector of telangiectasia (Figure 10.24). There may be evidence of extensive laser treatment.

Microscopic

Serial sections are required to identify areas of abnormal vasculature. These are recognised by spaces around the endothelium of the affected vessels. Endothelial dysfunction permits the leakage of red cells and plasma into the vessel wall and the adjacent retina. Inflammatory cell infiltration (macrophages and lymphocytes) is a secondary phenomenon (Figures 10.25–10.27).

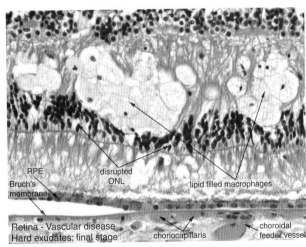

Figure 10.21

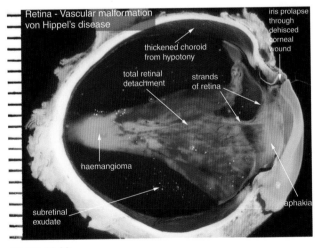

Figure 10.22

Figure 10.21 At a much later stage, the exudate is removed and clusters of foamy macrophages are present in the outer plexiform layer. Resolution is slow due to the inability of macrophages to migrate out of the retina. In this autopsy specimen, the photoreceptors are autolysed and the retinal pigment epithelium (RPE) is detached by artefact. ONL = outer nuclear layer.

Figure 10.22 A 7 year old boy known to be suffering from von Hippel's disease developed a cataract. Surgery was complicated by corneal wound dehiscence, iris prolapse, retinal detachment, and hypotonia. In this specimen, the angioma can be seen as an orange mass in the stalk of the detached and congested retina.

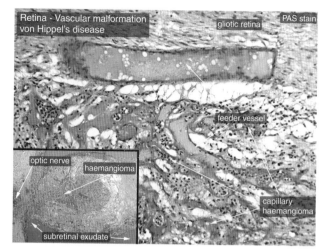

Figure 10.23

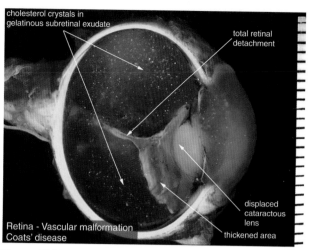

Figure 10.24

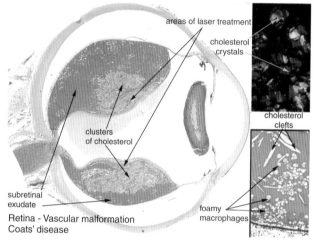

Figure 10.25

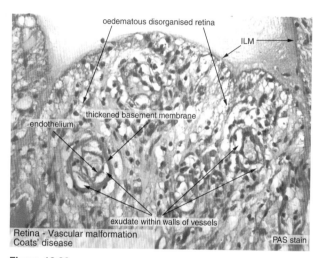

Figure 10.26

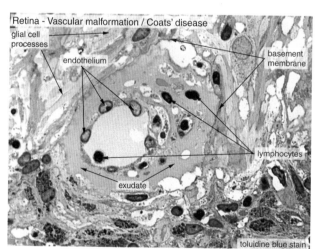

Figure 10.27

Figure 10.23 A section through the stalk illustrated in Figure 10.22 reveals the haemangioma within the detached retina (inset). The tumour mass consists of proliferating capillaries and feeder vessels. The PAS stain outlines the walls of the capillaries.

Figure 10.24 In the past, cases of Coats' disease were treated by enucleation to exclude the possibility of a retinoblastoma. A thickened area within the detached retina and a gelatinous subretinal exudate containing numerous cholesterol crystals are strongly suggestive of the diagnosis of Coats' disease.

Figure 10.25 Laser treatment of telangiectatic areas in Coats' disease is not always successful. In this example, large masses of cholesterol and blood are located beneath the lasered retina. Cholesterol crystals are birefringent in polarised light: these crystals are obtained from the subretinal exudate (upper right). Processing for paraffin wax histology uses fat solvents which remove the cholesterol crystals leaving cleft-like spaces in the eosinophilic exudate. Foamy macrophages ingest the lipids within the exudate and this pattern is characteristic of lipoproteinaceous exudation from any cause (lower right).

Figure 10.26 The PAS stain demonstrates the thickening due to leakage in the vessel walls in Coats' disease. This produces characteristic clear spaces between the endothelium and the smooth muscle layer. Leakage of fluid into the retina results in massive oedema, disorganisation, and gliotic replacement of the normal architecture. ILM = inner limiting membrane.

Figure 10.27 In Coats' disease, the integrity of the endothelium of capillaries is compromised and protein rich fluid leaks into the adjacent tissue. The presence of inflammatory cell infiltration led Coats to believe that this is an inflammatory process. It is now accepted that sectorial endothelial dysfunction is the primary abnormality (plastic embedded section, stained with toluidine blue).

Acquired

Retinopathy of prematurity (ROP)

A vascular proliferative retinopathy of premature, low birth weight infants exposed to high and fluctuating levels of oxygen partial pressures. It is important to appreciate that in the developing premature infant, migration of the retinal vessels is incomplete, leaving an avascular zone in the periphery. The basis of this condition is an abnormal proliferation of the developing retinal blood vessels at the junction of vascularised and avascular retina.

Clinical presentation
The clinical ROP classification is summarised in Table 10.2.

Risk factors
1 Low birth weight (LBW) <1000 g.
2 Short gestational age <29 weeks.
3 Multiple births.
4 Race (there is a twofold increase in progression to severe disease in whites compared with blacks). Gender is *not* associated with progression.

Pathogenesis
Common theory (fluctuating oxygen)
1 Exposure to high O_2 partial pressures: suppresses stimuli for vessels to penetrate the avascular retina; vaso-obliteration of existing vessels.
2 Return to normal O_2 partial pressures: results in relative retinal hypoxia; upregulation of vascular endothelial growth factor (VEGF) production initiates vasoproliferation.

Alternate theory The common theory does not explain ROP in LBW infants who did not receive oxygen. In the alternate theory, free radicals of oxygen stimulate mesenchymal spindle cells and may be a source of angiogenic growth factors.

Possible modes of treatment
Depending on the severity of disease:
1 Observation.
2 Laser photocoagulation of peripheral non-vascularised retina.
3 Vitrectomy and retinal detachment surgery in selected cases.

Clinicopathological correlation
In the most severe form, blindness is the result. It is rare for the pathologist to receive specimens in the early stages of the disease. Most enucleations for ROP would follow failed treatment for the complications of longstanding detachment (Figures 10.28, 10.29). Compared with Coats' disease, in ROP the integrity of the endothelium in the vasculature is preserved so that exudation is absent.

Three main criteria determine the severity of ROP and the possible need for intervention (as recommended by the Committee for the Classification of Retinopathy of Prematurity and its Management, 1984 and 1988):
1 *Stage:* Table 10.2 shows the clinicopathological correlation of the five stages of ROP.
2 *Plus disease:* vascular shunting of blood causes posterior venous engorgement and arterial tortuosity involving one or more quadrants. This is seen clinically as:
   • dilatation and tortuosity of peripheral retinal vessels
   • iris vascular engorgement
   • pupillary rigidity
   • vitreous haze.
Plus disease is the hallmark of rapidly progressive disease.

Table 10.2 Clinicopathological correlation in the staging of retinopathy of prematurity.

Stage	Clinical appearance	Pathological findings
Stage I	Thin, flat white demarcation line between the vascular and avascular retina	Proliferation of immature endothelial cells occurs at the periphery of the avascular zone
Stage II	Development of a demarcation line into a ridge or mesenchymal shunt that forms an elevated thickened tissue between vascular and avascular retina	Further hyperplasia of spindle cells, with proliferation of endothelial cells of the rearguard mesenchymal tissue (Figure 10.30)
Stage III	Appearance of extraretinal fibrovascular proliferation	Extraretinal neovascular proliferation. Proliferation of endothelial cells occurs along small, thin-walled vessels
Stage IVa	Formation of a fibrovascular mass with resultant traction on the retina causes a subtotal retinal detachment	Fibrovascular bands and tractional detachment of the retina. Condensation of vitreous into sheets and strands orientated anteriorly toward the lens equator. Hence, tractional retinal detachment occurs with the peripheral retina drawn centrally and anteriorly The subretinal space contains serous exudate
Stage IVb	Involvement of the fovea	
Stage V	Total retinal detachment seen as a retrolental white mass (previous term, "retrolental fibroplasia")	Total (tabletop) retinal detachment (Figures 10.28, 10.29)

3 *Location:*
- zone 1: optic disc to radius twice the distance from the disc to the fovea
- zone 2: radius of zone 1 to temporal equator
- zone 3: temporal crescent of retina, not encompassed by the other zones.

NB: If nasal retina is vascularised fully, it is labelled zone 3 by convention.

Hypertension

Ocular disease from uncontrolled systemic hypertension is now rarely encountered as this condition is diagnosed early and treated effectively.

Clinical presentation

Although there is bilateral involvement, there may be asymmetry in progression. The patient is usually asymptomatic although decreased vision may be experienced.

The appearances of the fundus will depend on whether the onset is acute or chronic:

1 *Acute (malignant):* hard exudates/macular star, retinal oedema, cotton wool spots, flame haemorrhages, focal chorioretinal infarcts (Elschnig's spots), and disc oedema. In extreme cases, there may be retinal detachment and vitreous haemorrhage.

2 *Chronic:* arteriovenous (AV) nipping with retinal arteriolar sclerosis ("copper" or "silver" wiring), retinal oedema and cotton wool spots, disc oedema, flame haemorrhages, and arterial macroaneurysms. Hypertension may be complicated by thrombotic occlusion of the central retinal vein (CRVO) or a branch retinal vein (BRVO).

Aetiology/pathogenesis

Most cases of hypertension are of the essential variety and of unknown aetiology. Acute hypertension is rare but preeclampsia/eclampsia would be the commonest association. Other causes include phaeochromocytoma, chronic renal failure, and renal artery stenosis.

It is speculated that the high pressure in the retinal arterioles leads to spasm and endothelial damage in the acute disease. In the chronic disease, the vessels become hyalinised and less prone to spasm.

Possible modes of treatment

Any underlying cause should be determined and treated with antihypertensive drug therapy.

Macroscopic

Acute malignant hypertension has been encountered in autopsy cases by pathologists (Figure 10.16). The appearances mirror those outlined in the clinical description.

Microscopic

Fibrinoid necrosis as seen in the renal arterioles is not a feature of retinal arteriolar disease, although the choroidal vessels undergo fibrinoid necrosis. The secondary effects of retinal arteriolar spasm (haemorrhage and microinfarction) have already been described (see Table 10.1).

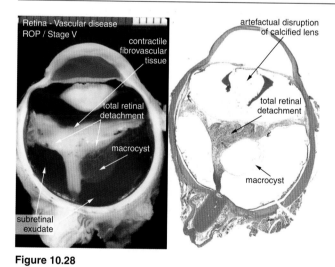

Figure 10.28

Figure 10.28 Stage V pathology in retinopathy of prematurity (ROP) is based on proliferation of fibrovascular tissue on the inner surface of the retina (see Figure 10.29). Macroscopic examination (left) reveals a retinal stalk beneath a thickened band of white tissue extending from ora to ora. Often, in longstanding retinal detachments, large cysts (macrocysts) form within the retina. In a section from the same globe (right), the detached retina is thrown into folds beneath an epiretinal fibrovascular membrane. Calcification in the lens is common in ocular disorders in childhood and results in artefactual tissue disruption when the sections are prepared.

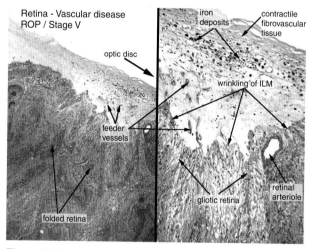

Figure 10.29

Figure 10.29 Contraction of the epiretinal fibrovascular tissue seen in Figure 10.28 causes marked distortion of the retina which is thrown into folds seen as circular and linear bands of the outer nuclear layer (left). At a higher power (right), small vessels extend from the inner retina into the fibrovascular mass. It is likely that these vessels are fragile and bleed, and this explains the breakdown products of blood (in the form of iron deposits) in the membrane. ILM = inner limiting membrane.

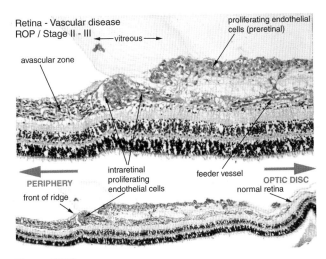

Figure 10.30

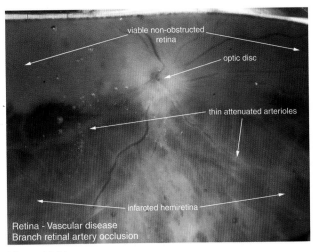

Figure 10.31

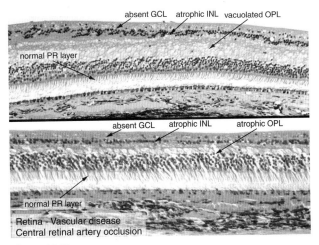

Figure 10.32

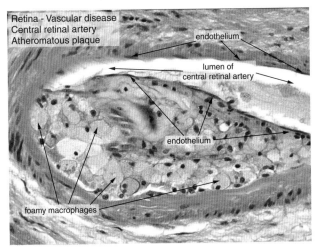

Figure 10.33

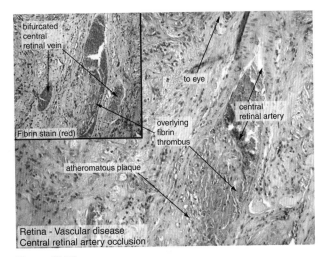

Figure 10.34

Figure 10.30 In retinopathy of prematurity (ROP), precise clinicopathological correlation between histopathology and indirect ophthalmoscopy has proved difficult. In this example from the retinal periphery in stage II–III, a cluster of endothelial cells resembling a renal glomerulus is present at the edge of the avascular and vascular zones. Behind this, there is a thick band of preretinal fibrovascular proliferation.

Figure 10.31 A branch retinal artery occlusion was chosen to illustrate the appearance in autopsy material of infarcted and non-infarcted tissue. With formalin fixation, the viable retina is grey and opaque. In the infarcted tissue, it is possible to see the underlying choroid.

Figure 10.32 Interruption of retinal arterial blood flow affects primarily the inner retinal layers. In an early example (upper), the outer plexiform layer (OPL) is vacuolated and is oedematous. The inner nuclear layer (INL) is markedly reduced in thickness and some of the cells may be microglial macrophages which remove necrotic tissue. In a late stage (lower), the inner retinal layers have vanished leaving only a thin line of residual nuclei in the INL. The photoreceptor (PR) layer, which is maintained by the choroidal circulation, is preserved. GCL = ganglion cell layer.

Figure 10.33 This is an example of an atheromatous plaque which consists of foamy macrophages lined by endothelium within the central retinal artery. Such plaques can arise *de novo* in the central retinal artery or may represent an atheromatous embolus from the internal carotid artery – it is not possible to make the distinction at this stage.

Figure 10.34 An organising thrombus in the central retinal artery contains fibrin which is best demonstrated by a special stain (Masson trichrome) as brick-red material (inset). The source is probably that of a thrombus arising on an atheromatous plaque. The bifurcated central retinal veins are patent (inset).

Central retinal artery occlusion (CRAO)/branch retinal artery occlusion (BRAO)

This is a rare condition where there is interruption in the blood supply to the retina by a thrombus or an embolus. In the case of CRAO, the artery is obstructed behind the lamina cribrosa. Obstruction of a branch arteriole can occur anywhere along the vascular bed.

Clinical presentation

A CRAO presents with unilateral sudden painless loss of vision and is more common in males.

Depending on the extent of vascular occlusion, there may be a relative afferent pupillary defect.

The retina is initially normal in appearance but gradually opacifies after several hours. The underlying choroidal vasculature beneath the macula may be visible ("cherry red spot"). The arterioles are attenuated. The opacified retina progressively resolves over 4–6 weeks and optic disc pallor ensues (in the case of CRAO).

Secondary neovascularisation (intraretinal or rubeosis iridis) may occur but is rare.

Further investigations with fundus fluorescein angiography and electrophysiology (ERG) may be necessary in atypical cases.

It is essential to investigate for primary causes of embolism and to include laboratory tests for giant cell arteritis and systemic vascular disease.

The sector of infarcted retina to occlusion of a branch retinal artery is initially opaque but later becomes atrophic.

Pathogenesis

Atheromatous or thrombotic emboli are the commonest causes of occlusion.

Possible modes of treatment

1 *Acute:* controversial but involves decompression of globe, anticoagulation, steroid therapy, and locoregional fibrinolysis.
2 *Chronic:* treatment of secondary retinal neovascularisation and neovascular glaucoma.

Macroscopic

Enucleation specimens, autopsy, or surgery for neovascular glaucoma in CRAO/BRAO are rare. In autopsy material, the appearances are never as striking as those seen *in vivo*. A BRAO in a well demarcated area of infarction that can be distinguished from the non-ischaemic tissue is shown in Figure 10.31.

Microscopic

Retina Initially, the inner layers of the retina are oedematous and this is followed by a total atrophy of the inner retinal layers as far as the inner nuclear layer (Figure 10.32).

Central retinal vessels Occasionally, it is possible to identify an atheromatous embolus in the central retinal artery (Figure 10.33) or an organising thrombus (Figure 10.34).

Central retinal vein occlusion (CRVO)/branch retinal vein occlusion (BRVO)

Retinal venous occlusive disease is relatively common, with incidence rising with age. CRVOs are subdivided into ischaemic and non-ischaemic groups; the latter patients have a better visual prognosis. BRVOs usually originate at the sites of arteriovenous crossings. Ischaemic central retinal venous disease is more commonly encountered by the pathologist and will form the main basis of the following description.

Clinical presentation

Painless loss of vision in the acute event – this is almost always unilateral. A relative afferent pupillary defect may be present. Late presentations may be in the form of neovascular glaucoma.

Fundus examination reveals dilated tortuous veins, intraretinal haemorrhages, macular and retinal oedema, microinfarcts (cotton wool spots), and optic disc swelling. Neovascularisation within and on the surface of the retina can lead to tractional retinal detachment.

Regular follow-up, including gonioscopy of the angle for neovascularisation in ischaemic cases of CRVO, is essential.

Further investigations with a fluorescein angiogram (to determine the extent of ischaemia) and electrophysiology may be necessary.

It is important to consider the following associated disorders:
1 Ocular associations: open angle glaucoma.
2 Systemic associations: diabetes, hypertension, serum hyperlipidaemia, and hyperviscosity syndromes.

Pathogenesis

The precise nature is unknown as investigation of CRV pathology is limited to end-stage disease. At this stage, evidence of CRA and arteriolar occlusive degenerative disease is present so that underperfusion and venous stasis could initiate thrombus formation in the vein within or behind the lamina cribrosa. The normal vein narrows within the lamina cribrosa and two of the criteria for thrombus formation are fulfilled – stasis and turbulence. The thrombosed vein is recanalised later and collaterals within the optic nerve head open so that some blood flow is re-established. The haemorrhages are eventually cleared from the retina by macrophages.

In the case of BRVO, disease of the adjacent arterial wall may be responsible for compression of the venous wall at the AV crossing.

Possible modes of treatment

Treatment of glaucoma and any underlying medical disorders are essential.

Panretinal photocoagulation (PRP) for neovascularisation has markedly reduced the incidence of enucleation. Macular oedema generally does not respond well to grid laser therapy.

Macroscopic

The pathological appearances of the retina and vitreous following CRVO vary quite markedly depending on the extent of haemorrhage and the interval between the acute event and enucleation. Haemorrhage within the retina can vary from the small dot blot varieties (Figures 10.35, 10.36) to massive involvement (Figure 10.37), often with evidence of longstanding glaucoma.

Retinal neovascularisation often follows an ischaemic vein occlusion. Preretinal neovascular fronds arise in the walls of hyalinised blood vessels and spread across the posterior hyaloid face to form sheets or nodules (Figure 10.38). Bleeding from these vessels into the vitreous produces complicated fibrovascular proliferations depending on the state of organisation of the blood (Figures 10.39, 10.40).

Microscopic – retina

Acute stage Haemorrhage follows the patterns described previously (Figure 10.13, 10.41), but is mainly restricted to the inner retinal layers. Resolution of a massive retinal haemorrhage leads to deposition of haemosiderin within a gliotic retina (Figure 10.42).

Late stage Ischaemia of the inner retinal layers stimulates vasoproliferation with the release of VEGF and other vasoformative factors. Endothelial cell proliferation can take the form of small capillary buds within and on the surface of the retina (Figure 10.43). Commonly, the endothelial cell proliferation arises in the walls of hyalinised blood vessels (Figures 10.44, 10.45). Progression of the ischaemia and endothelial cell damage result in the formation of lipoproteinaceous (hard) exudates and microcysts in the posterior retina. Ultimately, contraction of the fibrovascular membranes distorts the retina with progression to tractional retinal detachment (Figure 10.46).

Microscopic – central retinal vein within the optic nerve

The opportunity to study the central retinal vein in the initial occlusion has arisen only rarely in autopsy material. Thrombus formation occurs in the vein at the level of or behind the lamina cribrosa. The thrombosed vessel becomes recanalised and this is the usual appearance by the time a surgical enucleation becomes necessary (Figure 10.47).

Pathological evidence of treatment

There may be evidence of panretinal photocoagulation (Figure 10.48) and surgery to treat neovascular glaucoma.

Diabetes

Although diabetes is a metabolic disorder, involvement of the eye has the characteristics of a vascular disease. Previously, diabetic eye disease was one of the commoner conditions submitted to the pathologist. Effective screening, metabolic control, and prompt treatment with panretinal laser photocoagulation have reduced the incidence of enucleation. Nonetheless, the topic is dealt with in detail owing to the increasing prevalence of the disorder and the implications for clinical practice.

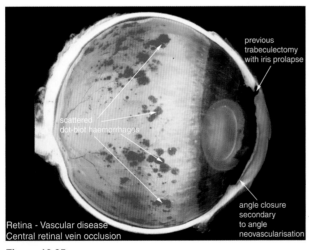

Figure 10.35

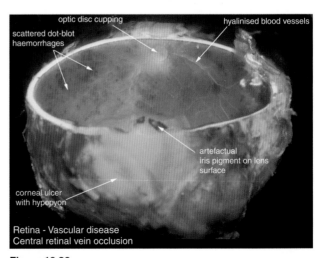

Figure 10.36

Figure 10.35 Pathological experience in central retinal vein occlusion is most commonly obtained from globes which are enucleated for intractable neovascular glaucoma. In this case, an iris prolapse is an indication of failed glaucoma surgery. Many of the original retinal haemorrhages have resolved, with those remaining confined to dots and blots in the mid-periphery.

Figure 10.36 Corneal decompensation with ulcerative keratitis is a common sequel to end-stage neovascular glaucoma in ischaemic central retinal vein occlusion. In this example, the disc is cupped and, as is often the case, the retinal vessels are hyalinised. Most of the haemorrhage has resolved leaving sparse dots and blots.

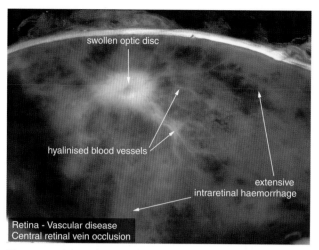

Figure 10.37

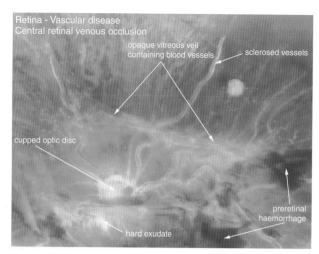

Figure 10.38

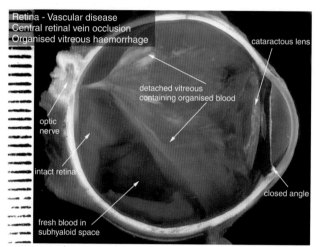

Figure 10.39

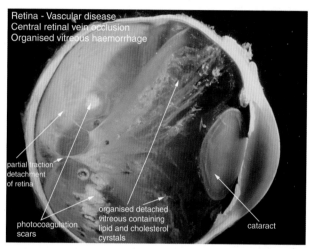

Figure 10.40

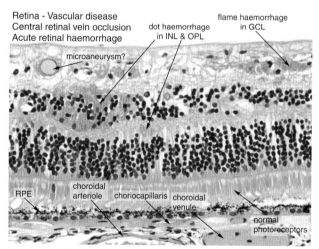

Figure 10.41

Figure 10.37 In this example of central retinal vein occlusion, the haemorrhage is so massive as to involve the entire retina. Again, the retinal vessels are sclerotic.

Figure 10.38 In the fundus at a later stage of ischaemic central retinal vein occlusion, intraretinal haemorrhage clears and neovascularisation dominates the picture. Further bleeding from preretinal neovascularisation is present. The retinal vessels are sclerosed to an advanced degree.

Figure 10.39 At a late stage in the pathology of untreated ischaemic central retinal vein occlusion, it is common to see massive bleeding into the vitreous from preretinal neovascularisation. In this specimen, there were two phases of haemorrhage – the first was into the vitreous, and at this stage there was early organisation which has led to vitreous detachment, and the second was a recent haemorrhage in the subhyaloid space

Figure 10.40 In the vitreous, blood eventually clears to leave behind lipid and cholesterol deposits. Pale white areas in the retina indicate photocoagulation, which was probably limited due to the late presentation of the patient with obscuration by the opaque vitreous. This eye was enucleated due to intractable pain from neovascular glaucoma.

Figure 10.41 In a recent retinal vein occlusion, the outer retina and choroid are preserved and haemorrhages are present in the nerve fibre layer, ganglion cell layer (GCL), inner nuclear layer (INL), and outer plexiform layer (OPL). RPE = retinal pigment epithelium.

Retina - Vascular disease
Central retinal vein occlusion
Resolving haemorrhage

Prussian blue stain

iron deposits in gliotic
inner retina

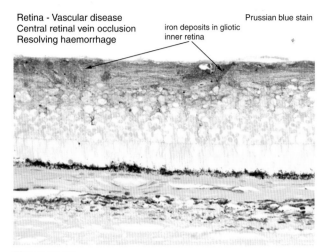

Figure 10.42

proliferating endothelial
cells within retina

ILM

tuft of preretinal
endothelial cells

gliotic
inner retina

feeder vessel

artefactual
cleft

Retina - Vascular disease
Central retinal vein occlusion
Early neovascularisation

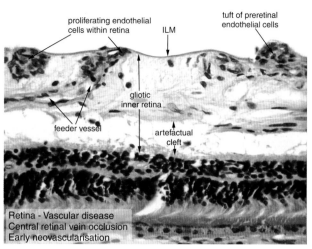

Figure 10.43

Retina - Vascular disease
Central retinal vein occlusion
Late stage / Neovascularisation

vitreous

fibrovascular membrane
on inner surface of retina

proliferating endothelial
cells within retina

gliotic inner retina

hyalinised feeder vessel

cyst

artefactual cleft in
photoreceptor layer

lipoproteinacious
(hard) exudates

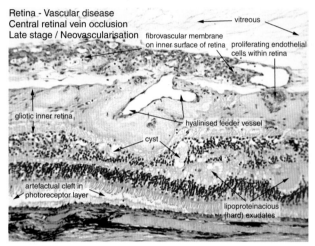

Figure 10.44

Retina - Vascular disease
Central retinal vein occlusion
Late stage / Neovascularisation

tree-like proliferation
of fibrovascular tissue
within the vitreous

vitreous strands

retinal cysts containing
exudates in OPL layer

hyalinised
feeder vessel

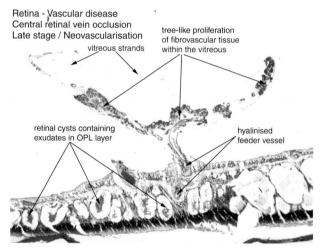

Figure 10.45

Retina - Vascular disease
Central retinal vein occlusion
Neovascularisation of optic disc

blood vessels in organised vitreous

hyalinised blood vessels

cyst formation in outer retinal layer

subretinal
exudate

reactionary
proliferation
of RPE

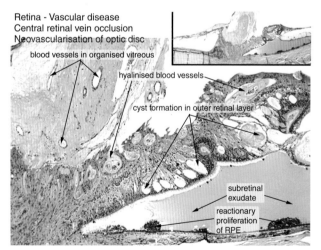

Figure 10.46

Figure 10.42 The red cells break down leaving haemosiderin, which stains positively for iron salts (Prussian blue stain). At this stage, there is atrophy and gliosis of the inner retina. The magnifications are identical in Figures 10.41 and 10.42 – compare the relative thickness of the inner retina in each.

Figure 10.43 Early neovascularisation within an ischaemic retina is manifest as buds of proliferating endothelial cells arising in the walls of blood vessels. ILM = inner limiting membrane.

Figure 10.44 In elderly patients following ischaemic central retinal vein occlusion, fibrovascular membranes arise from hyalinised feeder vessels (venules and arterioles). This fibrovascular membrane appears to extend into the subhyaloid space between the inner limiting membrane and the posterior vitreous face.

Figure 10.45 The detached vitreous can form a scaffold for the proliferating fibrovascular tissue so that a tree-like configuration is adopted. In this end-stage central retinal vein occlusion, there is extensive cyst formation in the outer plexiform layer (OPL). The inner retina is atrophic but in this and the above examples, the photoreceptor layer is preserved.

Figure 10.46 In many pathological specimens in central retinal vein occlusion, neovascularisation of the optic disc is a major feature. In this example there is tractional retinal detachment at the peripapillary retina accompanied by subretinal exudation. The disorganised cystic retina contains hyalinised blood vessels. Atrophy of the photoreceptors and proliferation of the retinal pigment epithelium (RPE) provides evidence of prolonged retinal detachment. The inset shows a low magnification of the optic nerve head and peripapillary retina.

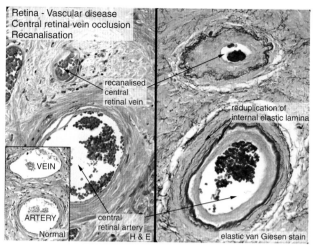

Figure 10.47

Figure 10.47 Transverse sections behind the lamina cribrosa in a late stage central retinal vein occlusion reveal a recanalised central retinal vein. The original vein wall is highlighted by a stain for the internal elastic lamina (right). The central retinal artery is recognisable by the smooth muscle cells in the vessel wall. Because such patients are elderly, the artery often shows reduplication of the internal elastic lamina. The inset shows the relative dimensions of the normal central retinal vessels.

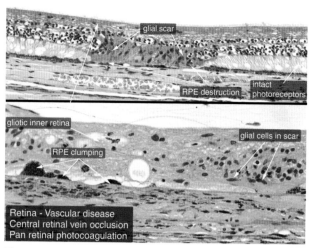

Figure 10.48

Figure 10.48 Evidence of photocoagulation is often obtained in cases of neovascularisation in central retinal vein occlusion (and diabetic retinopathy, see below). These appear as sectors of outer retinal destruction (upper) or total retinal destruction (lower) depending on the energy level and wavelength employed. Müller cells are thought to be the source of the glial cells in the scars: these cells have large irregular nuclei.

Clinical presentation

Diabetes may involve many ocular tissues and the cranial nerves:

1 *Cornea:* recurrent surface erosions secondary to decreased sensitivity and reduced epithelial adhesion to the underlying basement membrane.

2 *Glaucoma:* increased incidence of primary open angle glaucoma and neovascular glaucoma.

3 *Lens:* earlier onset of cataract (subcapsular). NB: An acute elevation in the blood glucose level may give rise to a temporary cataract.

4 *Optic neuropathy:* acute disc oedema can occur in young diabetics. A subclinical optic neuropathy may be evident in visual-evoked potential studies.

5 *Cranial neuropathy:* neuropathy involving cranial nerves (CN) III, IV, and VI may result in an extraocular muscle palsy. This condition is due to a localised infarction in the surrounding myelin sheath (mononeuritis multiplex). In cases involving CN III, there may be sparing of the pupillary reflex.

6 *Retinopathy:* this is the most significant ocular pathology and is classified in four stages:
   (a) *Early non-proliferative diabetic retinopathy (NPDR):* microaneurysms, dot blot haemorrhages, and hard exudates. Macular oedema may occur at any stage of retinopathy, and when hard exudates and cyst formation occur there is a sharp decrease in visual acuity.
   (b) *Moderate NPDR:* as above plus cotton wool spots, venous beading, or loops.
   (c) *Severe NPDR:* as above with four quadrants of intraretinal haemorrhages, two quadrants of venous beading, or one quadrant of intraretinal microvascular abnormalities (IRMA). The features of IRMA are flat retinal neovascularisations with absence of leakage on fluorescein angiography.
   (d) *Proliferative diabetic retinopathy:* as above with neovascularisation of the disc (NVD) or elsewhere (NVE). The preretinal fibrovascular tissue may result in tractional retinal detachment or vitreal haemorrhage. Secondary glaucoma may occur with neovascularisation of the angle (NVA) or iris (NVI).

Further investigations will include fluorescein angiography to determine areas of capillary non-perfusion, neovascularisation and exudation.

In the differential diagnosis, CRVO (which may be secondary to diabetes), radiation retinopathy, and hypertension should be considered.

Pathogenesis

The incidence and severity of diabetic eye disease is dependent upon the following factors:

1 Duration of condition post puberty.

2 Degree of metabolic control – good control delays the onset and decreases the severity of the disease.

3 Other exacerbating factors: pregnancy, hypertension, hyperlipidaemia, cigarette smoking, and renal disease.

Diabetes affects the retinal vasculature in several ways. The arterioles undergo degenerative changes with sclerosis (luminal narrowing and reduction in blood flow) and there is also arteriolar occlusion, both of which lead to patchy areas of non-perfusion. The precise mechanism of vascular occlusion is not understood.

Metabolic disturbances selectively affect the capillary pericytes (see below).

The most important results of the diabetic vasculopathy are exudation and neovascularisation. The latter leads to vitreous haemorrhage, vitreous traction, and retinal detachment.

The abnormal metabolic pathways in the development of diabetic retinopathy are poorly understood, as exhibited by the various theories of pathogenesis:

1 *Vasoproliferative factors:* release of VEGF from the hypoxic retina has been theorised to be the stimulant for neovascularisation. This theory has formed the basis of panretinal photocoagulation which attempts to control the level of VEGF by the destruction of ischaemic cells. There is currently much interest in the development of agents that may suppress the effects of VEGF.

2 *Aldose reductase:* an intracellular enzyme which converts sugars to alcohol and is found in high quantities in lens epithelium, pericytes, and Schwann cells. The increased glucose load in diabetes may damage pericytes, leading ultimately to cell death.

3 *Growth hormone:* remission has been obtained in patients subjected to hypophysectomy, but this procedure has been abandoned due to a high mortality.

4 *Platelets and blood viscosity:* altered platelet adhesion characteristics may cause focal capillary occlusion and retinal ischaemia.

5 *Apoptosis:* large fluctuations in blood glucose levels cause pericyte death *in vitro.*

6 *Autoimmune disease:* levels of circulating antibodies to pericytes are raised in patients with diabetes.

Possible modes of treatment

1 *Prophylaxis:* careful metabolic control.

2 *Treatment:* timely argon laser panretinal photocoagulation for proliferative disease. Clinically significant macular oedema is treated with focal/grid argon laser therapy. Vitreoretinal surgery is employed for persistent vitreous haemorrhage, removal of epiretinal membranes, and for tractional retinal detachment.

Cataract surgery is performed if required.

Macroscopic

Most of the specimens submitted to the pathologist are globes complicated by extensive treatment for neovascular glaucoma or tractional retinal detachment. In many specimens, the effects of diabetic retinopathy (Figure 10.49) resemble those illustrated in CRVO, and indeed CRVO may be an accompaniment. In diabetes, there is, however, a greater tendency to leakage of lipoproteinaceous exudate, which may be predominant (Figure 10.50). The macula is especially prone to oedema and exudation (Figure 10.51). Venous congestion with preretinal traction of dilated vessels into the vitreous (omega loops) is an uncommon pathological finding (Figure 10.52).

It is now more frequent to perform a vitrectomy or membrane peel procedure for sight-threatening cases of tractional retinal detachment or epiretinal membrane formation.

Microscopic

Non-specific features These are secondary to focal arteriolar ischaemia, for example microinfarction, haemorrhage (see above), and neovascularisation.

Microaneurysms Microaneurysms located in the posterior pole are characteristic of diabetes. These are easily identified clinically and by fluorescein angiography but only with difficulty in routine paraffin sections (Figure 10.53). Previously, retinal digest preparations were useful in demonstrating the distribution of microaneurysms and changes in the relative density of the endothelial cells and pericytes (Figure 10.54). There is a preferential loss of pericytes in diabetes, although some capillaries are totally acellular (Figures 10.55, 10.56).

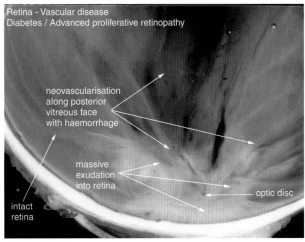

Figure 10.49

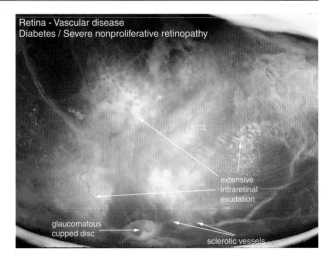

Figure 10.50

Figure 10.49 Neovascularisation arising from the optic disc and penetrating the vitreous with secondary haemorrhage is common to central retinal vein occlusion and diabetes. The presence of massive exudation into the peripapillary retina is suggestive of a diabetic aetiology.

Figure 10.50 In some cases of severe exudative diabetic retinopathy, extensive areas of the retina contain yellow exudates.

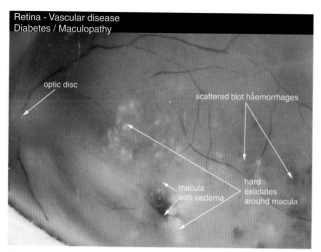

Figure 10.51

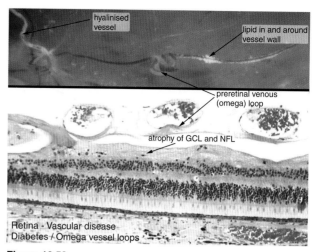

Figure 10.52

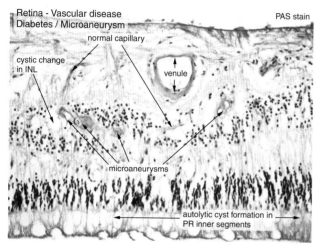

Figure 10.53

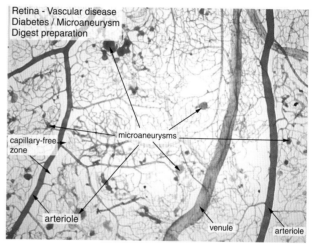

Figure 10.54

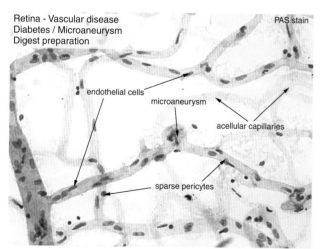

Figure 10.55

Figure 10.51 The macula is especially prone to the effects of exudation and oedema (it acts like a sponge) in diabetic retinopathy. In this autopsy specimen, some of the retinal opacification and thickening adjacent to the macula is due to autolysis and formalin fixation.

Figure 10.52 The macroscopic and microscopic appearances of one of the consequences of venous congestion in diabetic retinopathy. The enlarged vessels break through the inner limiting membrane and form loops into the vitreous (omega loops). The upper illustration also shows lipid around the wall of a sclerotic vessel (see Figure 10.57). GCL = ganglion cell layer, NFL = nerve fibre layer.

Figure 10.53 The retinal capillaries loop down into the inner nuclear layer (INL). In this diabetic retina, microaneurysms can be identified by their larger size in comparison with normal capillaries. The INL is disrupted, presumably due to leakage from the microaneurysms (autopsy material, PAS stain). PR = photoreceptor.

Figure 10.54 This is a retinal digest at low power to show the arterioles (thinner) and venules (thicker) with the intervening capillary network in a diabetic retina (PAS stain). Arterioles are identified by the relative absence of adjacent capillaries. Microaneurysms are scattered throughout the capillary bed. Compare with Figure 10.9 but note that the control tissue is from the peripheral retina where the capillary bed is sparser.

Figure 10.55 At an early stage in diabetic retinopathy, small microaneurysms form (possibly as capillary loops) and pericyte numbers are reduced by comparison with the normal endothelial cell density. Some of the capillaries are acellular. Compare with Figure 10.10.

Precapillary arteriolar disease Although microaneurysms and pericyte loss are pathognomonic of diabetes, it is important to appreciate that degenerative disease (hyalinisation, thrombus formation, and embolisation) in the precapillary arterioles contributes significantly to retinal ischaemia (Figure 10.57). Not all arterioles are affected to the same degree, which accounts for the patchy distribution of ischaemic damage.

Neovascularisation The vitreous forms a scaffold for preretinal neovascularisation. Separation and movement of the vitreous lead to vascular disruption and haemorrhage, which stimulates further fibrovascular proliferation. Subsequent fibrosis and contraction result in distortion of the retinal surface (Figure 10.58) and tractional retinal detachment (Figures 10.49, 10.59, 10.60). Membranes removed surgically in diabetic vasoproliferative retinopathy consist of a fibrous mass containing numerous capillaries (Figure 10.60). The absence of an inner limiting membrane on the surface of the optic disc gives free access for blood vessels to grow into the vitreous. The consequent distortion is identical to that seen in CRVO (Figure 10.46).

Diabetic maculopathy This abnormality is attributed to the fact that the capillaries, derived from the surrounding arteriolar arcades do not extend to the macula ("capillary free zone"). Diabetic vasculopathy in surrounding vessels (see above) results in leakage into the macula, a site where fluid resorption is ineffective due to avascularity. Hard exudate formation (Figure 10.61) is especially significant at the macula where intraretinal oedema and cyst formation are additional complications (Figure 10.62).

Specific features For the pathologist, a histological diagnosis of diabetic eye disease can be made by examination of the iris pigment epithelium and the basement membrane of the ciliary body.

1 *Iris:* the pigment epithelium is vacuolated and the cystic spaces contain PAS positive glycoprotein (Figures 10.63, 10.64).
2 *Ciliary body:* the basement membrane thickening is best recognised with a PAS stain (Figure 10.65).

Pathological evidence of treatment – laser burn pathology The appearances of the treated outer retina are identical to those seen in CRVO (Figure 10.48).

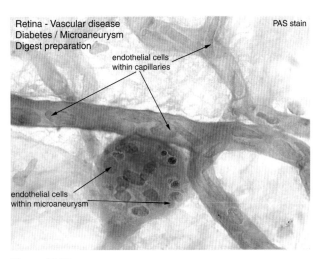

Figure 10.56

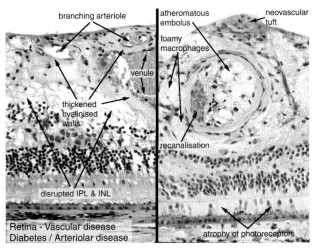

Figure 10.57

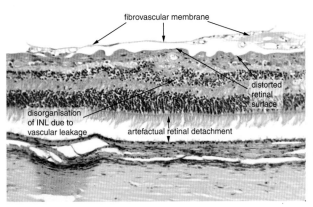

Figure 10.58

Figure 10.56 In the evolution of a microaneurysm, a sack-like "blowout" of the capillary is filled by endothelial cells. Later, the content is replaced by basement membrane material. In this advanced diabetic state, pericytes are not identified.

Figure 10.57 Two of the possible causes of retinal underperfusion are illustrated: (i) arteriolar walls become thickened (left) and there is potential damage to the lining endothelial cells which may predispose to thrombus formation; (ii) it is also possible that lipid emboli could occlude the vessel which later recanalises (right). The effect of ischaemia is seen at this stage as oedematous disruption of the inner nuclear layer (INL, left) and leakage of lipid into the surrounding retina (manifest as accumulation of foamy macrophages, right). The figure on the right was taken from an area of perivascular lipid exudation shown in Figure 10.52. IPL = inner plexiform layer.

Figure 10.58 Despite an innocuous appearance, contraction of a fibrovascular membrane on the retinal surface can lead to significant tissue distortion. In this diabetic retina, exudation from the hyalinised vessels in the centre of the image has led to leakage with disruption of the inner nuclear layer (INL). The apparent retinal detachment is an artefact – fragments of photoreceptor tips are present in the inner surface of the retinal pigment epithelium.

Retina - Vascular disease
Diabetes / Neovascularisation

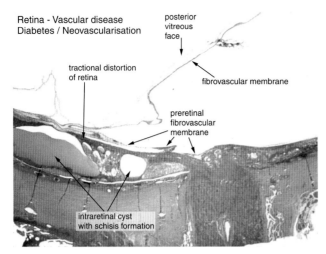

Figure 10.59

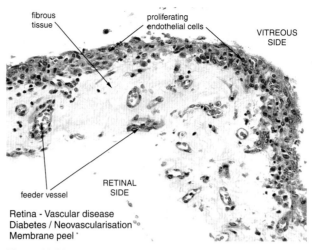

Retina - Vascular disease
Diabetes / Neovascularisation
Membrane peel

Figure 10.60

Retina - Vascular disease
Diabetes / Hard exudates

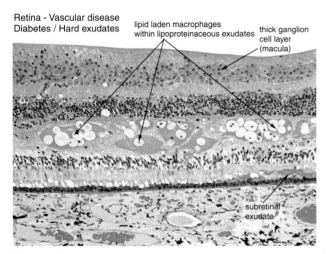

Figure 10.61

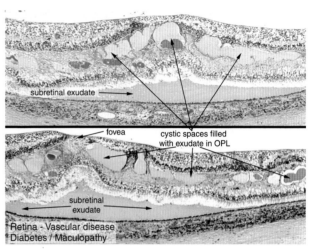

Retina - Vascular disease
Diabetes / Maculopathy

Figure 10.62

Iris - Vascular disease
Diabetes / Iridopathy

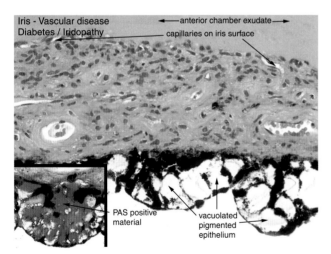

Figure 10.63

Figure 10.59 Gross distortion of the retina and disc occurs when fibrovascular tissue extends across the retinal surface and into the posterior vitreous face. Contraction of the tissue has led to secondary cyst formation and splitting of the outer plexiform layer (retinoschisis).

Figure 10.60 Vitreoretinal surgery is often employed to remove the tractional fibrovascular bands which are submitted for pathological examination. These specimens are formed by fibrovascular tissue and the inner aspect is lined by a hypercellular layer formed by proliferating endothelial cells and capillaries.

Figure 10.61 At an early stage of diabetic maculopathy, the inner retinal layers are preserved and the outer plexiform layer is disrupted by leakage of lipoproteinaceous exudate with subretinal extension. The lipoprotein has attracted macrophages which are identified by their large size, small nuclei, and clear or foamy cytoplasms.

Figure 10.62 In advanced diabetic maculopathy, there is extensive cystic degeneration in the outer plexiform layer (OPL) and secondary degeneration of the photoreceptors over a subfoveal proteinaceous exudate. The concentration of lipoprotein varies within the cysts – condensation in some cysts forms darker red structures. The upper and lower figures are taken at different levels through the macula.

Figure 10.63 Vacuolation of the iris pigment epithelium (diabetic iridopathy) is a well recognised feature of diabetes but the aetiology is poorly understood. The material within the vacuoles stains positively with PAS (inset). More importantly, the presence of a vascular membrane on the iris surface with loss of crypts indicates neovascularisation and implies the presence of neovascular glaucoma.

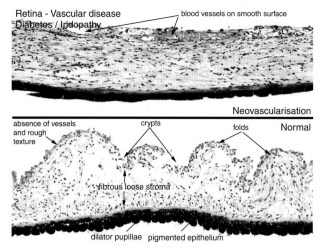

Figure 10.64

Figure 10.64 Very few cases of diabetic iridopathy show vacuolation of the pigment epithelium. In pathological material, in almost every case there will be a well developed fibrovascular membrane on the anterior surface (upper). Compare this with the crypts and loose stroma of a normal iris (lower).

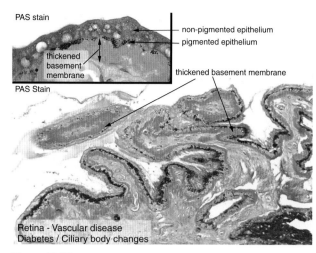

Figure 10.65

Figure 10.65 A thickened basement membrane beneath the epithelium of the ciliary processes is a pathognomonic feature of diabetes (PAS stain). The inset shows the membrane at a higher magnification.

Radiation

Radiation retinopathy is discussed in Chapter 9.

Sickle cell disease

Within the family of haemoglobinopathies, sickle cell disease is the most important in ophthalmology. This inherited condition results in the replacement of either one or both alleles of adult haemoglobin (Hb AA) by abnormal Hb S and/or C. Individuals of African origin are most commonly affected, and the resultant retinal pathology is a consequence of ischaemia. The pathogenesis is based on the decreased malleability of red cells under certain conditions (such as reduced oxygen tension) leading to microvascular occlusion. The patient is usually visually asymptomatic unless there is direct involvement of the macula or the visual axis.

Retinal pathology is most commonly seen clinically as macular ischaemia, peripheral vascular non-perfusion, and neovascularisation.

Severe complications are rare and an enucleation would be exceptional.

The five stages of proliferative sickle cell retinopathy are:
1 *Peripheral arteriolar occlusions:* characteristic retinal haemorrhages may be present:
   • black sunbursts: subretinal haemorrhage with disruption of the RPE layer located in the equator
   • salmon patches: intraretinal and preretinal haemorrhages with tracking along a retinal arteriole.
2 *Arteriolar–venular anastomoses.*
3 *Neovascular proliferation* ("sea fan appearance").
4 *Vitreous haemorrhage.*
5 *Retinal detachment.*

Dystrophies

Retinitis pigmentosa

The term "retinitis pigmentosa" (RP) is a misnomer in that the disease is a retinal dystrophy without evidence of inflammation. RP represents a group of inherited retinal disorders involving progressive dysfunction and death of photoreceptors (rods more than cones).

Clinical presentation

Typical RP is bilateral with symmetrical loss of rod photoreceptors. The following symptoms are common:
1 Nyctalopia: poor night vision with prolonged dark adaptation.
2 Loss of peripheral vision, which is explained by the fact that the density of rods is greater towards the periphery.
3 Loss of central vision at the final stage.
   Classic fundus findings are:
1 Bone spicules in the peripheral retina: there may be a preferential distribution to perivascular regions or to sectors of the retina; the degree of pigmentation varies among patients.
2 Retinal arteriolar attenuation.
3 Optic disc pallor.
4 Atrophy of RPE and choriocapillaris.
5 Vitreous cells in some cases.
   Other associated ocular findings are:
1 Maculopathy: cystoid macular oedema, epiretinal membrane formation, and/or macular atrophy.
2 Subcapsular cataract.

Management would include a full clinical work-up to confirm the diagnosis and, to identify the subgroups known to exist (see below for genetics), a careful family history is required. Visual field and electrophysiological investigations are useful, for example to show markedly reduced responses in affected rod photoreceptors. The following conditions are examples of disorders, which have a similar fundus appearance to classic RP and should be considered in the differential diagnosis:

1 Usher's syndrome: autosomal recessive associated with deafness.
2 Kearns–Sayre syndrome: a group of mitochondrial cytopathies associated with weakness of skeletal muscle.
3 Refsum's disease: skeletal abnormalities.
4 Hereditary abetalipoproteinaemia: fat intolerance and malabsorption resulting in fat-soluble vitamin (A and E) deficiency and neurological impairment.
5 Bardet–Biedl syndrome: polydactyly, obesity with short stature.

The reader should consult the clinical texts for a more extensive list.

Pathogenesis

The exact mechanisms of photoreceptor degeneration are unknown but the final pathway involves apoptosis of the rod photoreceptors with cone degeneration at a later stage. The RPE responds to photoreceptor atrophy by proliferation into the retina. The pigmented cells accumulate around atrophic retinal blood vessels, which explains the classical "bone-spicule" fundus appearance.

Genetics

Variants of RP are mostly inherited, with all forms represented (AD, AR, and X-linked). Isolated cases are usually attributable to autosomal recessive inheritance. Intensive research has been undertaken to identify genetic abnormalities in the different subgroups. The most significant are shown in Table 10.3.

Table 10.3 The most significant subgroups in retinal pigment epithelium.

Inheritance	Incidence	Prognosis	Commoner genetic mutations
Autosomal dominant (AD)	Commonest	Best	Rhodopsin mutation (3q) Peripherin gene (6p)
Autosomal recessive (AR)	Common	Medium	cGMP gate channels (4p) Rhodopsin mutation (3q)
X-linked (XL)	Rare	Worst	Xp 11 and Xp 21

Female carriers of X-linked disease may have patchy involvement of the retina due to random inactivation of one of the X chromosomes (Lyon hypothesis) and resultant cluster expression of RP.

Possible modes of treatment

There are no definitive treatments for RP. Systemic acetazolamide is often successful in treating selected cases of cystoid macular oedema. Intraocular surgery may be used to treat cataract and in certain cases of epiretinal membrane formation.

Dietary supplementation with vitamins A, E and other lipids (for example docosahexaenoic acid) have been recommended, but opinions and study results are varied, as are the potential side effects.

Macroscopic

RP sufferers are often willing to allow pathological examination of their eyes post mortem. The retina shows the typical perivascular bone spicule patterns with a variable degree and distribution of pigment clumping (Figures 10.66, 10.67).

Microscopic

From animal models, it is assumed that photoreceptor atrophy is the initial event and the study of human material suggests that this is also the case (Figure 10.68). The atrophic outer retina becomes gliotic and the hyperpigmented RPE migrates into the retina (Figure 10.69). The macula is often better preserved in pathological specimens (Figure 10.70), although there is marked loss of nuclei in the outer nuclear layer.

Degenerations

Central

Age-related macular degeneration (ARMD)

ARMD is the commonest cause of visual impairment in individuals aged over 50 years in developed countries. There are two variants: atrophic (dry) and neovascular (wet/exudative), with the latter being less common and accountable for more severe visual loss. Involvement is usually bilateral although there may be asymmetry in progression.

Clinical presentation

In both dry and wet forms, the disease may be detected in the following circumstances:
• Incidental finding and asymptomatic.
• Decreased visual acuity. The onset is usually gradual, although sudden loss implies haemorrhage from neovascular ARMD.
• Metamorphopsia. Distortions in the visual image – this is more common in the wet form.

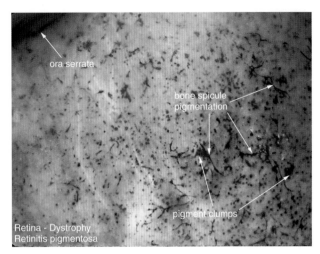

Figure 10.66

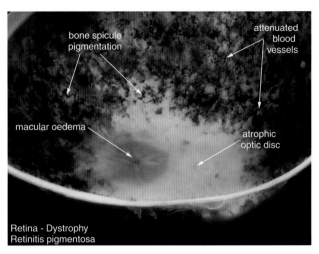

Figure 10.67

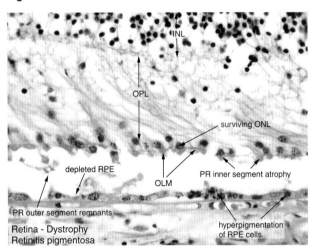

Figure 10.68

Retina - Dystrophy
Retinitis pigmentosa

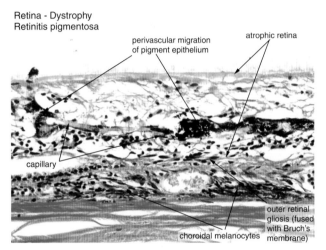

Figure 10.69

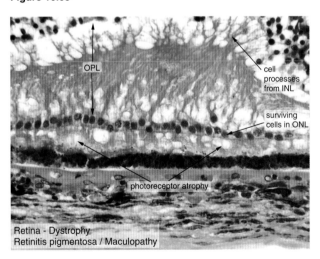

Figure 10.70

Figure 10.66 The atrophic retinal periphery in retinitis pigmentosa contains numerous retinal pigment epithelium clumps. The retinal vessels are surrounded by retinal pigment epithelial cells. The radiating appearance of the perivascular pigmented tissue resembles the osteocyte canaliculae in bone, hence the term "bone spicule".

Figure 10.67 The pigmentary disturbance progresses from the periphery towards the flat white atrophic disc but the macula is spared. However, there is maculopathy in the form of oedema.

Figure 10.68 At the stage when the pathologist has the opportunity to study retinitis pigmentosa, atrophy of the outer nuclear layer (ONL) is advanced with a residue of inner segments beneath the outer limiting membrane (OLM) of the retina. Hyperpigmentation of the retinal pigment epithelium (RPE) is patchy. INL = inner nuclear layer, OPL = outer plexiform layer, PR = photoreceptor.

Figure 10.69 Migration of hyperpigmented retinal pigment epithelial cells into the retina, particularly around blood vessels, is a characteristic feature of retinitis pigmentosa. In this example, gliosis has resulted in fusion between the retina and Bruch's membrane. Inner retinal atrophy is advanced.

Figure 10.70 The photoreceptor layer is best preserved at the macula although the density of nuclei is reduced markedly. In this example the retinal pigment epithelium is heavily pigmented but there is no evidence of migration into the avascular macula. (Abbreviations as in Figure 10.68.)

Appearance of the macula

1 *Atrophic ARMD:* geographic atrophy characterised by pale areas of patchy loss of the RPE. These areas may grow in size and coalesce.

2 *Exudative ARMD:* characterised by the presence of a subretinal neovascular membrane. There may be associated subretinal exudation, haemorrhage, or a fibrovascular (disciform) scar. The haemorrhage may track through the retina into the vitreous. Pigmented epithelial detachment (PED) may develop in subretinal neovascularisation with serous exudate or haemorrhage.

Associated findings

1 Drusen – subretinal pale areas are either small and discrete (hard) or are larger with indistinct edges (soft).

2 Irregular pigment hyperpigmentation (clumping).

Investigations may include the usage of fluorescein and indocyanine green angiography to diagnose and ascertain the severity of subretinal neovascularisation.

Aetiology and pathogenesis

Multiple aetiologies have been implicated including choroidal arteriosclerosis, oxidative stress, diet, inflammation, and genetics for both dry and wet forms of ARMD. Much interest has also centred on changes in Bruch's membrane (for example calcification and lipid accumulation) which could interfere with metabolism of the RPE cells.

The various pathological features of ARMD are introduced by means of diagrams (Figures 10.71–10.75).

Atrophic ARMD may involve choroidal sclerosis and obliteration of the choriocapillaris that could explain total photoreceptor atrophy (Figure 10.71).

Cigarette smoking and hypertension are risks factors for the development of neovascular ARMD.

The following deposits between Bruch's membrane and the retinal pigment epithelium are *commonly* found in ARMD.

1 *Hard drusen* are easily identified clinically as tiny, discrete, non-pigmented elevations beneath the retina between the *basement membrane and Bruch's membrane*, but are not considered to be precursors of neovascularisation (Figure 10.72).

2 *Soft drusen* possess indistinct borders and may be more easily identified with fluorescein angiography (Figure 10.73). These structures are located between the *cell basement membrane and Bruch's membrane* and are implicated in the attraction of blood vessels beneath the RPE (choroidal/subretinal neovascularisation).

3 A third deposit has been variously termed basal linear/basal laminar/basement membrane deposit (Figure 10.74). This material is located between the *cell membrane and the basement membrane* and is so thin that it can be difficult to identify clinically. This deposit is often found in relation to neovascular tissue proliferating beneath the macula.

Some authors use the term "basal linear deposit" as synonymous with confluent soft drusen which adds to confusion in the literature. For the purposes of this text, the terms "soft drusen" and "basement membrane deposit" are preferred.

Soft drusen and the basement membrane deposit stimulate cellular infiltration between Bruch's membrane and the RPE, and are therefore presumed to be the precursors of neovascular ARMD (Figure 10.75).

Neovascular ARMD (subretinal neovascular membrane – SRNVM) occurs after Bruch's membrane is penetrated by capillaries beneath the RPE (type 1 SRNVM). Plasma leakage and bleeding lead to progression of the RPE detachment and to rupture of the monolayer. Bleeding and neovascularisation then occur in the subretinal space (type 2 SRNVM).

Genetics

Unclear, although ARMD appears to favour white races, and family clusters can exist.

Retina - Central degeneration
ARMD
Dry/Geographic atrophy

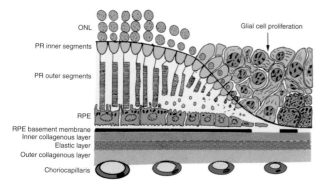

Figure 10.71

Figure 10.71 Diagram based on ultrastructural features. In atrophic age-related macular degeneration (ARMD), for reasons unknown, the photoreceptor layer in the macula disappears, and is replaced by glial tissue. The edge of the area of atrophy is sharply demarcated. The choroidal vessels and the choriocapillaris are atrophic in some cases. (Abbreviations as in Figure 10.68.)

Retina - Central degeneration
ARMD
Deposits - Hard drusen

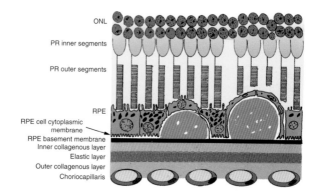

Figure 10.72

Figure 10.72 Diagram based on ultrastructural features. Hard drusen project as round or ovoid masses into the retinal pigment epithelium which becomes atrophic. The overlying photoreceptor outer segments are reduced in height but the adjacent photoreceptors are unaffected. (Abbreviations as in Figure 10.68.)

Possible modes of treatment

Prophylaxis and definitive treatment are not available for atrophic ARMD.

The argon laser is the only clinically proven treatment used to photoablate well demarcated subretinal neovascularisation (the reader should consult clinical texts with reference to the findings of the Macular Photocoagulation Study).

Other treatments with limited success include photodynamic therapy (PDT) and macular surgery.

Recurrence of neovascularisation is a problem with all current therapy. Preventative measures using dietary supplements such as zinc and fat-soluble vitamins have been suggested but much controversy exists.

Macroscopic and microscopic

ARMD is a common finding in elderly eyes enucleated for other conditions. Appearances vary according to progression of the disease and depend on whether the disease takes the form of dry atrophic or wet exudative ARMD.

NB: In the microscopic examination of a globe, location of abnormalities within the macular region can be confirmed by a thickened ganglion cell layer and the presence of the inferior oblique muscle on the adjacent sclera.

1 *Atrophic ARMD:* a well demarcated area of depigmentation is seen at the macula. The depigmented oval areas have a petaloid pattern and are surrounded by a rim of hyperpigmentation (Figure 10.76). At the histological level, there is total atrophy of the outer retina in the region of the fovea (Figure 10.77). Hard drusen (Figures 10.78, 10.79) are not a significant aetiological factor in dry ARMD and are commonly present throughout all ageing retinae.

2 *Exudative ARMD precursors:*
(a) *Soft drusen* (Figure 10.80) can be recognised by irregular tapering edges and a fluffy eosinophilic content.
(b) *Basement membrane deposits* (other names: basal linear, basal laminar – see above for explanation) are different to soft drusen in their location, staining characteristics, and ultrastructural appearance. The deposits form broad strips beneath the RPE and have a striated pattern (Figures 10.81–10.83).

3 *Exudative ARMD:* at the early stage, small capillaries are present between the RPE and Bruch's membrane (Figure 10.84). This abnormality is referred to as a type 1 SRNVM and progression takes the form of an established fibrovascular membrane in which arterioles and venules can be identified. A vicious circle arises when the small capillaries leak or burst with further inflammation and fibrovascular repair. Subsequently, interference with photoreceptor metabolism is followed by atrophy and degeneration of the outer retina (Figure 10.85).

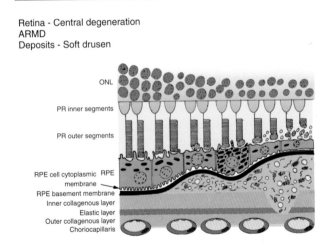

Retina - Central degeneration
ARMD
Deposits - Soft drusen

Figure 10.73

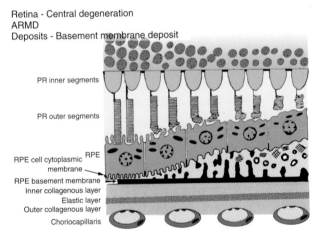

Retina - Central degeneration
ARMD
Deposits - Basement membrane deposit

Figure 10.74

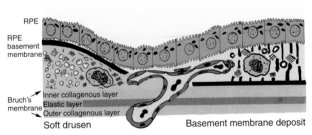

Retina - Central degeneration
ARMD - Wet/Neovascular
Sub-RPE (Type I)

Figure 10.75

Figure 10.73 Diagram based on ultrastructural features. The term soft drusen is used to describe the accumulation of what appears to be cell debris between the basement membrane of the retinal pigment epithelium and the inner collagenous layer. Compared with hard drusen, the area affected is wider and the photoreceptor outer segments are more severely affected. (Abbreviations as in Figure 10.68.)

Figure 10.74 Diagram based on ultrastructural features. Basement membrane deposit differs from soft drusen because the accumulating material is between the basal cytoplasmic membrane and the basement membrane of the retinal pigment epithelium (RPE) cells. One component takes the form of linear strands identical to the basement membrane, and the other component is cellular debris, presumably secreted by the RPE. PR = photoreceptor.

Figure 10.75 Diagram based on ultrastructural features. The presence of cell debris (in the case of soft drusen and basement membrane deposits) beneath the retinal pigment epithelium (RPE) appears to act as a chemoattractant for macrophages which, in turn, stimulate fibrovascular ingrowth. This initiates a vicious circle of plasma leakage, haemorrhage, and further neovascularisation.

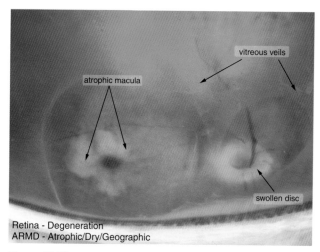

Figure 10.76

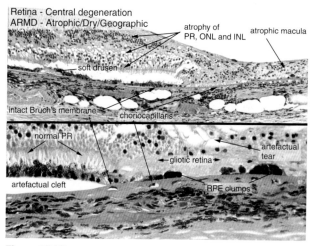

Figure 10.77

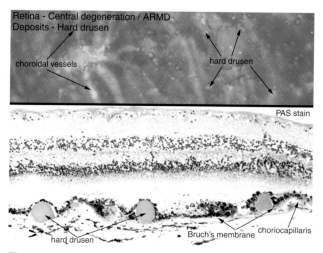

Figure 10.78

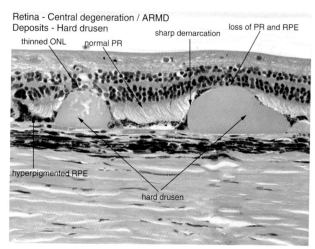

Figure 10.79

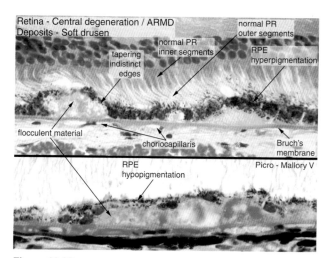

Figure 10.80

Figure 10.76 A corneal donor eye by chance was found to have a typical petaloid area of atrophic age-related macular degeneration (ARMD). Coincidentally the disc was swollen (cause unknown) and the vitreous contained veils.

Figure 10.77 This is a chance finding of atrophic (dry/areolar) age-related macular degeneration (ARMD) in a surgical enucleation for glaucoma – note the inner retinal atrophy (upper). In atrophic ARMD, the central macular region becomes completely atrophic and gliotic, and this is sharply demarcated from the adjacent normal outer retina (lower). In the atrophic region, the gliotic retina fuses with Bruch's membrane and residual retinal pigment epithelium cells are hyperplastic (lower). In this specimen, the choriocapillaris appears to be patent but the vessels are small – ischaemia is one of the proposed pathogenetic mechanisms. (Abbreviations as in Figure 10.68.)

Figure 10.78 In autopsy material it is possible to strip off the retina to expose the underlying hard drusen, which appear as small, discrete, pale areas (upper). A PAS stain demonstrates the glycoprotein within small hard drusen beneath the macula with relative sparing of the photoreceptor layer (lower). The apparent overlying retinal detachment is artefactual due to autolysis.

Figure 10.79 Hard drusen are also present in the peripheral retina. As they increase in size, there is more focal damage to the outer retina. Note the homogeneous pink appearance with sharp edges in comparison with soft drusen (see below). (Abbreviations as in Figure 10.68.)

Figure 10.80 Soft drusen appear as elevations of the retinal pigment epithelium (RPE) over dome-shaped spaces containing flocculent material (upper). The RPE may be hypo- or hyperpigmented. The edges are indistinct in comparison to hard drusen. The Picro-Mallory V stain (lower) demonstrates a pink appearance within the soft drusen compared with the blue appearance of basement membrane deposit (see below). PR = photoreceptor.

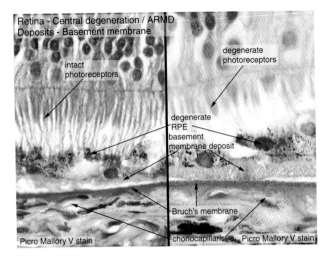

Figure 10.81

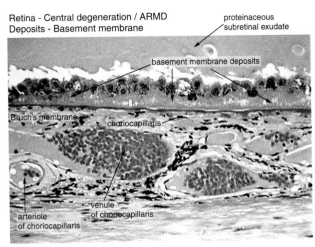

Figure 10.82

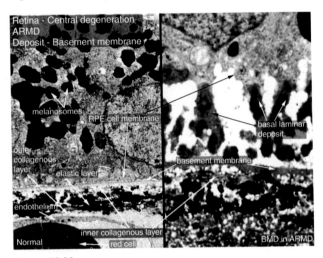

Figure 10.83

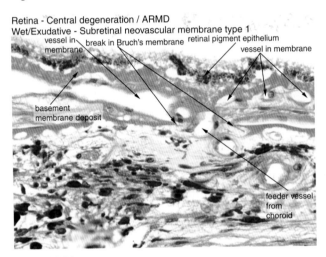

Figure 10.84

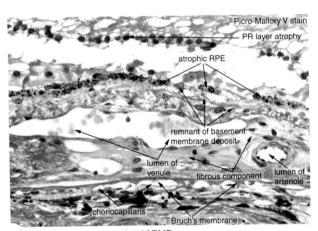

Retina - Central degeneration / ARMD
Wet/Exudative - Subretinal neovascular membrane type 1

Figure 10.85

Figure 10.81 Basement membrane deposit (BMD) is best identified with a special stain (Picro-Mallory V). The deposit is blue and appears striated and the overlying retinal pigment epithelium (RPE) is degenerate. This is associated with degeneration of photoreceptors. On the left, the BMD is thin and the photoreceptors are preserved. On the right, the deposit is thick and the photoreceptors are atrophic.

Figure 10.82 Advanced basement membrane deposits have a striated appearance in light microscopy. In this example, the retinal pigment epithelium cells are swollen beneath a proteinaceous subretinal exudate.

Figure 10.83 By electron microscopy, the "spiky" appearance of the basement membrane deposit (BMD) is apparent between the cell membrane of the retinal pigment epithelium and the basement membrane (right). The left figure is that of the normal appearance in a young individual for comparison.

Figure 10.84 In the early stages of neovascular age-related macular degeneration (ARMD), fibrovascular tissue is located between the retinal pigment epithelium and Bruch's membrane. In many cases, it is possible to identify basement membrane deposit beneath the retinal pigment epithelium.

Figure 10.85 Organisation of the subretinal pigment epithelial fibrovascular membrane (subretinal neovascular membrane type 1) which contains arterioles and venules is associated with atrophy of the overlying photoreceptor (PR) layer (Picro-Mallory V stain).

A type 2 subretinal neovascular membrane in exudative ARMD refers to an extension of fibrovascular proliferation between the RPE and the neural retina (subretinal space). This potential space provides an easy extension of haemorrhage from the fragile capillaries (Figure 10.86). Continuing leakage and haemorrhage from the capillaries lead to large submacular fibrous scars (Figure 10.87). This is termed a *disciform scar*. Continuous subretinal traction may lead to retinal distortion and rupture of the retina and its blood vessels may be followed by bleeding into the vitreous.

Haemorrhage may be complicated by a massive retinal detachment (Figure 10.88) which, in the past, has lead to enucleation because the subretinal mass simulated a melanoma (Figure 10.89).

Submacular surgery

It is increasingly frequent for a pathologist to receive specimens from submacular surgery for assumed subretinal neovascularisation. It is a common understanding that the removal of type 2 membranes has a better prognosis than type 1. Histology of excised membranes reveals fibrovascular tissue lined by RPE cells or containing strips of RPE cells (Figure 10.90).

Differential diagnosis of subretinal neovascularisation in ARMD

1 Trauma (civil or iatrogenic including overzealous panretinal photocoagulation).
2 Presumed ocular histoplasmosis syndrome (POHS).
3 High myopia (see below).
4 Angioid streaks.
5 Any condition that disrupts Bruch's membrane or the retinal pigment epithelium can potentially lead to subretinal neovascularisation (Figure 10.91).

Epiretinal membrane

Other names: cellophane maculopathy, macular pucker, premacular gliosis.

These are thin contractile membranes derived from intraretinal glial cells which distort the inner limiting membrane of the retina. This condition is often asymptomatic but increasing severity of membrane contracture may lead to decrease or distortion of vision, particularly when the macula is involved (Figure 10.92). A lower threshold for vitreoretinal surgical intervention means that more specimens are submitted to pathology.

Numerous aetiologies have been associated with the formation of an epiretinal membrane:
• idiopathic
• uveitis
• previous trauma including surgery
• diabetes and other vascular diseases.

The composition of the excised membranes will depend on the aetiology but the tissue usually consists primarily of glial cells (Figure 10.92). This entity differs from proliferative vitreoretinopathy (PVR) which is secondary to a previous retinal break with or without rhegmatogenous retinal detachment. In PVR, the membrane contains pigmented cells derived from RPE (see below).

Myopia

This condition occurs when the plane of focus of the image is in front of the retina. There are two types:
1 *Index:* when the globe dimensions are normal.
2 *Axial:* when it is secondary to elongation of the globe.

In the latter variant, elongation of the globe is thought to be due to factors influencing the stretching of the sclera, but the precise mechanisms are debatable – hereditary, reading, and close work.

Depending on the severity, the clinical features of axial myopia are variable and include: elongation of the globe with possible posterior staphyloma, lacquer cracks, and disc changes (tilting and temporal peripapillary atrophy in the form of a white crescent) due to posterior stretching of the sclera. The pathological features of the optic nerve head are shown in Figures 10.93 and 10.94. Myopic eyes are at a higher risk of rhegmatogenous retinal detachment due to an earlier onset of peripheral retinal degeneration, vitreous syneresis, and detachment (see below).

Peripheral

This section deals with the changes which are seen in the peripheral retina by indirect ophthalmoscopy and in pathology as incidental findings in enucleated globes. These degenerations are usually innocuous but some may progress to retinal detachment.

Lattice

This form of peripheral degeneration has the greatest association with retinal detachment. Small, sharply demarcated linear areas contain an overlying network of white lines (Figure 10.95). Foci of lattice degeneration are patchy in distribution and are most common in the upper temporal quadrant. Histology reveals retinal thinning and hole formation in the region of a hyalinised retinal arteriole (Figure 10.96). There is an absence of vitreous over the defect, although attachments appear to be firm at the edge.

Cobblestone/pavingstone

Indirect ophthalmoscopy and macroscopic pathological examination demonstrate cobblestone degeneration as discrete, yellow, circular areas of chorioretinal atrophy with speckled clumps of hyperpigmentation. These areas expand slowly and may merge with other areas of degeneration (Figure 10.97). At the histological level, the atrophic gliotic retina is fused with Bruch's membrane and the choroid and choriocapillaris are atrophic. The RPE is absent in the scarred area but is hyperplastic at the periphery where there may be intraretinal proliferation (Figure 10.97). This form of degeneration is found most commonly in the inferior peripheral retina and is innocuous.

Retina - Central degeneration / ARMD
Wet/Exudative - Subretinal neovascular membrane type 2

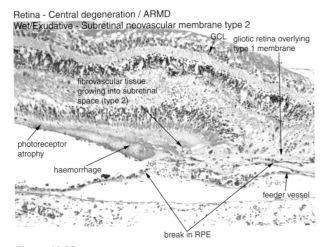

Figure 10.86

Retina - Central degeneration / ARMD
Wet/Exudative - Disciform scar

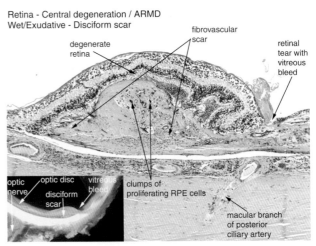

Figure 10.87

Retina - Central degeneration
ARMD
Wet/Exudative - Disciform scar

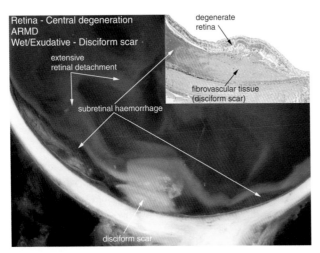

Figure 10.88

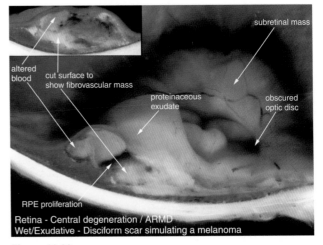

Retina - Central degeneration / ARMD
Wet/Exudative - Disciform scar simulating a melanoma

Figure 10.89

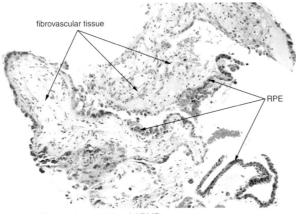

Retina - Central degeneration / ARMD
Wet/Exudative - Excision of subretinal neovascular membrane

Figure 10.90

Figure 10.86 This type 2 subretinal neovascular membrane (SRNVM) in wet ARMD has arisen from the edge of a type 1 SRNVM in which there is a disruption in the retinal pigment epithelium (RPE). Neovascularisation and haemorrhage have extended between the RPE and a normal outer retina. The presence of a thickened ganglion cell layer (GCL) confirms that the location is the macula area.

Figure 10.87 Contraction of fibrous tissue within this disciform scar leads to macular distortion and tears in the retina from which there is bleeding into the vitreous. The macroscopic appearances are shown in the inset.

Figure 10.88 Bleeding from a relatively small disciform scar leads to extensive haemorrhagic detachment of the retina. The inset shows the histological appearance in this specimen.

Figure 10.89 This archival specimen was an enucleation for a presumed peripapillary choroidal melanoma. Examination of the cut surface (inset) reveals a disciform scar, altered blood, and exudation. The hyperpigmented areas are due to a reactionary proliferation of the retinal pigment epithelium.

Figure 10.90 It is of clinical interest that an excised subretinal neovascular membrane is identified as type 1 or type 2. As can be seen in this specimen, a considerable degree of expertise (and inspired guesswork!) is required to answer this question. However, considering the close relationship between the continuous monolayer of retinal pigment epithelium (RPE) and the fibrovascular tissue, it is likely that this is a type 1 subretinal neovascular membrane (see Figure 10.85 – type 1 SRNVM).

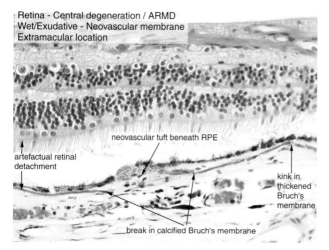

Retina - Central degeneration / ARMD
Wet/Exudative - Neovascular membrane
Extramacular location

neovascular tuft beneath RPE

artefactual retinal detachment

kink in thickened Bruch's membrane

break in calcified Bruch's membrane

Figure 10.91

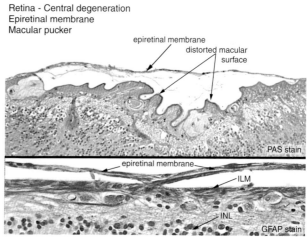

Retina - Central degeneration
Epiretinal membrane
Macular pucker

epiretinal membrane

distorted macular surface

PAS stain

epiretinal membrane

ILM

INL

GFAP stain

Figure 10.92

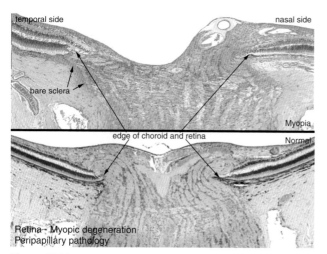

temporal side

nasal side

bare sclera

Myopia

edge of choroid and retina

Normal

Retina - Myopic degeneration
Peripapillary pathology

Figure 10.93

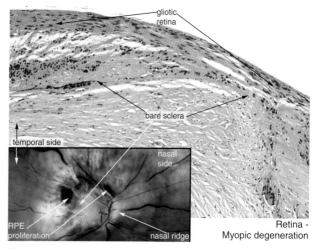

gliotic retina

bare sclera

temporal side

nasal side

RPE proliferation

nasal ridge

Retina - Myopic degeneration

Figure 10.94

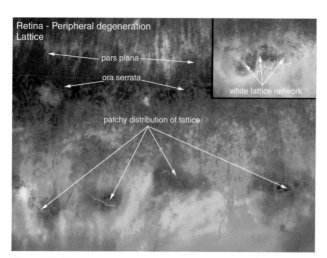

Retina - Peripheral degeneration
Lattice

pars plana

ora serrata

white lattice network

patchy distribution of lattice

Figure 10.95

Figure 10.91 This example of subretinal neovascular membrane type 1 was a chance finding. The Bruch's membrane is purple in colour and this is assumed by pathologists to represent calcification. When there is kinking, a break in Bruch's membrane stimulates subretinal pigment epithelial neovascularisation. This appearance is similar to breaks observed in pseudoxanthoma elasticum, Paget's disease, and angioid streaks.

Figure 10.92 The effects of contraction on the inner retina by a thin glial membrane are shown in this figure (upper, PAS stain). Secondary degenerative changes are present in the inner layers of the macula. The lower figure illustrates glial cell proliferation within an epiretinal membrane and within the inner retina. The immunohistochemical identification of glial cells is by an antibody label for a contractile glial protein (glial fibrillary acidic protein – GFAP) using a brown chromogen. ILM = inner limiting membrane, INL = inner nuclear layer.

Figure 10.93 An appreciation of the abnormal histological configuration of the optic disc in myopia is better understood when the normal disc is included for comparison (lower). On the temporal side of the myopic disc (upper), the choroid and retina are displaced away from the scleral canal. The temporal peripapillary retina overlies bare sclera and this corresponds to the temporal crescent seen on ophthalmoscopy. On the nasal side, the nerve fibre layer is formed into a prominent ridge. Clinically the myopic abnormality is termed a tilted disc.

Figure 10.94 The inset shows the macroscopic appearance of a myopic disc in which there is considerable temporal atrophy and retinal pigment epithelial (RPE) reactionary proliferation. The main histopathological feature of a myopic disc is the presence of gliotic retina on the temporal side overlying "bare" sclera.

Figure 10.95 Lattice degeneration is easily identified in a pathological specimen as linear oval defects in the peripheral retina. These areas are crossed by fine white lines which represent hyalinised peripheral retinal arcades. The inset shows a detail of an area of lattice degeneration.

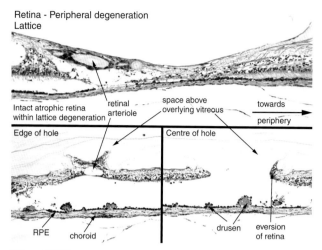

Retina - Peripheral degeneration
Lattice

Intact atrophic retina within lattice degeneration · retinal arteriole · space above overlying vitreous · towards periphery

Edge of hole · Centre of hole

RPE · choroid · drusen · eversion of retina

Figure 10.96

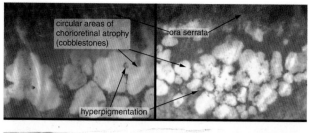

circular areas of chorioretinal atrophy (cobblestones) · ora serrata · hyperpigmentation

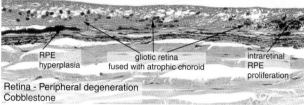

RPE hyperplasia · gliotic retina fused with atrophic choroid · intraretinal RPE proliferation

Retina - Peripheral degeneration
Cobblestone

Figure 10.97

Figure 10.96 A composite illustration of different levels taken from the area of lattice degeneration shown in the inset in Figure 10.95. At the edge of the lattice, the retina is thinned and gliotic anterior to a hyalinised blood vessel which is surrounded by retinal pigment epithelium (RPE) cells (upper). The lower left illustration shows a deeper level in the lattice to reveal the changes of detachment and hole formation with photoreceptor atrophy and the effects of vitreous traction on the glial cells on the inner surface of the hyalinised vessel. Lower right, in the

centre of the lattice, there is a retinal hole and a defect in the overlying vitreous. Traction on the edge of the retina hole has produced eversion of the gliotic retina.
Figure 10.97 Irregular circular areas of depigmentation occur in the peripheral retina and do not predispose to any complication. Pigmentation is seen at the periphery as well as within the white areas (upper left and right). Histology reveals a gliotic retina fused with an atrophic choroid (lower) – this corresponds with the pale areas seen macroscopically and by indirect ophthalmoscopy.

Peripheral microcystoid

Sheets of microcysts may be present in the retina just posterior to the ora serrata (Figures 10.7, 10.98). The presumed pathogenesis is ischaemia due to degenerative occlusive disease in the peripheral retinal arterioles. The only complication is that the cysts may break down to form a retinoschisis in the outer plexiform layer (Figure 10.99) or, as an extreme rarity, a giant cyst (Figure 10.100).

Retinal breaks (holes/tears/dialysis)

Retinal breaks are full thickness defects in the retina that may result in a rhegmatogenous retinal detachment (see below).

Holes

Holes are full thickness defects of the retina in the absence of vitreous traction. They are usually the result of peripheral atrophic changes (Figure 10.101) and rarely progress to detachment.

Tears

In the ageing eye, the vitreous liquefies (syneresis) and the remaining condensed gel detaches from the posterior retina and disc. Tears are full thickness defects of the retina resulting from persistent traction on focal adhesions between the vitreous and the retinal surface. The break often possesses an overlying flap (operculum) with attached vitreous (Figure 10.102).

Unrelieved traction at the edge of the tear often results in further progression of this condition.

Dialysis

Breaks along the edge between the retina and the ora serrata are called dialyses and are usually large at the time of diagnosis.

Retinal detachment

This is defined as the separation of the neurosensory retina from the underlying RPE.

There are three types of retinal detachment:
1 Rhegmatogenous.
2 Exudative.
3 Tractional – see text on diabetic retinopathy in the section "Diabetes" above.

Rhegmatogenous retinal detachment

Rhegmatogenous (Gk *rhegma:* a tear) retinal detachment is the result of a full thickness tear in the retina permitting egress of vitreal fluid into the space between the neural retina and the RPE.

Clinical presentation
1 *Symptoms:* predetachment symptoms include increased visual floaters and/or flashes. With detachment, a partial scotoma is experienced which, if untreated, leads to total loss of vision.
2 *Signs:* fundus examination shows a mobile detached retina. A break or multiple breaks may also be visible, most commonly in the upper temporal quadrant. The contralateral eye may show peripheral retinal breaks or lattice degeneration in the corresponding quadrant.

If the fundus cannot be visualised, an ultrasound investigation may be necessary.

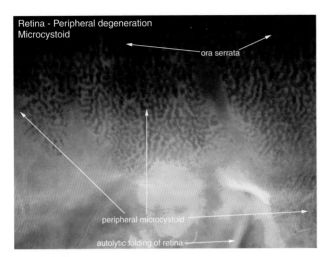

Retina - Peripheral degeneration
Microcystoid

ora serrata

peripheral microcystoid

autolytic folding of retina

Figure 10.98

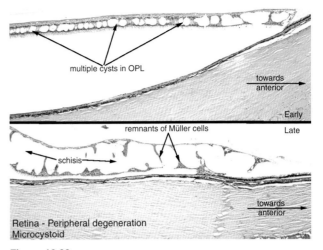

multiple cysts in OPL

towards anterior

Early

remnants of Müller cells

Late

schisis

towards anterior

Retina - Peripheral degeneration
Microcystoid

Figure 10.99

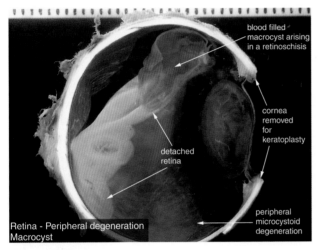

blood filled macrocyst arising in a retinoschisis

cornea removed for keratoplasty

detached retina

peripheral microcystoid degeneration

Retina - Peripheral degeneration
Macrocyst

Figure 10.100

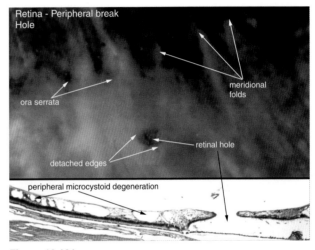

Retina - Peripheral break
Hole

meridional folds

ora serrata

retinal hole

detached edges

peripheral microcystoid degeneration

Figure 10.101

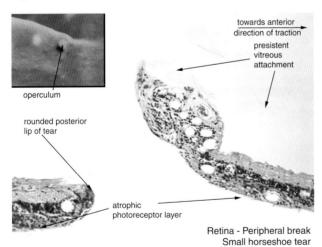

operculum

rounded posterior lip of tear

atrophic photoreceptor layer

towards anterior direction of traction

presistent vitreous attachment

Retina - Peripheral break
Small horseshoe tear

Figure 10.102

Figure 10.98 In microcystoid degeneration, the cysts adopt a honeycomb pattern particularly when an autopsy globe is fixed in formal saline, which makes the retina opaque.

Figure 10.99 The tiny cysts of microcystoid degeneration form in the outer plexiform layer (OPL) and are located in the peripheral retina. The cysts become smaller in the posterior part of the abnormality (upper). As the cysts enlarge, the inner and outer retinal layers are bridged by surviving Müller cells. When these break down, the two retinal layers split to form a retinoschisis (lower).

Figure 10.100 This archival specimen illustrates a blood-filled retinal macrocyst which was erroneously diagnosed as a malignant melanoma. The practice at that time was to use the cornea for donor purposes.

Figure 10.101 Retinal holes are occasional findings in eyes enucleated for other disorders. In this example, folds of retina project onto the pars plana – so-called meridional folds (upper). Histologically, the edge of a retinal hole is rounded and there is an associated small retinal detachment – note the peripheral microcystoid degeneration (lower).

Figure 10.102 In a rhegmatogenous retinal detachment (see below), it is sometimes possible for a pathologist to identify a retinal tear (inset) with an overlying flap (operculum). In this example, histology through the tear reveals persisting vitreous attachment to the anterior lip of the operculum. The atrophic photoreceptor layer, the rounded edge of the tear, and small cysts within the gliotic anterior lip each indicate longstanding detachment.

Aetiology and pathogenesis

Predisposing factors include:

- increasing age
- myopia
- lattice degeneration of the retina
- mechanical trauma (civil and surgical).

In the absence of predisposing factors, the incidence of retinal detachment is 1:10 000.

The pathogenesis of rhegmatogenous retinal detachment is based on the following factors:

- syneresis with liquefaction of vitreous gel
- persistent vitreous traction
- retinal break
- fluid movement from vitreous into the subretinal space.

Possible modes of treatment

The principles involve surgery to close the retinal break, reattachment of the retina, and relief of vitreous traction. The different procedures are multiple and complex – see the relevant clinical texts.

Surgery is subdivided into the following categories:

1 *Conventional:* involving explant material to indent the globe.
2 *Vitrectomy:* removal of vitreous, hence reducing tractional forces. The vitreous may be replaced with silicone oil or with gas (for example air, SF_6, C_3F_8) in order to tamponade the break.

See below for the pathology of retinal detachment surgery.

Macroscopic

The most common rhegmatogenous detachment specimen presented to the pathologist would be a globe following multiple failed reattachment procedures that was enucleated for secondary complications such as neovascular glaucoma (Figure 10.103).

Microscopic

It is important to appreciate that the retina commonly detaches by artefact and this is recognised by attachment of photoreceptor fragments to the RPE (Figure 10.104). A pre-existing retinal detachment can be recognised by the presence of photoreceptor atrophy and a reduction in the number of nuclei in the outer nuclear layer (Figures 10.102, 10.104). The photoreceptor layer will not recover after detachment of longer than 6 weeks, and there is a strong case to be made for early surgical intervention. As the detachment progresses over months and years, the retina becomes contracted with a linear appearance (Figure 10.105). At the end stage, the detached retina shows ischaemic atrophy, gliosis, and cyst formation (Figure 10.106). Evidence of neovascular glaucoma may be present.

Pathology of retinal detachment treatment

Conventional surgery The principle of conventional surgery is to close the retinal break by placing the RPE in direct contact with the sensory retina and to relieve the vitreous traction.

The explant is easily recognised macroscopically and may be either localised (radial and segmental circumferential) or encircling (Figure 10.107). Different materials have been used including sponge (Figures 10.107, 10.108) and solid silicone (Figures 10.108, 10.109). It is important to note that the explant is removed prior to paraffin sectioning; the site of the explant appears as an oval space forming an indentation in the sclera (Figure 10.110).

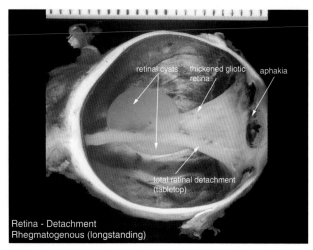

Figure 10.103

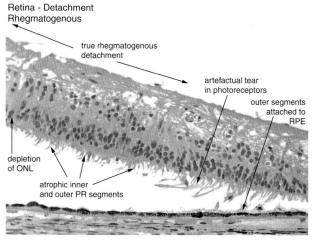

Figure 10.104

Figure 10.103 This globe had an uncomplicated intracapsular lens extraction which was later complicated by retinal detachment. The patient did not report his visual loss until several years later when he presented with neovascular glaucoma. The retina is thickened (by gliosis) and large cysts have formed in the outer retina: this is a common secondary finding in longstanding retinal detachment.

Figure 10.104 At the edge of a rhegmatogenous detachment, there may be artefactual tearing of the photoreceptors. This appears as a residue of photoreceptor (PR) tips on the retinal pigment epithelium (RPE). After the retina is detached for a period of weeks, the PR inner segments become atrophic and the outer nuclear layer (ONL) is depleted. In this example, there is also atrophy of the inner retina from longstanding glaucoma.

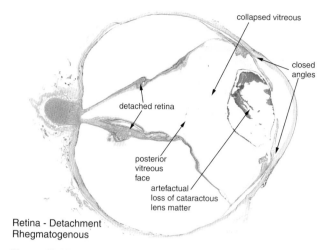

Retina - Detachment
Rhegmatogenous

Figure 10.105

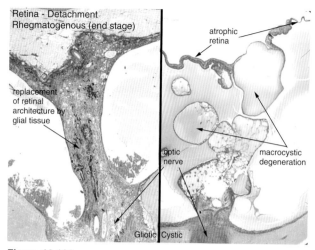

Figure 10.106

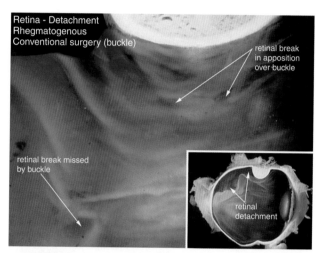

Figure 10.107

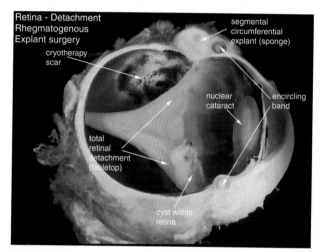

Figure 10.108

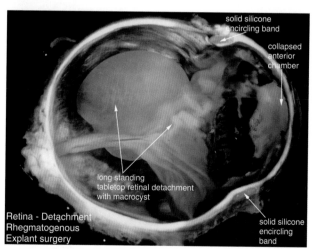

Figure 10.109

Figure 10.105 This archival material illustrates untreated rhegmatogenous retinal detachment. Presumably, the cataractous lens had obscured vision for the patient and the fundus view for the clinician. The retinal detachment was not discovered until secondary angle closure (neovascular glaucoma) had ensued. Note that the optic disc is not cupped; this is a common finding in retinal detachment followed by glaucoma.

Figure 10.106 At the end stage of longstanding detachment, there may be total gliotic replacement of the normal retinal layers (left). Cyst formation (right) may progress to the formation of a macrocyst – see Figure 10.103.

Figure 10.107 An indentation explant consisting of a sponge was used to approximate the retinal pigment epithelium to the retinal break, and to relieve vitreous traction in rhegmatogenous detachment. The breaks are not closed by the explant, suggesting the possibility of pre-existing proliferative vitreoretinopathy (see below). There are also retinal breaks posterior to the explant that are not apposed. The inset shows the complete specimen – the absence of blood in the episcleral tissue is a feature of autopsy material.

Figure 10.108 In this specimen, it may be assumed that the encircling and segmental explants have slipped anteriorly because of the posterior proximity of the cryotherapy burns and the location of the band on the pars plana. The anterior segment structures appear normal apart from a dense nuclear cataract.

Figure 10.109 One complication of an encircling band is that the sclera can be eroded, as in this specimen in which retinal detachment followed surgery for a congenital cataract.

Retinopexy – laser photocoagulation and cryotherapy
Current procedures utilise either laser photocoagulation or cryopexy to induce scarring between the retinal break and the underlying RPE in order to seal the retinal defect and promote adhesion (Figures 10.108, 10.111). The appearances of laser photocoagulation are identical to panretinal photocoagulation in ischaemic retinopathy but are on a larger scale. Both types of burn are easily identified as large pale areas of RPE atrophy with patchy hyperpigmentation due to reactionary proliferation of the RPE (Figures 10.48, 10.108, 10.111).

Proliferative vitreoretinopathy (PVR) PVR is the most common cause of failure in retinal detachment surgery. Clinically and pathologically, this is recognised by a distorted, stiffened, and folded retina with or without detachment. A pale membrane with patchy pigmentation may be identified on the inner surface of the retina (Figure 10.112).

This condition is the result of proliferation of glial and RPE cells, usually on the inner retinal surface. RPE cells may also proliferate as strands or cords within the subretinal space (Figure 10.113). The RPE cells undergo metaplasia to fibroblast-like cells with contractile properties. The resultant tissue fibrosis and contracture distorts the inner retina with

further redetachment. The diagnosis of PVR would assume a previous history of either a rhegmatogenous retinal detachment (at least 4–6 weeks postoperative) or a penetrating trauma with access of RPE to the vitreous cavity.

In the enucleated globe, the macroscopic appearance is that of a thickened distorted retina (Figure 10.112). Subretinal strands of proliferating RPE are identified by the presence of retinal folds in the absence of traction (Figure 10.113). Microscopically, the outer retina is atrophic and clumps of RPE cells are present on the inner surface (Figure 10.114, upper). The process continues with fibrous metaplasia of the RPE and the formation of contractile fibrous tissue (Figure 10.114, lower).

If left untreated, tissue contracture from PVR may result in retinal redetachment with formation of new retinal breaks or from reopening of a previous break. Apart from the complications of long term retinal detachment (see above), other features of PVR may include ocular hypotony and shrinkage of the globe (phthisis bulbi).

The pathologist will have previously encountered PVR in globes following unsuccessful retinal detachment surgery complicated by glaucoma. Currently it is more common to receive excised membranes (Figure 10.115) or excised retina removed in the surgical procedure of retinectomy.

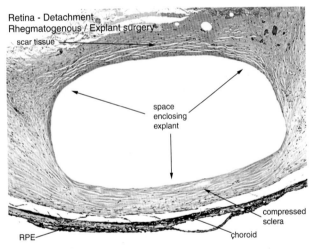

Figure 10.110

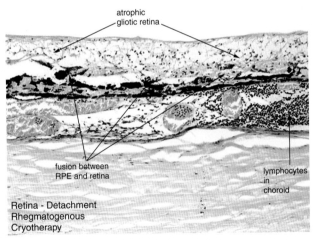

Figure 10.111

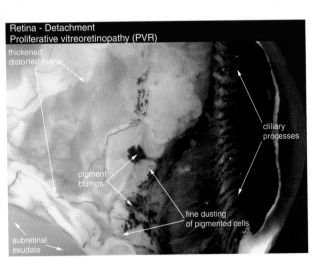

Figure 10.112

Figure 10.110 Encircling silicone bands are biologically inert. The adjacent scleral tissue is free from inflammatory cell infiltration. In this example, the retina is detached and is not included. A thin strip of choroid lined by proliferating retinal pigment epithelium (RPE) cells underlies the compressed sclera and the encircling band.

Figure 10.111 This is an example of cryotherapy in the treatment of rhegmatogenous retinal detachment. Proliferating retinal pigment epithelium (RPE) cells have migrated into the gliotic retina within the adhesion. Inflammatory cell infiltration is present in the choroid.

Figure 10.112 Proliferation of retinal pigment epithelium cells on the inner surface of the retina is a characteristic feature of proliferative vitreoretinopathy although the extent of the membrane can only be surmised by folds within the detached retina. In this example of end-stage detachment, there is a secondary subretinal exudate and the angles are closed. At this stage it is often impossible to identify a pre-existing break in the peripheral retina.

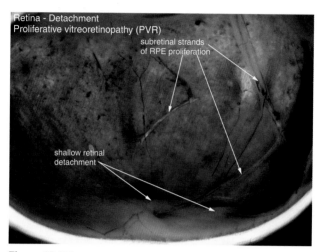

Retina - Detachment
Proliferative vitreoretinopathy (PVR)

subretinal strands
of RPE proliferation

shallow retinal
detachment

Figure 10.113

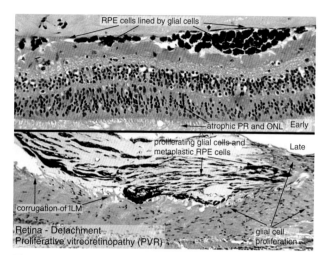

RPE cells lined by glial cells

atrophic PR and ONL   Early

proliferating glial cells and
metaplastic RPE cells   Late

corrugation of ILM

Retina - Detachment
Proliferative vitreoretinopathy (PVR)

glial cell
proliferation

Figure 10.114

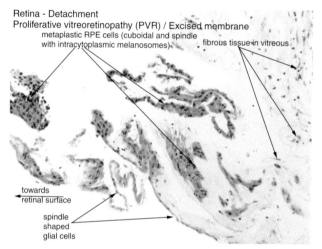

Retina - Detachment
Proliferative vitreoretinopathy (PVR) / Excised membrane

metaplastic RPE cells (cuboidal and spindle
with intracytoplasmic melanosomes)

fibrous tissue in vitreous

towards
retinal surface

spindle
shaped
glial cells

Figure 10.115

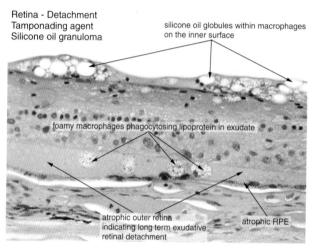

Retina - Detachment
Tamponading agent
Silicone oil granuloma

silicone oil globules within macrophages
on the inner surface

foamy macrophages phagocytosing lipoprotein in exudate

atrophic outer retina
indicating long term exudative
retinal detachment

atrophic RPE

Figure 10.116

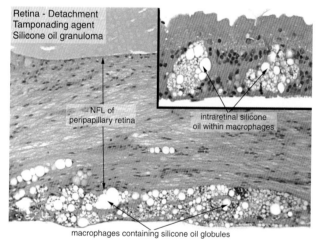

Retina - Detachment
Tamponading agent
Silicone oil granuloma

NFL of
peripapillary retina

intraretinal silicone
oil within macrophages

macrophages containing silicone oil globules

Figure 10.117

Figure 10.113 In this example of a longstanding retinal detachment, the initial appearances are deceptive as the retina appears to be attached. Close observation reveals a shallow retinal detachment. Strands of partially pigmented tissue beneath the retina are indicative of subretinal proliferation of retinal pigment epithelium (RPE). The subretinal location of the ridges is confirmed by the relationship to the overlying retinal vessels.

Figure 10.114 After migration of retinal pigment epithelium (RPE) cells into the vitreous through a retinal break, the cells form clusters on the inner surface of the detached retina (upper). The process continues with spindle cell metaplasia and the formation of fibrous tissue which results in corrugation of the inner limiting membrane (ILM) and contributes to the retinal rigidity (lower). ONL = outer nuclear layer, PR = photoreceptors.

Figure 10.115 An excised epiretinal membrane typically consists of metaplastic retinal pigment epithelium (RPE) cells and glial cells embedded in fibrous connective tissue. The RPE cells assume a spindle shape but still possess intracytoplasmic melanosomes.

Figure 10.116 Silicone oil is removed during processing for paraffin histology but the location of the emulsified oil droplets is identified by large empty circular spaces within the epiretinal macrophages. Compare this appearance with the foamy macrophages present in the subretinal exudate. The retina is atrophic due to a longstanding detachment.

Figure 10.117 Emulsified silicone oil can pass through a break in the retina and disperse within the subretinal space. In this example a band of oil laden macrophages is found on the outer surface of the peripapillary retina. The inset shows the presence of oil laden macrophages within the outer part of an atrophic retina – presumably, the outer limiting membrane is less of a barrier to these cells. NFL = nerve fibre layer.

Tomponading agents Tomponading agents are often used to facilitate retinal detachment surgery. Silicone oil (and expanding gases such as SF_6 and C_3F_8) may also be left postoperatively to aid internal closure of the retinal break. In the case of silicone oil, the viscous oily fluid extrudes from the enucleated eye on macroscopic examination.

1 *Silicone oil:* success of tamponade by silicone oil will depend on the depot maintaining surface tension in the form of a sphere. The oil is lighter than water and is useful for the tamponade of superior breaks. However, silicone oil can emulsify and this stimulates a lipogranulomatous reaction against the oil droplets wherever they are dispersed. Clusters of macrophages distended by silicone oil globules are present most commonly on the inner and outer surfaces and within the retina (Figures 10.116, 10.117). If the emulsified silicone enters the anterior chamber, it appears as a crescentic white layer in the upper quadrant of the angle (the silicone oil being lighter than aqueous). A section through the superior angle will show a massive lipomacrophagic infiltrate in the iris stroma and trabecular meshwork (Figure 10.118). The corneal endothelium also has the ability to phagocytose oil droplets (Figure 10.118).

2 *Heavy liquids:* being heavier than water, heavy liquids have the advantage of flattening a detached retina. Heavy liquid is usually removed at the end of detachment surgery, but in an exceptional specimen a small quantity may be present beneath the retina and appears as an ovoid mound that shifts with gravity (Figure 10.119).

Exudative retinal detachment

Other names: serous retinal detachment.

Definition: a retinal detachment that occurs with an accumulation of subretinal fluid in the absence of a retinal break.

Any condition that disrupts the blood–ocular barrier or damages the RPE may potentially lead to an accumulation of subretinal fluid and hence an exudative retinal detachment.

See the relevant chapters for examples of exudative retinal detachment:

- *neoplastic:* choroidal melanoma, retinoblastoma, and choroidal haemangioma
- *inflammatory:* sympathetic ophthalmia, posterior scleritis
- *vascular:* wet ARMD, Coats' disease
- *idiopathic:* uveal effusion syndrome (see below)
- *trauma:* hypotonia (e.g. detachment of the ciliary body).

Clinically, exudative retinal detachment is recognised by gravitational shifting of subretinal fluid in the absence of a retinal break. The pathologist regularly encounters exudative retinal detachment in enucleated globes that are affected by the conditions listed above.

After fixation, an exudative detachment is readily recognised by a solid brown proteinaceous gel beneath the retina (Figure 10.120). Histologically, the proteinaceous exudate is pink in colour with the H&E stain (Figure 10.121).

Uveal effusion syndrome

This is a unique cause of exudative retinal detachment. In some cases, rheumatoid disease is an association, but many are idiopathic and bilaterality is common. In addition to the retinal detachment, there is also exudation into the ciliary body and anterior choroid (Figure 10.122).

The main histological features (Figure 10.123) are:

1 Detachment of the ciliary body, choroid, and retina by exudation.

2 Absence of inflammatory or neoplastic disease.

3 Thickening of the sclera is thought to be of importance. Currently, resection of part of the anterior sclera is considered a means of improving fluid diffusion. As an alternative, posterior sclerectomy is employed to decompress the vortex veins.

4 Ultimately, hypotonia and phthisis is due to ciliary body shutdown from chronic detachment, which compromises the blood supply to the ciliary processes.

It is important to note the potential difficulties in the clinical differential diagnosis of this condition (for example uveal melanoma and metastatic tumour), especially when high resolution ultrasound facilities are not available.

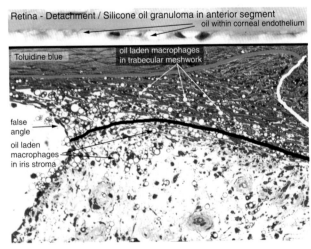

Figure 10.118

Figure 10.118 When emulsified silicone oil enters the anterior segment, oil spaces can be seen within the corneal endothelium (upper) and within numerous macrophages in the superior angle, iris stroma, and trabecular meshwork (toluidine blue – lower). The coloured lines indicate the scleral sulcus (red), the scleral spur (white), and the anterior border of the iris (black).

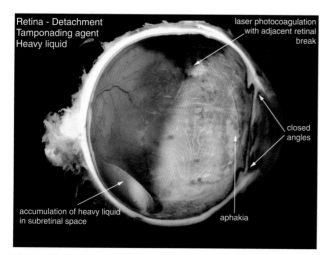

Figure 10.119

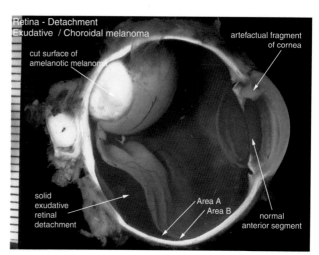

Figure 10.120

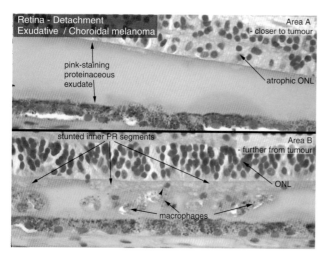

Figure 10.121

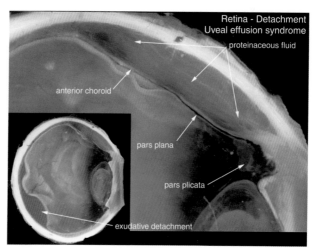

Figure 10.122

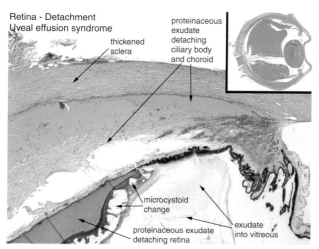

Figure 10.123

Figure 10.119 Cataract surgery was performed on this eye and later was complicated by retinal detachment. Detachment surgery was performed using a heavy liquid tamponade intraoperatively and retinopexy using laser photocoagulation. Presumably, some heavy liquid had passed through the retinal break into the subretinal space and, with gravity, had migrated inferiorly. The patient unfortunately developed neovascular glaucoma with a painful keratopathy that necessitated enucleation.

Figure 10.120 An exudative retinal detachment is appropriately illustrated by a globe containing a malignant melanoma. Leakage of proteinaceous fluid from the superior tumour has led to an extensive inferior detachment (and this may be the presenting sign). Areas marked A and B are the sites for the histology shown in Figure 10.121.

Figure 10.121 As the exudate extends beneath the retina, there is progressive photoreceptor atrophy. The upper figure is the area shown as A in the previous figure and here there is total photoreceptor (PR) atrophy due to prolonged detachment. By contrast, in the more anterior area B (lower) there are some remaining PR inner segments, owing to the more recent detachment. The content of nuclei in the outer nuclear layer (ONL) is closer to normal in area B. Macrophages are present within the subretinal exudate.

Figure 10.122 The presence of a mass in the anterior uvea and a posterior exudative detachment led to the erroneous diagnosis of malignant melanoma. The eye was enucleated and the cornea was used for donor penetrating keratoplasty. The mass in the ciliary body is, in fact, the anterior uvea detached by proteinaceous exudation with a similar exudate beneath the detached retina (inset). These findings are consistent with the uveal effusion syndrome.

Figure 10.123 Histological examination in the uveal effusion syndrome demonstrates pink-staining proteinaceous fluid between the ciliary body and sclera with extension beneath the anterior choroid. The retina is detached by a more condensed exudate and, as an incidental finding, there is microcystoid change within the retina. This case was also misdiagnosed as a malignant melanoma. The inset is a low power image of the whole globe to show the extent of the retinal detachment.

Chapter 11
Intraocular tumours

The commonest primary intraocular tumours in *adult life* are derived from melanocytes, for example naevi and malignant melanoma. Melanocytes are spindle shaped and have branching cytoplasmic processes (dendritic); the cytoplasmic melanosomes are round. Embryologically, these cells are derived from the neural crest and both benign and malignant variants possess a similar antigenic profile. Malignant melanomas have a tendency to metastasise to the liver.

In *childhood*, a retinoblastoma is the most important primary malignant intraocular tumour: the histogenesis is based on an origin from primitive embryonic neuroretinal cells. Although rare, it forms an important part of the differential diagnosis of leucocoria. Retinoblastomas metastasise to the CNS via the optic nerve and systemically by the bloodstream.

A rare group of tumours are derived from embryonic neuroepithelium and these are most commonly located in the ciliary epithelium, for example adenomas and adenocarcinomas.

For a description of ocular embryology, see Chapter 6.

Metastatic tumours are common in autopsy material but are rare in clinical practice.

Systemic diseases can involve any part of the eye, for example metastasis, lymphoma, and leukaemia.

Primary intraocular tumours are most conveniently described in an anatomical format:

- iris
- ciliary body
- choroid
- retina
- panophthalmic neoplasia.

Iris

The following are the most commonly encountered iris abnormalities (Table 11.1):

- naevus
- melanoma
- cysts
- metastasis
- other spindle cell tumours.

Table 11.1 Differential diagnosis of common iris tumours.

Pigmented	Non-pigmented
Freckle/naevus	Amelanotic melanoma
Malignant melanoma	Lymphoma
Cyst	Metastasis

Iris naevus

This tumour may be static or enlarge slowly over decades. Approximately 1 in 4000–5000 undergoes malignant transformation. The incidence is increased in Down's syndrome and in neurofibromatosis (NF1).

Clinical presentation

Cosmetic – abnormal iris appearance. The tumour is flat, usually pigmented, and static. In rare situations, an iris naevus may be associated with secondary glaucoma (see text on iris naevus syndrome under "Macroscopic" below).

Possible modes of treatment

1 Conservative by means of observation for growth/change.
2 Excision in the form of a broad iridectomy may be performed if the tumour increases in size or alters pigmentation.

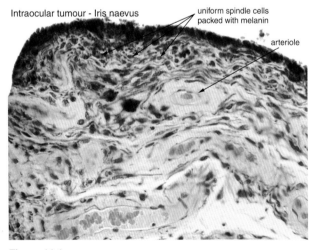

Figure 11.1

Figure 11.1 Spindle cells in an iris naevus are heavily pigmented and are packed in the anterior stroma. Nucleoli are not easily identified in the cell nuclei. Compare with the normal iris in Figures 1.8, 1.9, 10.64.

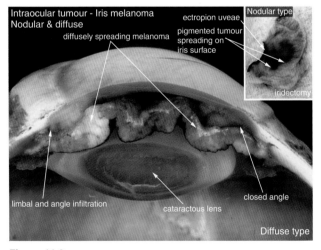

Figure 11.2

Figure 11.2 The two types of iris melanoma: nodular and diffuse. The inset shows a nodular melanoma of the iris spreading across the surface of a blue iris in an iridectomy specimen. Surface spread and contraction lead to an ectropion uveae. A diffuse melanoma involves the whole iris and tumour infiltration of the angle results in secondary glaucoma. Enucleation is the only option.

Macroscopic

Most examples of an iris naevus are encountered in globes enucleated for other reasons. In suspicious cases, a specimen may be submitted in the form of an iridectomy or fine needle aspiration biopsy. A naevus appears as a flat heavily pigmented patch occupying a sector or an even larger area, usually <3 mm diameter and <0.5 mm thickness.

Iris naevus syndrome is pigmentation of the entire iris stroma (causing heterochromia) with secondary glaucoma, due to degeneration of the trabecular endothelial cells when overburdened with melanin.

Microscopic

The tumour is formed by heavily pigmented spindle-shaped melanocytes. The uniform nuclei possess an even distribution of condensed chromatin and inconspicuous nucleoli. The major part of the tumour is in the anterior stroma (Figure 11.1).

Iris melanoma

In the iris, a malignant proliferation of melanocytes does not carry the serious propensity for metastatic disease recognised in melanomas in the remainder of the uveal tract. An iris melanoma can arise *de novo* or from a pre-existing naevus that may have been present for many years.

Clinical presentation

An iris mass that increases in size and/or changes in appearance should be viewed with suspicion. The colour may be variable – black, white, pale brown, or patchily pigmented. The tumour may be nodular or spread diffusely on the iris surface.

Circumferential growth around the chamber angle (ring melanoma) causes secondary glaucoma by lining and subsequently infiltrating the trabecular meshwork.

Possible modes of treatment

The treatment is variable depending on the clinical behaviour of the tumour. Basic management involves observation, local excision, brachytherapy, or enucleation (in cases of an untreatable primary, a recurrence or secondary glaucoma). Complications can occur after surgical intervention (for example cataract and extraocular spread); the metastatic rate is <2%.

Macroscopic

In the nodular form of iris melanoma, the tumour will be submitted within an iridectomy specimen (Figure 11.2) or as an iridocyclectomy with a partial sclerectomy (block excision). The diffuse form is often not amenable to eye conservation treatment and thus an enucleation is performed (Figure 11.2).

After unsuccessful local resection, tumour recurrence is often widespread in an enucleation specimen (Figure 11.3).

Microscopic

The cytological features of an iris melanoma are rarely those typical of a malignant tumour. The cells are small and spindle shaped, with uniform nuclei which do not possess conspicuous nucleoli (Figure 11.4). The nature of the spread on the surface and into the stroma governs the diagnosis of malignancy. Pigmentation is variable and mitotic figures are extremely rare. Invasion of the outflow system is a helpful indicator of aggressive behaviour which establishes the malignant nature of the tumour. Erosion of the iris pigment epithelium is a common feature (Figure 11.5).

In recurrent tumours, the cells may transform into large, oval "epithelioid cells" and tumour giant cells.

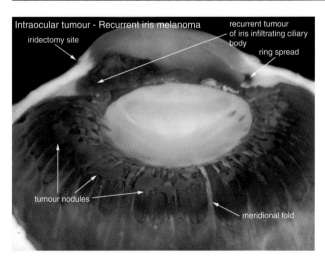

Figure 11.3

Figure 11.3 After an incomplete resection of an iris melanoma, a large tumour recurrence with ring spread and secondary cataract formation was the indication for an enucleation. Nodules are also present on the ciliary processes. Note the meridional fold on the pars plana.

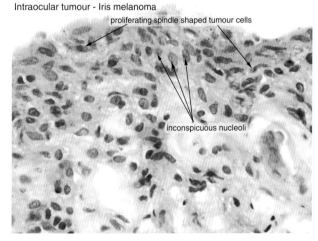

Figure 11.4

Figure 11.4 In this amelanotic melanoma, the nuclei possess inconspicuous nucleoli.

Immunohistochemistry

Markers for a neural crest origin: A103 (anti-Mart-1/Melan A) are most commonly used. S 100 (anti-gp100), HMB45, and T311 (anti-tyrosinase) were used previously.

Proliferation markers (for example Ki 67) may be helpful in indicating the degree of proliferative activity, but most iris melanomas have a low proliferation rate.

Iris cysts

Cystic structures within the iris can be lined by cells of two derivations:

1 *Corneal or conjunctival epithelium:* this tissue may be implanted after surgical and non-surgical penetrating trauma (acquired). The location is usually on the anterior surface of the iris, and often at the point of contact with the corneal wound (Figure 11.6).

2 *Iris pigment epithelium:* separation of the two embryonic layers (see Chapter 6) leads to the formation of a cyst on the posterior surface. Such cysts are either congenital or acquired, in the latter case especially after long term miotic therapy. This can be misdiagnosed as an iris melanoma. Such specimens are rare.

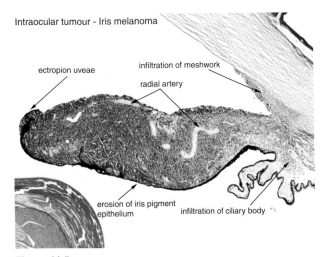

Figure 11.5

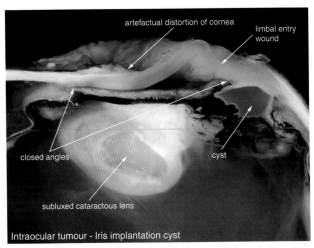

Figure 11.6

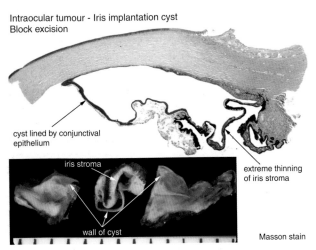

Figure 11.7

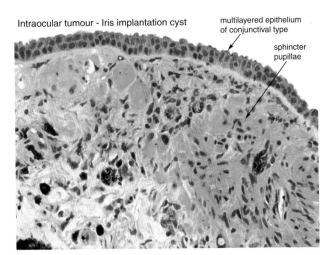

Figure 11.8

Figure 11.5 In this malignant melanoma of the iris, the stroma is totally infiltrated by melanoma cells which are eroding the pigment epithelium. The melanoma is also infiltrating the trabecular meshwork and the anterior part of the ciliary body. The lens cortex is undergoing non-specific degenerative changes.

Figure 11.6 After non-surgical trauma at the limbus, an implantation cyst had formed in the peripheral iris which had led to angle closure glaucoma. An appropriate level though the enucleated globe reveals the cyst and subluxation of a cataractous lens. The corneal distortion is due to a fixation artefact.

Figure 11.7 Currently, the treatment for an implantation cyst in the anterior segment is a total block excision including the sclera and ciliary body. In the Masson stain, the collagen is green and the epithelium is red. The inset shows an iridectomy specimen containing an epithelial inclusion cyst. Detail of the epithelium lining the cyst in the inset is shown in Figure 11.8.

Figure 11.8 The histological detail in an implantation cyst reveals a multilayered epithelium on the surface of the iris at the pupil margin. The cyst epithelium is of conjunctival type.

Clinical presentation

An iris cyst presents as a unilateral pigmented spherical ovoid mass that may transilluminate. Visual obscuration may be caused by a large cyst. Secondary angle closure glaucoma can occur if the cyst is large enough to compress the iris against the angle. Spontaneous rupture of epithelial inclusion cyst will result in acute uveitis and glaucoma.

Possible modes of treatment

Pigment epithelial cysts are usually stationary, although treatment has included surgery (excisional and incisional) and laser.

In epithelial implantation cysts, block excision is usually preferred (Figure 11.7). An incomplete excision can result in extensive epithelial spreading over the surface of the anterior segment tissues.

Macroscopic

Within iridectomy and iridocyclectomy specimens, an epithelial inclusion cyst may appear as a thin walled cystic structure located on the anterior surface of the iris (Figure 11.7, inset).

An iris stromal cyst appears as a swelling within the iris stroma.

Microscopic

An epithelial inclusion cyst is located on the anterior surface of the iris, and is characteristically lined by either corneal or conjunctival epithelium (Figures 11.7, 11.8).

A congenital stromal cyst is located within the iris stroma and is lined with pigment epithelium.

Metastasis to the iris

The most common primary source is of a pulmonary or mammary origin. Deposits of lymphoma, leukaemia, and metastatic carcinoid have also been reported.

Clinical presentation

If single or multiple iris nodules of variable colour and size are present, metastatic disease should be suspected.

Possible modes of treatment

The treatment varies depending on the primary source. A fine needle aspiration biopsy (FNAB) diagnosis is more frequently employed than in the past. Modalities include observation, radiotherapy, chemotherapy, and surgery (block excision and enucleation).

Pathology

A diagnostic iridectomy/biopsy will contain single or multiple amelanotic masses of variable size and form. An enucleation specimen will be received if there is angle involvement with secondary glaucoma. There may be multiple metastases within the eye. The microscopic features of metastatic tumours are described in the section on metastatic diseases under "Panophthalmic neoplasia" (p. 264).

Other spindle cell tumours of the iris

Spindle cell tumours which are not of melanocytic origin (for example leiomyoma, schwannoma) are extremely rare, as are vascular tumours.

Ciliary body

The following are the most commonly encountered abnormalities of the ciliary body:
- naevus
- melanoma
- melanocytoma
- other spindle cell tumours
- adenoma/adenocarcinoma of non-pigmented/pigmented ciliary epithelium.

Naevus

The true incidence of ciliary body naevi is unknown. The histological features are identical to those in the iris and choroid.

Melanoma

The incidence of melanoma in the ciliary body (12%) lies between that of the iris (8%) and the choroid (80%), which is in proportion to the numbers of melanocytes in each structure.

Clinical presentation

Displacement of the lens leads to visual disturbance (blurred vision). Invasion of the iris simulates an iris melanoma. Secondary glaucoma is caused by angle closure, invasion of trabecular meshwork, or pupil block. When the tumour extends to the posterior segment, flashes and floaters may be the symptom. With larger tumours, a uniocular visual field defect may occur. Localised episcleral vascular congestion (sentinel vessel) or transcleral extension of tumour may be the first indication of disease.

Possible modes of treatment

The modes of treatment will depend on the size and location of the tumour:
1 Surgery: iridocyclectomy (external resection).
2 Brachytherapy ([109]Ru and ^{125}I).
3 External beam radiotherapy.
4 Enucleation/exenteration.

Macroscopic

Most specimens will be submitted in the form of an enucleation, although in some centres a local eye-wall excision may be performed. These tumours appear as solid and well circumscribed masses. The cut surface may be amelanotic, variegated, or heavily pigmented (Figure 11.9). Exudative retinal detachment and extraocular spread are important features: Spontaneous necrosis may cause secondary open angle melanomalytic glaucoma (see Chapter 7). Infiltration of the angle and outflow system can occur and the tumour may extend posteriorly (Figure 11.10).

There may be evidence of previous surgical or radiotherapeutic treatment.

Microscopic

The cytological features are identical to those described in melanomas of the choroid (see below).

Melanocytoma (magnocellular naevus)

This is a rare benign form of melanocytic proliferation but is an important component in the differential diagnosis of melanoma.

Clinical presentation

The presentation of a melanocytoma is similar to those described for a malignant melanoma but the tumour is heavily pigmented and there is often episcleral involvement.

Possible modes of treatment

Observation if the diagnosis is certain. The diagnosis is often made after surgical excision (iridocyclectomy with sclerectomy if there is scleral involvement).

Macroscopic and microscopic

The tumour appears as an intensely black mass in the ciliary body and episclera. Histologically, the tumour cells are large, heavily pigmented, and oval with small, uniform nuclei. Mitotic figures are not seen.

Other rare spindle cell tumours not derived from melanocytes

For completion, other very rare tumours are listed:
- leiomyoma/leiomyosarcoma/schwannoma
- mesectodermal leiomyoma.

Tumours of the epithelium of the ciliary processes and pars plana – adenoma/adenocarcinoma of the non-pigmented and pigmented epithelium (NPE and PE)

The two layers (pigmented and non-pigmented) of epithelium of the ciliary processes are sources of rare low grade tumours, but the most aggressive variants may destroy the ocular tissues. Adenomas are the commonest variant encountered.

Clinical presentation

The patient will present with similar signs and symptoms of a ciliary body melanoma. Lens displacement by the mass effect causes visual disturbance.

Possible modes of treatment

These tumours are commonly treated by local eye-wall resection.

Macroscopic and microscopic

The tumour forms solid nodular masses within and projecting from the ciliary body. The cut surface is most frequently sparsely pigmented. A local resection specimen will include a wide rim of normal uveal tissue (Figure 11.12, inset).

The histogenesis is based on the normal architecture of the ciliary epithelium (Figure 11.11). Some tumours consist predominantly of amelanotic cuboidal cells with uniform nuclei (Figure 11.12), others are heavily pigmented (Figure 11.13), and often the tumour is formed from both cell types (Figure 11.14).

Figure 11.9 A patient presented with visual disturbance; on examination a pigmented iris tumour was observed in the angle. Ultrasonic investigation revealed a mass in the ciliary body causing lens displacement. An appropriate section through the enucleated globe shows a variegated melanoma in the ciliary body with lens displacement and pupil block. The adjacent angle is invaded and there is evidence of bleeding from the surface of the tumour into the vitreous. The lens cortex adjacent to the tumour is opaque.

Figure 11.10 A patient suddenly became aware of loss of vision in one eye. Clinical examination revealed raised intraocular pressure due to closed angles and opaque media. On ultrasonic investigation, there was a large tumour in the ciliary body and an enucleation was carried out. This large malignant melanoma of the ciliary body is growing posteriorly into a vortex vein, which worsens the prognosis. Leakage of plasma from the tumour results in an exudative detachment of the retina. Leakage of plasma into the vitreous is a consequence of retinal penetration. As can be seen, the changes could not have been "sudden".

Figure 11.11 The pathology of tumours of the ciliary epithelium relates to normal histology. The normal ciliary epithelium is bilayered. The inner layer is not pigmented and is continuous with the neuroretina. The outer layer is pigmented and is continuous with the retinal pigment epithelium. The normal ciliary epithelium basement membrane is illustrated – compare with changes in diabetes (see Figure 10.65).

Figure 11.12 Small tumours of the ciliary body can be excised by local resection. This example of an adenoma is formed by non-pigmented ciliary epithelium. The inset shows the surface of the tumour which appears to be black and could be mistaken for a melanoma. The pigmentation is due to proliferation of pigmented cells on the surface of the tumour.

Figure 11.13 A local resection of a ciliary body mass reveals on histology to be a heavily pigmented ciliary body adenoma (derived from the outer layer of the ciliary epithelium).

Figure 11.14 Detail of cells in a ciliary body adenoma to show juxtaposition of pigmented cells and non-pigmented cells.

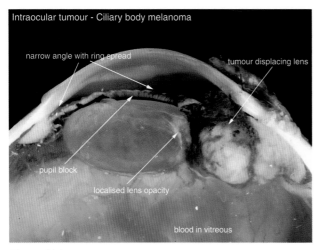

Intraocular tumour - Ciliary body melanoma

narrow angle with ring spread

tumour displacing lens

pupil block

localised lens opacity

blood in vitreous

Figure 11.9

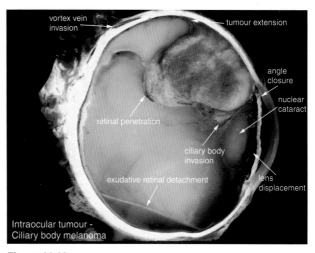

vortex vein invasion

tumour extension

angle closure

nuclear cataract

retinal penetration

ciliary body invasion

lens displacement

exudative retinal detachment

Intraocular tumour - Ciliary body melanoma

Figure 11.10

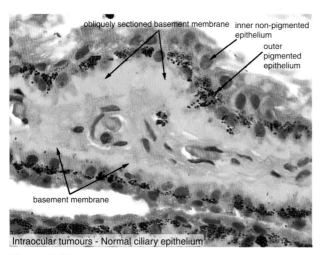

obliquely sectioned basement membrane

inner non-pigmented epithelium

outer pigmented epithelium

basement membrane

Intraocular tumours - Normal ciliary epithelium

Figure 11.11

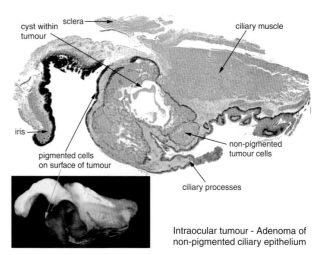

cyst within tumour

sclera

ciliary muscle

iris

pigmented cells on surface of tumour

non-pigmented tumour cells

ciliary processes

Intraocular tumour - Adenoma of non-pigmented ciliary epithelium

Figure 11.12

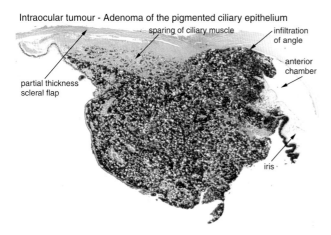

Intraocular tumour - Adenoma of the pigmented ciliary epithelium

sparing of ciliary muscle

infiltration of angle

anterior chamber

partial thickness scleral flap

iris

Figure 11.13

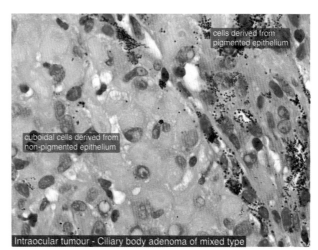

cells derived from pigmented epithelium

cuboidal cells derived from non-pigmented epithelium

Intraocular tumour - Ciliary body adenoma of mixed type

Figure 11.14

Choroid

The following are the most commonly encountered choroidal and retinal pigment epithelium (RPE) abnormalities:

- naevus
- melanoma
- ocular melanosis
- melanocytoma of the optic nerve head
- vascular hamartoma: cavernous haemangioma
- RPE hamartoma: congenital hypertrophy and hyperplasia of the RPE (CHRPE)
- choristoma: choroidal osteoma.

Table 11.2 lists the differential diagnoses in common choroidal pathology.

Naevus

Choroidal naevi by clinical definition are flat circular brown or slate grey in appearance with a size of less than 5 mm diameter and a thickness of less than 1 mm. Twenty per cent of Caucasian eyes contain naevi.

Clinical presentation

Naevi are usually asymptomatic and are noted on routine fundoscopy. Rarely, an associated exudative retinal detachment may cause a visual field loss.

Only infrequently does a naevus progress to malignancy (estimated as 1 in 10 000–15 000).

Macroscopic and microscopic

As a chance finding in an enucleated globe, a naevus appears as a flat, brown mass in the choroid (Figure 11.15). Drusen may be present on the surface (see Chapter 10) and, in rare cases, there may be a shallow exudative detachment of the retina.

The cells in a choroidal naevus are normally of small spindle cell type and are heavily pigmented. The nuclei are uniform and mitotic figures are absent (Figure 11.16).

Table 11.2 Differential diagnosis in common choroidal pathology.

Pigmented	Non-pigmented
Melanoma	Amelanotic melanoma
Naevus	Metastasis
"Wet" macular degeneration (see Chapter 10)	Choroidal haemangioma
	Chroidal osteoma
Choroidal haemorrhage (see Chapter 9)	Naevus
Retinal macrocyst (see Chapter 10)	Uveal effusion syndrome (see Chapter 10)
CHRPE	
Melanocytoma	
RPE adenoma/carcinoma	

CHRPE = congenital hypertrophy and hyperplasia of the RPE, RPE = retinal pigment epithelium.

Immunohistochemistry

Markers for cells of neural crest origin (melan-A, S100, HMB45) are not useful in distinguishing an active naevus from a melanoma.

Melanoma

Ocular melanomas are the commonest unilateral intraocular tumours in adults. They are most frequent in Caucasians (7 per 1 000 000) but occasionally occur in blacks, Indians, and Asians. The histology is applicable to melanomas of both the ciliary body and the choroid.

Clinical presentation

The presentation of this condition is variable:

1 A melanoma may be a chance finding in an asymptomatic individual.
2 Visual disturbance results when the tumour affects the macula (Figure 11.17).
3 Peripheral field loss may be the result of a peripheral tumour and may be exacerbated by exudative retinal detachment.
4 Secondary glaucoma may follow angle neovascularisation.
5 Proptosis may be the presentation if extraocular extension occurs.
6 Extraocular metastases have a preferential spread to the liver – the patient may present with hepatomegaly.

Possible modes of treatment

The treatment modalities of choroidal melanoma are variable depending on the size and location of the tumour and the clinical centre:

1 *Radiotherapy:* brachytherapy (using ^{60}cobalt, ^{125}iodine, ^{109}ruthenium, or ^{103}palladium plaques). Teletherapy employs proton, helium ion, or gamma radiation.
2 *Laser:* photocoagulation and transpupillary thermal therapy (TTT).
3 *Surgery:* local eye-wall resection, endoresection, and enucleation/exenteration.
4 *Chemotherapy and palliative care* for liver metastasis.

Paradigm shifts

In the last two decades, significant progress has been made in refining prognostic indicators for metastatic disease.

Cytogenetic studies Cytogenetic studies have revealed that monosomy of chromosome 3, when combined with multiplication of chromosome 8q, carries a worse prognosis, while aberrations of chromosome 6 may be associated with a better prognosis in uveal melanomas.

Microcirculation The vascular patterns in melanomas as assessed by PAS staining can be subdivided into those that resemble naevi and those that are more typical of malignant melanomas – it is possible to show that the latter carry a worse prognosis when there is a network pattern or a closed loop pattern involving three loops. The presence and quantity of vascular endothelial growth factor(s) are not an indicator of metastatic potential.

Cell proliferation indices

1 Study of nucleolar organiser regions (AgNOR technique) showed some promise in prognostication but this technique is no longer applied.

2 Measurement of the nucleolar area has been shown to be of some value in survival prognostication, particularly when the standard deviation of nucleolar area is considered in relation to the mean value of the area.

3 DNA synthesis. The synthetic phase (or S phase) can be identified by monoclonal antibodies such as Ki-67/Mib-1 or cyclin/proliferating cell nuclear antigen (PCNA) and these can to some extent be used as prognostic indicators. The use of the cell cycling marker PC-10 has also been investigated and found to be of value in combination with other prognostic indicators.

Ploidy analysis If there is a normal amount of DNA in a cell it is euploid, diploid, or tetraploid. Cells, especially many that are malignant, with grossly abnormal amounts of DNA, are classified as aneuploid. Flow cytometry when applied to choroidal melanomas has shown that spindle A cells are diploid and that epithelioid cells are tetraploid and aneuploid or hypertetraploid. There is currently some controversy whether tumour recurrence and metastases correlate with the distribution of the amount of DNA in a tumour population using ploidy analysis on fixed tissue.

Macroscopic

The appearances of the tumour can vary considerably and are subgrouped to nodular or diffuse. Most tumours are nodular, with an ovoid shape, and are only lightly pigmented measuring between 10 and 15 mm diameter with a minimum thickness of at least 2 mm. A heavily pigmented tumour is the rarest encountered (Figure 11.17).

The classic partially pigmented mushroom shape of a melanoma is due to penetration of Bruch's membrane. Tumour proliferation beneath the retina forms the collarstud or mushroom shape (Figures 11.18, 11.19). The periphery of the tumour may be well circumscribed or there may be a thin extension for a considerable distance into the adjacent choroid and sclera. These growth patterns make treatment by surgery or radiotherapy inaccurate, as the tumour limits cannot be defined (Figure 11.10).

Identification of tumour in a vortex vein carries a poor prognosis (Figures 11.20, 11.21).

With increasing size, there is a greater tendency to spontaneous necrosis (Figures 11.22, 11.23) and/or transcleral spread (Figures 11.24, 11.25).

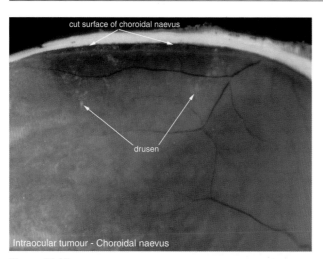

Figure 11.15

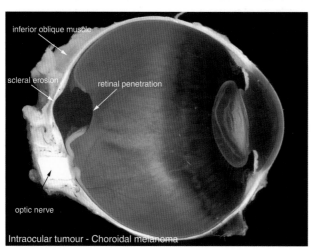

Figure 11.17

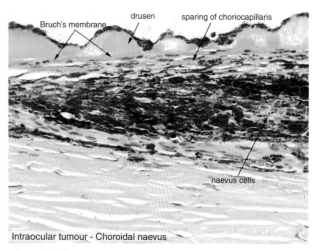

Figure 11.16

Figure 11.15 A chance finding in an autopsy globe shows a choroidal naevus. Naevi appear as flat, brown or dark grey circular tumours. Drusen are commonly present on the surface of a naevus. The retina is flat over the tumour.

Figure 11.16 Microscopic examination of a choroidal naevus reveals uniform heavily pigmented spindle cells in the stroma with sparing of the choriocapillaris. Hard drusen are ovoid structures on the inner surface of Bruch's membrane (see Chapter 10) and are lined internally by retinal pigment epithelial cells.

Figure 11.17 A young patient presented with visual loss in one eye. A small heavily pigmented nodular choroidal melanoma was identified behind the macula (confirmed by the location of the overlying inferior oblique muscle). This is an archival case – currently, the tumour would be treated by methods to conserve the eye (e.g. endoresection, proton beam).

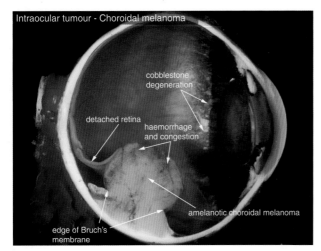

Intraocular tumour - Choroidal melanoma

cobblestone degeneration

detached retina

haemorrhage and congestion

amelanotic choroidal melanoma

edge of Bruch's membrane

Figure 11.18

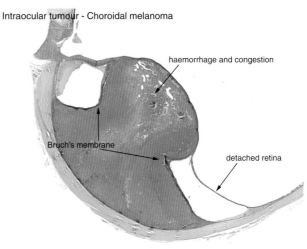

Intraocular tumour - Choroidal melanoma

haemorrhage and congestion

Bruch's membrane

detached retina

Figure 11.19

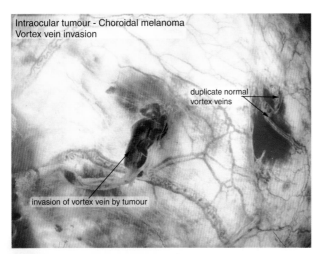

Intraocular tumour - Choroidal melanoma
Vortex vein invasion

duplicate normal vortex veins

invasion of vortex vein by tumour

Figure 11.20

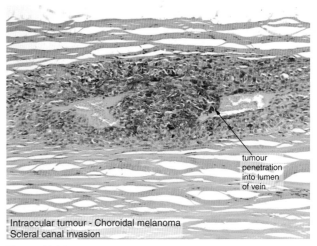

tumour penetration into lumen of vein

Intraocular tumour - Choroidal melanoma
Scleral canal invasion

Figure 11.21

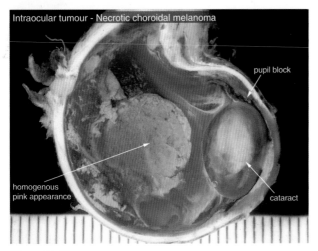

Intraocular tumour - Necrotic choroidal melanoma

pupil block

homogenous pink appearance

cataract

Figure 11.22

Figure 11.18 The "classic" mushroom shape in choroidal melanomas is the result of constriction of the base by Bruch's membrane. The tumour is amelanotic and a secondary exudative detachment is an indication of malignancy.

Figure 11.19 Low power microscopic appearance of the tumour shown in Figure 11.18. Haemorrhage and congestion in the apical part of the tumour are due to constriction of the blood supply. The detached retina is atrophic. The subretinal exudate seen macroscopically has been artefactually removed in processing.

Figure 11.20 Routine macroscopic examination of the surface of the globe occasionally reveals melanoma in the lumen of a vortex vein. This carries a poorer prognosis.

Figure 11.21 The histological appearance of melanoma cells infiltrating along a scleral canal with penetration into the lumen of a vortex vein.

Figure 11.22 A patient with a longstanding blind eye presented when it became acutely painful due to secondary pupil block and angle closure glaucoma. A large pre-existing malignant melanoma had undergone spontaneous necrosis with rapid expansion and secondary lens displacement. Necrosis within a melanoma is recognised by the presence of pink amorphous areas, tissue fragmentation, and haemorrhage.

Diffuse melanomas spread throughout the uveal tract and carry a very poor prognosis (Figures 11.26, 11.27).

Penetration of the retina with seeding into the vitreous is rare.

Enucleated globes are often complicated by the following: exudative retinal detachment, extraocular spread, glaucoma secondary to pupil block or neovascularisation, and cataract.

Microscopic

Cell type classification is based on nuclear morphology, melanin content varies in different regions of a melanoma and between individual cells:

1 *Spindle cell melanomas* can be divided into two types, A and B, but this practice is not uniform amongst pathologists. The cytoplasmic membrane is indistinct and the nuclei overlap. Mitotic figures are rare. Spindle A cells are closely packed and have elongated oval nuclei with small nucleoli and a longitudinal fold in the nuclear membrane – pure spindle A tumours are small and are rare (Figure 11.28). Spindle B cells are larger than type A cells and have a rounder nucleus in which the nucleolus is prominent (Figure 11.29).

2 *Epithelioid cell melanomas:* these tumour cells are larger than spindle cells and the cytoplasm is more eosinophilic; their presence carries a poorer prognosis. The cell boundaries are distinct and the cells appear to be separated by intercellular spaces. The nuclei of the cells, compared with spindle, do not overlap (Figures 11.30, 11.31). Mitotic figures are more easily found in epithelioid tumours that in rare instances may dedifferentiate into an anaplastic variant with giant nuclei and multinucleate cells. (Tumours consisting only of epithelioid cells are rare (<5%).)

3 *Mixed cell melanomas* contain both spindle cells and epithelioid cells and this variant represents the majority of choroidal melanomas (Figure 11.32).

Although the mitotic rate is low in melanomas, pyknotic cells showing apoptosis are often scattered throughout the tumour and focal necrosis is common.

Immunohistochemistry

Melanoma cells react positively with melan A (anti-S-100 and HMB45 were more commonly used previously) irrespective of cell type, but the expression of the epitopes in individual cells is variable.

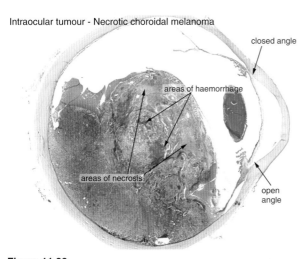

Figure 11.23

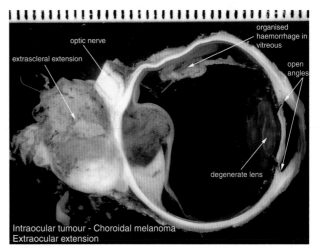

Figure 11.24

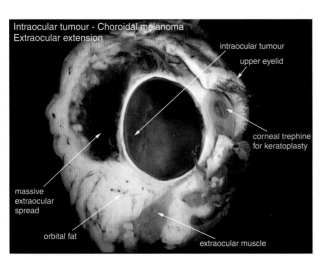

Figure 11.25

Figure 11.23 Cytoplasmic and nuclear detail is lost in a necrotic melanoma in which there is prominent haemorrhage. The lens appears small because the section is taken away from the midline. The upper part of the retina was lost in sectioning. Over the tumour, the retina is necrotic.

Figure 11.24 Ultrasound investigation revealed a retro-ocular mass in a patient presenting with choroidal melanoma. The globe and retro-ocular tumour were excised. Cuts into the specimen demonstrated a partially pigmented intraocular melanoma of moderate size with a considerably larger retro-ocular extension. This specimen is the central block after removal of the calottes.

Figure 11.25 A patient periodically reviewed for a flat pigmented tumour at the posterior pole presented with proptosis. Ultrasound and MRI revealed a large retro-ocular mass and an exenteration was performed. Note that the primary choroidal tumour is relatively small and the partially pigmented retro-ocular extension is the size of the globe.

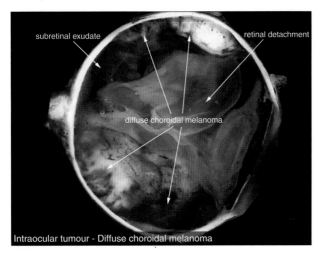

Figure 11.26

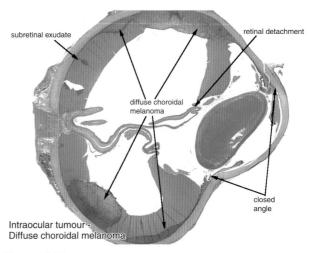

Figure 11.27

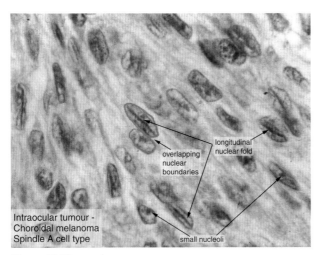

Figure 11.28

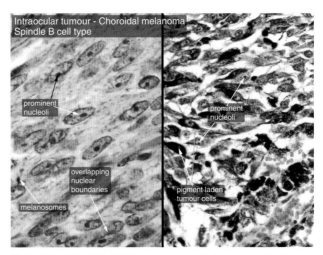

Figure 11.29

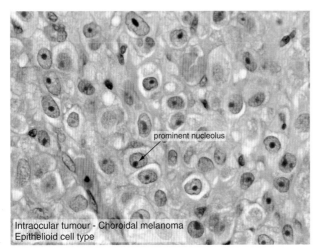

Figure 11.30

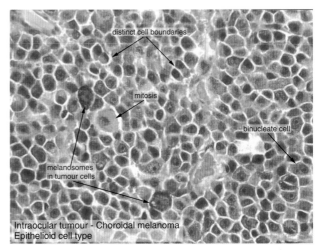

Figure 11.31

Figure 11.26 A patient presented with a blind painful eye. Clinical examination revealed a retinal detachment and, on diagnostic ultrasound, multiple choroidal masses were detected. Nodules of a diffuse malignant melanoma showing varying degrees of pigmentation are present throughout the choroid.

Figure 11.27 A low power histological preparation from the specimen shown in Figure 11.26. Exudation from the melanoma nodules diffusely scattered in the choroid has caused a total retinal detachment. Much of the subretinal exudate is absent due to artefact.

Figures 11.28 The morphology of spindle A melanoma cells is characterised by overlapping nuclei with longitudinal folds.

Figures 11.29 Spindle B melanoma cells possess larger nuclei than spindle A and have prominent nucleoli (left). In some spindle melanomas there is hyperpigmentation (right).

Figures 11.30 Epithelioid melanoma cells are larger and more circular in outline than the spindle cell variants; the nucleoli are prominent.

Figures 11.31 In some epithelioid melanomas, the intercellular spaces are distinct, hence the similarity to epithelial cells. Melanomas in the cytoplasm are diagnostic of a melanoma and exclude a metastatic tumour.

Prognostic indicators

Malignant melanoma of the uvea is characterised by a long time interval between clinical detection and metastatic death. After 5 years, 50% of the patients are alive, and after 25 years, 20% are alive. Traditionally, the following features were considered to be of prognostic importance:

1 *Cell type:* spindle A carries the best prognosis which worsens with progression through spindle B, mixed, and epithelioid.
2 *Size of tumour:* larger tumours carry a worse prognosis.
3 *Location of tumour:* ciliary body location carries a worse prognosis compared with choroid.
4 *Evidence of invasion:* extrascleral or vortex vein involvement.
5 *Age of patient:* prognosis worsens with increasing age.
6 *Cytology:* nucleolar size variation, vascular loops, and mitotic activity.
7 *Genetics:* see above.

Pathological evidence of treatment

Local "eye-wall" resection A local resection specimen is recognised by the solitary tumour attached to a thin layer of sclera and surrounded by a frill of choroid. The margins should be inspected carefully for clearance. In an enucleated globe that had previous local excision surgery, a large coloboma is evident. Enucleation in such cases is likely for tumour recurrence.

Ionising radiation Radiotherapy as listed above may be delivered in the form of plaque brachytherapy, proton or gamma teletherapy techniques. In eyes enucleated after unsuccessful radiotherapy, the resultant tumour histology ranges from no apparent effect to complete necrosis and infarction. The histological findings include that of tumour recurrence, neovascular glaucoma, cataract, and radiation retinopathy (see Chapter 9).

Ocular melanocytosis (melanosis oculi)

This is a congenital disorder in which there is an abnormal migration of melanocytes which accumulate in the episclera, sclera, and uvea. An ipsilateral intradermal naevus of the eyelid may be present (oculodermal melanocytosis – naevus of Ota). This disorder affects all races.

Clinical examination reveals hyperpigmentation of the episclera and sclera. There is an increased risk of intraocular tumours (uveal naevus or melanoma) and glaucoma.

Enucleation is most likely to be required if the globe contains a melanoma. Macroscopically, the globe shows extensive brown pigmentation of the episclera, sclera, and uveal tract (Figure 11.33).

Histological examination reveals dendritic melanocytes in abundance throughout the uveal tract and the scleral envelope. Involvement of the trabecular meshwork results in secondary glaucoma.

Melanocytoma of the optic nerve head

This tumour is a static hamartomatous proliferation of large uniform round or oval heavily pigmented melanocytes that occur within the anterior part of the optic nerve and in the peripapillary retina.

The patient is usually asymptomatic and the tumour is discovered on routine fundus examination appearing as an intensely black thickening of the optic disc with a feathery periphery. Regular observation is required to assess for changes in size and appearance which may suggest a misdiagnosis of a melanoma.

Enucleation is not required and histological studies are rare. These reveal melanocytic cells which are closely packed among the axons in the optic disc and anterior optic nerve. The cells are oval and packed with melanosomes; the nuclei are small, round, and inconspicuous. Bleaching of melanin is essential to show nuclear detail.

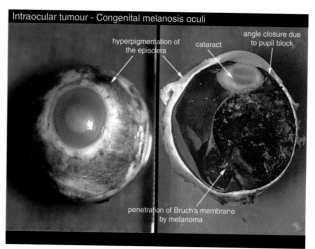

Intraocular tumour - Choroidal melanoma
Mixed cell type

apoptotic pigmented epithelioid cell

spindle B cell

epithelioid cell

Figure 11.32

Figure 11.32 The majority of uveal melanomas contain spindle B and epithelioid cells.

Intraocular tumour - Congenital melanosis oculi

hyperpigmentation of the episclera

cataract

angle closure due to pupil block

penetration of Bruch's membrane by melanoma

Figure 11.33

Figure 11.33 A patient with a history of oculodermal melanocytosis presented with unilateral loss of vision. A large intraocular mass was evident on clinical examination. A diagnosis of choroidal melanoma was made and an enucleation was performed. The ocular surface of the globe shows hyperpigmentation (left). A large pigmented choroidal melanoma is apparent on dissection (right).

Hamartomas

Hamartomas are benign proliferations of cells and tissues of the type that are normally present at the site.

Vascular

Cavernous haemangioma and Sturge–Weber syndrome

This is a benign congenital tumour of the choroid. There are two forms:

1 *Solitary cavernous haemangioma* localised to the choroid.
2 *Multifocal diffuse angiomas* in the Sturge–Weber syndrome in which vascular hamartomas are also found in the face, scalp, meninges, and brain.

Clinical presentation

The patient may be either asymptomatic or have visual symptoms from accumulation of subretinal fluid with possible progression to an exudative retinal detachment. A patient with Sturge–Weber syndrome will have a coexisting ipsilateral facial naevus flammeus and meningohaemangiomatosis. Glaucoma may be present and is secondary to episcleral tumour and venous congestion.

Genetics

There is no apparent hereditary link.

Possible modes of treatment

1 *Laser:* photocoagulation or transpupillary thermotherapy.
2 *Radiotherapy:* brachytherapy or external beam irradiation.
3 *Medical:* glaucoma medications.

Macroscopic

A cavernous haemangioma appears as an elliptical dark red mass with interlacing fibrous septae in the cut surface. Subretinal exudation with retinal detachment is a complication (Figure 11.34). Cupping of the optic disc and evidence of glaucoma surgery may be present in the Sturge–Weber syndrome (Figure 11.35).

Microscopic

The intraocular tumour consists of large vascular channels formed by fibrous septae which are lined by endothelium. The haemangioma fills the choroid and extends to Bruch's membrane (Figures 11.36, 11.37). Circumscribed tumours end abruptly, whereas the diffuse multifocal form blends imperceptibly into the peripheral tissue.

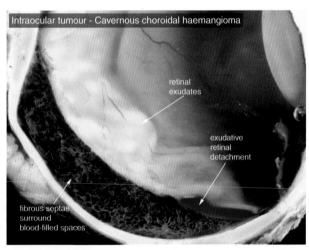

Figure 11.34

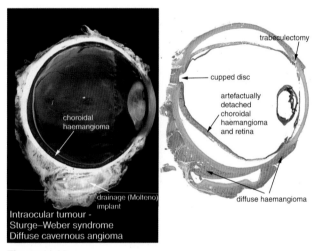

Figure 11.35

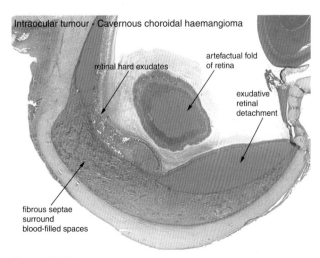

Figure 11.36

Figure 11.34 This globe was enucleated after an intraocular tumour was suspected. The choroid is thickened by a large vascular tumour which contains prominent fibrous septae – these are typical features of a cavernous choroidal haemangioma. The overlying retina is detached.

Figure 11.35 A 14 year old boy disfigured by naevus flammeus involving half the face developed secondary glaucoma which is a complication of the Sturge–Weber syndrome. Treatment was by trabeculectomy and drainage surgery included the insertion of a tube draining into a plastic plate (Molteno implant) which failed to control the intraocular pressure. Episcleral haemangiomas interfere with aqueous drainage, and this explains the secondary open angle glaucoma.

Figure 11.36 A cavernous haemangioma in the choroid has led to an exudative detachment of the retina. Retinal ischaemia has resulted in the formation of hard exudates.

The overlying neural retina may be cystic and thickened due to fibrous transformation of the underlying RPE giving rise to impairment of metabolic exchange with the outer retina.

Glaucoma and radiation retinopathy may be evident.

Retinal pigment epithelium (RPE)

The RPE is derived from neuroepithelium and very rarely is the source of neoplasms such as adenomas and adenocarcinomas. More commonly, areas of the hypertrophic RPE appear in normal fundi as brown patches.

Congenital hypertrophy and hyperplasia of the RPE (CHRPE)

This abnormality is a chance finding and appears as circular flat black or brown areas in the fundus that result from hypertrophy or hyperplasia of the RPE.

Clinically, these abnormalities are asymptomatic and are chance findings. There are several forms:

1 *Typical:*
   • solitary, unifocal, and unilateral
   • grouped (or multifocal) and unilateral – "bear tracks". Hereditary patterns are unknown in the typical forms and are not associated with systemic conditions.
2 *Atypical:* these are bilateral multiple ovaloid pigmentations with a hypopigmented "tail". This group is associated with *familial adenomatous polyposis.* The variant of familial polyposis with extracolonic involvement in the form of osteomas and soft tissue tumours is defined as *Gardiner's syndrome* and has an autosomal dominant inheritance pattern. In addition, atypical CHRPE also has associations with neuroepithelial tumours of the CNS (*Turçot syndrome*). It is thought that all three conditions are related to the same genetic disorder.

In a pathological specimen, a typical solitary CHRPE appears as a flat, heavily pigmented area of variable size and irregular outline. A halo may be seen at the periphery and areas of depigmentation (lacunae) are present (Figure 11.38).

In grouped pigmentation, the smaller and lighter patches occur in the retinal periphery (Figure 11.38).

Hypertrophy of the RPE cells is common in both the isolated and grouped forms of typical CHRPE. In the isolated form, the cells are hyperplastic and multilayered and the melanosomes are much larger than normal (Figure 11.39). Areas of lacunae and the halo indicate loss of RPE.

The histology of atypical CHRPE is not well documented.

Adenomas/adenocarcinomas of the RPE

Adenomas and adenocarcinomas of the RPE are much rarer than those in the ciliary body. The proliferating tumour cells have the characteristics of RPE cells with oval melanocytes and similar cytoplasmic adhesion systems. RPE tumours can be misdiagnosed as choroidal melanomas. There have been very few cases reported in the literature.

Choristoma

A benign congenital tumour composed of cellular elements and tissues not normally present at that site.

Choroidal osteoma

A choroidal osteoma is an excellent example of a choristoma. The tumours are benign static masses formed from compact and cancellous bone in the posterior choroid and are of unknown aetiology. These tumours are extremely rare and the majority of cases are female. As this tumour can be reliably diagnosed using ultrasound and CT, it is highly unlikely that this tumour will be studied pathologically.

A patient will present with a slowly progressive and painless visual loss or disturbance, especially when the macula is affected. The alternative is a chance finding in an asymptomatic individual. There may be a family history in autosomal dominant cases.

In the reported cases, mature cancellous bone is found within the choroid. The overlying RPE and retina are atrophic combined with subretinal neovascularisation.

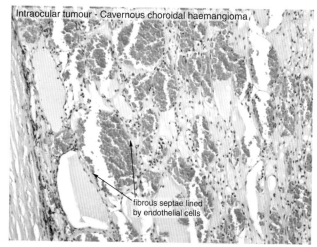

Figure 11.37

Figure 11.37 A cavernous haemangioma of the choroid consists of vascular channels formed by thin walled septae lined by endothelium.

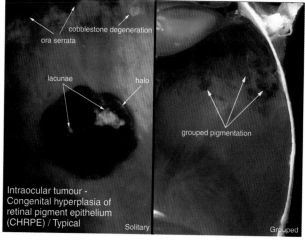

Figure 11.38

Figure 11.38 Congenital hyperplasia of the retinal pigment epithelium may take the form of a solitary heavily pigmented disc (left) or smaller irregular areas of pigmentation (grouped, right). These abnormalities are usually incidental findings in globes enucleated for other conditions.

Intraocular tumour - CHRPE
Solitary

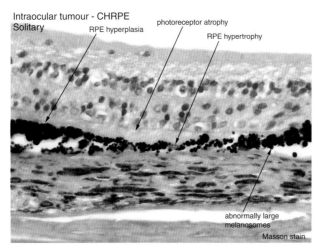

Figure 11.39

Intraocular tumour -
Retina astrocytic hamartoma

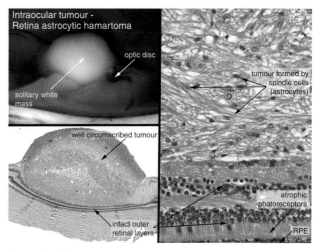

Figure 11.40

Intraocular tumour - Retinoblastoma

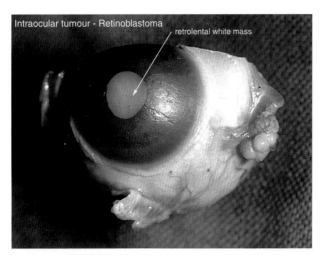

Figure 11.41

Intraocular tumour - Retinoblastoma
Spread into optic nerve

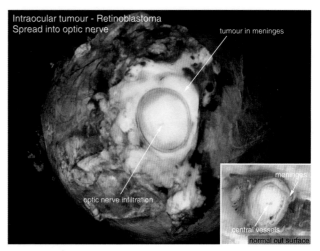

Figure 11.42

Intraocular tumour - Retinoblastoma

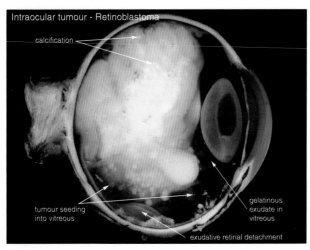

Figure 11.43

Figure 11.39 Histology taken from the solitary retinal pigment epithelium (RPE) hyperplasia shown in the left side of Figure 11.38 reveals simple hypertrophy and hyperplasia of the RPE with atrophy of the overlying photoreceptor layer. The melanosomes in the hyperplastic cells are four times larger than those in the normal RPE (Masson stain).

Figure 11.40 A small white tumour adjacent to the optic disc in an otherwise normal child was misdiagnosed as a retinoblastoma (upper left). On histological examination, the mass was formed by a well circumscribed proliferation of spindle cells (lower left), which by electron microscopy and immunohistochemistry had the characteristics of astrocytes. Detail of the spindle-shaped tumour cells is shown on the right. RPE = retinal pigment epithelium.

Figure 11.41 Leucocoria as seen by an ophthalmic pathologist.

Figure 11.42 In dealing with a retinoblastoma specimen, it is standard practice to take 2 mm slices across the optic nerve from the surgical limit to the back of the globe. In this specimen, the cut closest to the globe reveals tumour infiltration seen as solid white areas within and around the optic nerve. The inset shows the normal cut surface of the optic nerve.

Figure 11.43 A large endophytic retinoblastoma fills the posterior part of the globe and there is seeding into the vitreous cavity. The cut surface of the tumour contains white flecks of calcification.

Retina

Tumours of the retina in *childhood* are rare. Clinical awareness of such tumours is overshadowed by the fact that one form of retinal neoplasia, retinoblastoma, is lethal if untreated. At the other end of the spectrum, there are hamartomatous astrocytic tumours which may resemble a small retinoblastoma, but which remain static. A hamartomatous vascular malformation is seen in the von Hippel–Lindau syndrome (see Chapter 10).

Astrocytic hamartoma/retinal astrocytoma

Tumours derived from retinal glial cells may be static, "astrocytic hamartomas", or slowly growing neoplasms, "astrocytomas". Clinically, both variants appear as white mulberry shaped masses which when multifocal and bilateral are features of tuberous sclerosis. An isolated tumour is non-syndromic.

On pathological examination, histology of a solitary astrocytic hamartoma (Figure 11.40) reveals a well circumscribed mass formed by astrocytes in the inner retina.

Retinoblastoma

This is the most common malignant ocular tumour of childhood. Originating from embryonal retinal cells, this tumour can be unilateral or bilateral, although it is often asymmetrical in size in the latter case. The tumour is rare with an incidence of 1 in 20 000 live births and is an extreme rarity in adults. The fact that in some cases this tumour may be inherited makes it of great interest in molecular genetics (see below).

Clinical presentation
Initial features
1 *Abnormal appearance of eye:* leucocoria and strabismus.
2 *Ophthalmoscopy:* shows whitish-pink tumour nodules projecting from the retina into the vitreous (endophytic growth) or a retinal detachment due to subretinal tumour proliferation and exudation (exophytic growth).

Late features
1 *Apparent uveitis:* tumour expansion with accompanying necrosis into the vitreous and anterior chamber results in an accumulation of cellular material simulating an inflammatory process (pseudohypopyon).
2 *Secondary neovascular glaucoma:* focal necrosis within a tumour causes the release of vascular endothelial growth factor with neovascularisation in the retina and iris accompanied by secondary angle closure glaucoma.
3 *Orbital involvement:* massive necrosis of tumour within the globe is associated with an acute orbital cellulitis. Note that this tumour is supplied by a single central retinal artery. Tumour spread along the optic nerve reaches the cranial cavity and transcleral spread into the orbit causes a proptosis.

Investigations may include an ultrasound of the eye and a cranial CT scan if extension is suspected.

If left untreated as in some societies, the tumour proliferates within the globe and extends along the optic nerve to the intracranial meninges. Perforation of the corneoscleral envelope leads to intraorbital spread and death is the result of blood borne visceral and skeletal metastases.

Possible modes of treatment
Treatment will depend on the size and extent of involvement of the tumour, whether it is unilateral or bilateral, and the treatment centre. Treatment options include:
* enucleation
* photocoagulation
* cryotherapy
* irradiation: external beam or brachytherapy
* chemotherapy: used to shrink tumours to facilitate other modes of treatment.

Cure rates with early diagnosis and treatment are in excess of 90%.

Macroscopic
External examination of the globe reveals a white retrolental tumour (Figure 11.41), but precise localisation by transillumination is difficult. Optic nerve involvement may be evident when initial cuts are made across the optic nerve (Figure 11.42). Trans-scleral tumour spread is uncommon in cases occurring in developed societies but is not infrequently encountered in developing countries.

Two forms of growth are recognised:
1 *Endophytic tumours* (i.e. those growing into the vitreous) are grey-white and smooth surfaced. Vitreous seeding may be evident (Figure 11.43). Larger tumours exhibit darker grey areas of necrosis, brown foci of haemorrhage, and firm white granules or flecks of dystrophic calcification. Further growth fills the interior of the globe and (as the tumour is supplied by a single artery) necrosis becomes more extensive (Figure 11.44). The resultant reaction can lead to a misdiagnosis of orbital cellulitis due to the release of inflammatory mediators. In a rare "diffuse" form of retinoblastoma (Figure 11.45), the retina is totally infiltrated and this form usually carries a poor prognosis. The widespread nodular thickening of the retina may simulate a retinitis.
2 *Exophytic tumours* (Figures 11.46, 11.47) are tumour proliferations in the subretinal space and secondary exudation contributes to retinal detachment.

Extraocular spread will only be seen in advanced untreated cases.

Microscopic
At low power, it is possible to identify calcification within what appears to be a homogeneous basophilic tumour (Figure 11.48). Even at this level, it is possible to assess the extent of tumour spread within the retina.

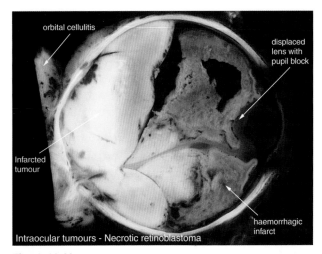

orbital cellulitis

displaced lens with pupil block

Infarcted tumour

haemorrhagic infarct

Intraocular tumours - Necrotic retinoblastoma

Figure 11.44

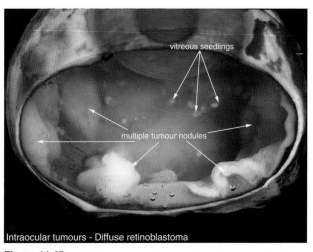

vitreous seedlings

multiple tumour nodules

Intraocular tumours - Diffuse retinoblastoma

Figure 11.45

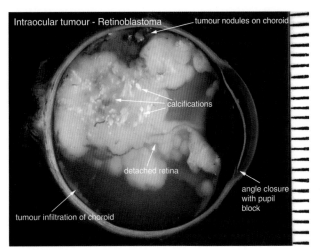

Intraocular tumour - Retinoblastoma

tumour nodules on choroid

calcifications

detached retina

tumour infiltration of choroid

angle closure with pupil block

Figure 11.46

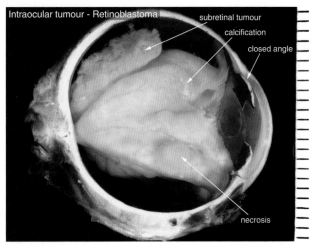

Intraocular tumour - Retinoblastoma

subretinal tumour

calcification

closed angle

necrosis

Figure 11.47

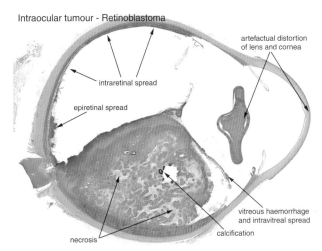

Intraocular tumour - Retinoblastoma

artefactual distortion of lens and cornea

intraretinal spread

epiretinal spread

vitreous haemorrhage and intravitreal spread

necrosis

calcification

Figure 11.48

Figure 11.44 On religious grounds, the parents of a child refused treatment until massive intraocular spread led to secondary glaucoma and orbital cellulitis. The infarcted tumour has a brown homogeneous appearance in the anterior part (haemorrhagic infarction). Episcleral thickening was the result of an orbital cellulitis. Surprisingly, no tumour was found in the orbital tissue.

Figure 11.45 In the diffuse form of retinoblastoma, tumour nodules and areas of thickening are present throughout the retina. Tumour seedlings are present in the vitreous.

Figure 11.46 In this exophytic retinoblastoma, white flecks of calcification are prominent in the cut surface of the tumour. A solid subretinal proteinaceous exudate is present. The tumour is seeding onto the inner surface of the choroid which may be invaded (a bad prognostic feature).

Figure 11.47 In this exophytic retinoblastoma, extensive infiltration obliterates the retina. Lens displacement has led to angle closure.

Figure 11.48 A low power view of a globe containing an exophytic retinoblastoma. Within the tumour mass, the paler areas represent necrosis and the dark blue granules represent calcification. NB: In the epiretinal nodules and in the diffusely spreading tumour in the retina, the tumour tissue is more basophilic because there is less necrosis.

At high magnification, the tumour cells are small and round with scanty cytoplasm (Figure 11.49). The nuclei are round or oval and the nuclear chromatin is finely granular. Nucleoli are inconspicuous and the cytoplasm and cell membranes are poorly defined. Mitotic figures can be easily identified.

The dependence on blood supply for survival is manifest as rings of viable cells around widely spaced blood vessels – "pseudorosettes" (Figure 11.50). Tumour calcification is a prominent feature (Figure 11.50). Without immersion in decalcifying fluids prior to processing, the calcification appears as basophilic granules which have a tendency to fragment on microtomy.

Widespread necrosis of the tumour cells also leads to precipitation of DNA in the walls of blood vessels and as pools in necrotic tissue (Figure 11.51). The DNA is basophilic and stains positively with the Feulgen stain (not used routinely).

Cell differentiation within retinoblastomas is seen in the following:

1 *Flexner–Wintersteiner rosettes* consist of a circle of cells limited internally by a continuous membrane and united by adherent junctions (Figure 11.52). The lumen of this type of rosette contains acid mucopolysaccharides which can be identified by special stains but are optically empty in routine H&E staining.

2 *Homer–Wright rosettes:* a multilayered circle of nuclei surrounds eosinophilic fibrillar material (Figure 11.49); this type of rosette in retinoblastomas is far less common than Flexner–Wintersteiner rosettes.

3 *Fleurettes:* a circular or oval group of cells in which cytoplasmic processes (resembling a fleur de lys) have the ultrastructural characteristics of inner segments of photoreceptors (Figure 11.53).

Effect of treatment

The tumour has a preferential spread along the optic nerve. Hence, it is important in an enucleation that the optic nerve is excised to provide the maximal length. Ophthalmic pathologists are well aware of the importance of examination of the surgical cut edge of the optic nerve stump (Figure 11.54).

Immunohistochemistry

Retinoblastoma cells stain positively with anti-S100, anti-NSE, and anti-GFAP antibodies. Antibodies against photoreceptor soluble retinal antigen (anti-S) label the cells in the differentiated tumours.

Genetics

A careful family history is essential for prognosis and genetic counselling.

The accepted theory for the development of retinoblastoma involves the deletion of both tumour suppressor genes (RB1) on 13q14 located on the two corresponding chromosomes of a retinal cell (Knudson two-hit hypothesis). There are two types:

1 *Hereditary form (40%):* a germ cell line mutation that involves the loss of one gene at the time of embryogenesis that was either inherited from an affected parent or by spontaneous mutation. Since this defect is reproduced throughout the cell line, the genetic defect can be inherited in an autosomal dominant manner by the offspring of the affected person. A retinoblastoma is manifest if there is loss of the second gene in the retinal cell and this involves 90% of affected individuals. This form of retinoblastoma usually presents bilaterally and earlier in life. Children with heritable bilateral retinoblastoma carry a high risk of a second malignancy: (a) within the first decade, of a midline cerebral tumour, for example a pinealoblastoma or trilateral retinoblastoma; (b) within the second to fourth decades, from a carcinoma or sarcomas of various types, for example fibrosarcoma, osteosarcoma, and rhabdomyosarcoma (embryonal or alveolar), most commonly arising in a limb or in the orbit. The second tumour may occur in an irradiated region, but more frequently the location is in untreated tissue.

2 *Non-hereditary form (60%):* involves a somatic cell mutation at the level of the retinal cell. In affected individuals, the tumour is usually unilateral and presents later in childhood.

Genetic counselling is an important part of the management of retinoblastoma and can be difficult. Whereas an individual with bilateral tumours or a clear family history probably has the hereditary form, the majority of cases are unilateral and sporadic (75%), of which 15% are known to be of the hereditary form. In these cases, Table 11.3 summarises the probability of the patient's offspring and siblings acquiring the genetic defect for retinoblastoma.

Differential diagnosis

- **C**oats' disease (see Chapter 10).
- **A**strocytic hamartoma.
- **R**etinopathy of prematurity (see Chapter 10).
- **P**ersistent hyperplastic primary vitreous (see Chapter 6).
- **E**ndophthalmitis (see Chapter 8).
- **T**oxocara retinitis (see Chapter 8).

The mnemonic is CARPET.

Table 11.3 Statistical risk of inheritance of the retinoblastoma gene from a single sporadic unilateral case.

	Unilateral	Bilateral
Offspring	7.5%	50%
Sibling	1%	5%

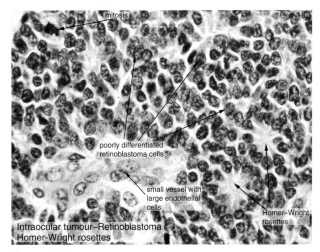

Figure 11.49

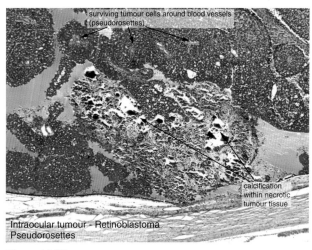

Figure 11.50

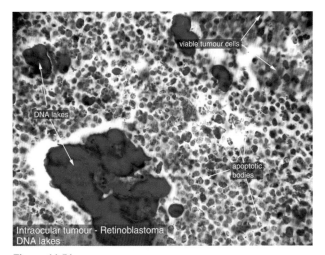

Figure 11.51

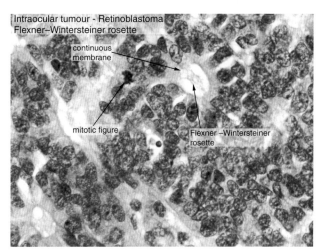

Figure 11.52

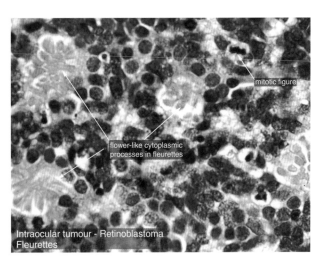

Figure 11.53

Figure 11.49 The tumour cells have scanty cytoplasm and nuclei which are irregular in size and shape, with a finely granular chromatin. In this example, the majority of cells are poorly differentiated but two rosettes (Homer–Wright) are present. Endothelial cells in blood vessels are stimulated by growth factors derived from the tumour.

Figure 11.50 Viable tumour survives around the blood vessels (pseudorosettes) against a background of extensive necrosis. In parts, there is calcification within the necrotic tissue.

Figure 11.51 Necrosis in retinoblastoma cells progresses to clumping of nuclear chromatin. The DNA which is released from necrotic cells forms lakes (large basophilic pools). Cells which resemble polymorphonuclear leucocytes due to nuclear fragmentation have the features of individual cell death (apoptosis).

Figure 11.52 The poorly differentiated cells have in one part formed a rosette (Flexner–Winndersteiner). A distinct limiting membrane is present on the inner surface of the circle of cells.

Figure 11.53 A rare variant of rosette takes the form of tumour cells which surround cytoplasmic processes resembling inner segments. Such arrangements are referred to as fleurettes. These are more commonly found in irradiated tumours.

Medulloepitheliomas – non-teratoid and teratoid

These are rare tumours in childhood which are derived from the embryonic tissue at the periphery of the retina and the pars plana and which differ in some respects from a retinoblastoma. The tumours contain cells that have the features of neoplastic ciliary epithelium in addition to areas resembling a retinoblastoma. Occasionally these tumours contain mesenchymal elements such as cartilage and are classified as *teratoid medulloepitheliomas*. Both non-teratoid and teratoid medulloepitheliomas arise in the ciliary body and are locally invasive within the globe.

These tumours are subclassified into benign and malignant variants but survival rates are high because the tumour is slow growing and is confined to the eye.

The child may present with visual impairment, iris heterochromia, or leucocoria. Occasionally, secondary neovascular glaucoma may be a final complication. Treatment is usually surgical in the form of an enucleation, although local eye-wall resection has been successful.

On pathological examination, a medulloepithelioma appears as a large white or partially pigmented mass arising in the ciliary body which permits the distinction from a retinoblastoma. The malignant variants are larger in size and more invasive (Figure 11.55). It is impossible to distinguish at the gross level whether the tumour is teratoid or non-teratoid, or to determine the degree of malignancy.

Microscopic features

Non-teratoid medulloepithelioma (benign and malignant)
The distinction between low grade and high grade malignant variants is somewhat subjective depending on mitotic activity and dedifferentiation in the tumour cells. At the more benign end of the spectrum, two cell types are present within these tumours (Figure 11.56):

1 Acinar tissue derived from ciliary epithelium consisting of cuboidal cells arranged in columns or circles.
2 Primitive neuroblastic tissue containing small cells in a random orientation with occasional rosette formation.

In malignant non-teratoid medulloepithelioma, both types of cells possess the features of active malignant proliferation with plentiful mitotic figures (Figure 11.57).

Teratoid medulloepithelioma Areas of neoplastic mesenchyme such as a malignant cartilaginous component may be easily identified within the teratoid subset (Figure 11.58). This variant contains cells of each histogenic origin (ciliary epithelium, neural retina, and mesenchyme).

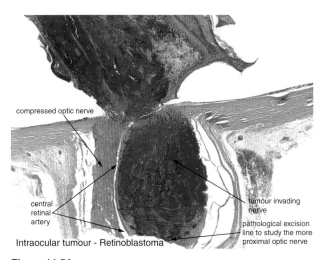

Figure 11.54

compressed optic nerve

central retinal artery

tumour invading nerve

pathological excision line to study the more proximal optic nerve

Intraocular tumour - Retinoblastoma

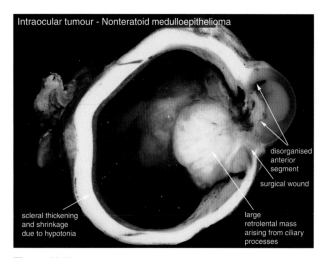

Figure 11.55

Intraocular tumour - Nonteratoid medulloepithelioma

scleral thickening and shrinkage due to hypotonia

disorganised anterior segment

surgical wound

large retrolental mass arising from ciliary processes

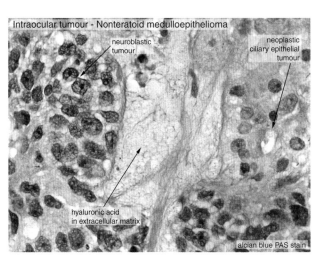

Figure 11.56

Intraocular tumour - Nonteratoid medulloepithelioma

neuroblastic tumour

neoplastic ciliary epithelial tumour

hyaluronic acid in extracellular matrix

alcian blue PAS stain

Figure 11.54 A low power micrograph showing invasion of part of the optic nerve (right) by a finger-like extension of a retinoblastoma. A compressed nerve is present on the left side. The posterior limit of the nerve has been removed during specimen grossing for serial sections to assess clearance at the proximal end.

Figure 11.55 A child presented with a unilateral leucocoria. A congenital cataract was diagnosed, and during cataract surgery a large retrolental mass was discovered. On sectioning the enucleated globe, a large mass with a white cut surface is seen arising from the ciliary body. The cut surface of these tumours is usually white. Histology of the tumour revealed a non-teratoid medulloepithelioma (see Figure 11.56).

Figure 11.56 The histology of the more benign variant of non-teratoid medulloepithelioma includes columnar cells which have an acinar pattern (ciliary epithelial origin) and neuroblastic cells which resemble embryonic neuroretina. This Alcian blue PAS stain demonstrates mucopolysaccharide within the tumour stroma – this substance is normally secreted by the ciliary epithelium.

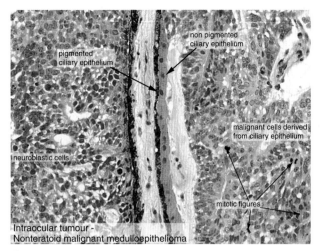

Figure 11.57

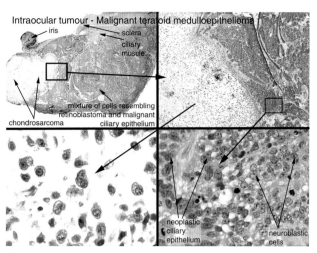

Figure 11.58

Figure 11.57 In this malignant non-teratoid medulloepithelioma, the neuroblastic and epithelial cells are poorly differentiated and mitotic figures are plentiful in the epithelial component.

Figure 11.58 A ciliary body tumour was considered on clinical examination to be an amelanotic melanoma. A local eye-wall resection was performed. The tumour at low power appears to contain compact masses of neuroblastic basophilic cells (upper left, upper right, lower right). The paler staining area consists of cartilaginous tissue which possesses the histological features of chondrosarcoma (lower left). The diagnosis was therefore "malignant teratoid medulloepithelioma".

Panophthalmic neoplasia

It is convenient in discussing metastatic disease to make a separation between metastases derived from viscera and those in which lymphoid neoplasia is the source.

Metastatic disease

Almost every known primary source has been reported to spread to the eye and, in the majority, to the choroid. In approximately 25% of patients with ocular metastasis, this is the presenting sign of generalised neoplasia. The growth of metastatic tumours is usually faster than that of ocular melanomas and is a useful clinical guide. The most common primary sources for ocular metastasis are pulmonary and mammary carcinomas with presumed blood borne metastasis. Bilateral involvement is a useful sign.

The clinical presentation is variable depending on the location of the tumours within the globe, and ranges from being asymptomatic to total visual loss. Involvement of the orbit would also lead to a proptosis. The treatment will depend on the primary source (for example surgery, chemotherapy, hormonal, and radiotherapy) and the histopathological diagnosis.

Macroscopic examination reveals single or multiple nodules of varying size throughout the uveal tract. With the exception of metastatic cutaneous melanoma, these tumours are usually amelanotic. There may be associated exudative retinal detachment and extraocular spread.

The microscopic features correspond to the primary tumour (Figures 11.59–11.62). Features of radiation retinopathy may be evident.

Lymphoid neoplasia

Primary lymphoid neoplasia takes the form of a massive infiltration of the retina and optic nerve with spillage into the vitreous. The CNS may be affected and the diagnosis is often made by vitrectomy or retinal biopsy.

In systemic lymphoid neoplasia, secondary tumour deposits can infiltrate any part of the uveal tract to form white tumours: a solitary mass may mimic amelanotic melanoma.

Clinical presentation
The presenting symptoms and signs are variable:
1 Painless loss of vision.
2 Apparent ocular inflammation (masquerade syndrome):
   - necrotising retinitis and vitritis (for example may mimic viral infections)
   - anterior or posterior uveitis (for example mimicking granulomatous inflammatory disorders).
3 Isolated tumour nodules in the uveal tract.

It is important to investigate for systemic involvement in the workup of an ocular lymphoid neoplasia.

Possible modes of treatment
Radiotherapy and/or chemotherapy.

Macroscopic and microscopic
Primary
1 *Macroscopic:* the retina is thickened by tumour cell infiltration which is accompanied by vascular occlusion and secondary haemorrhagic infarction (Figure 11.63). Tumour cells frequently spread into the vitreous and the diagnosis is often made by examination of a vitrectomy specimen.

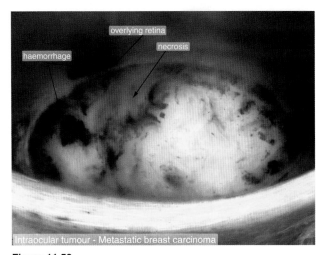

Intraocular tumour - Metastatic breast carcinoma

Figure 11.59

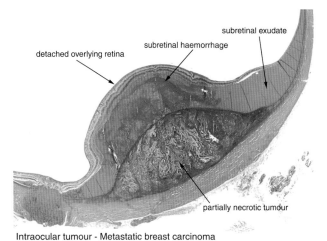

Intraocular tumour - Metastatic breast carcinoma

Figure 11.60

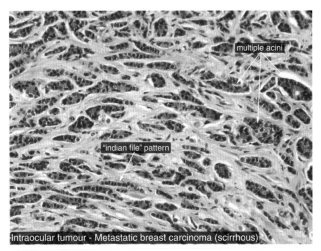

Intraocular tumour - Metastatic breast carcinoma (scirrhous)

Figure 11.61

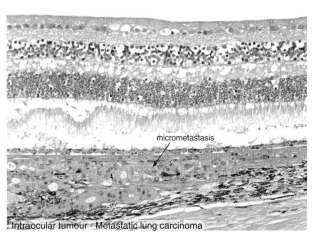

Intraocular tumour - Metastatic lung carcinoma

Figure 11.62

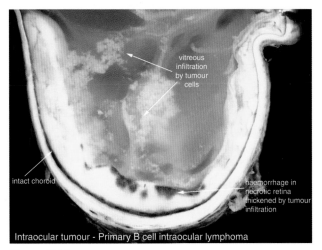

Intraocular tumour - Primary B cell intraocular lymphoma

Figure 11.63

Figure 11.59 An elderly female patient presented with unilateral visual disturbance which on fundus examination was found to be due to a solid choroidal mass. Routine questioning revealed a history of treatment for breast carcinoma. The globe was initially irradiated but continued growth led to the decision to enucleate. This metastatic tumour forms an ovoid mass in the choroid and contains areas of necrosis and haemorrhage. NB: It would be difficult to distinguish this solitary tumour from an amelanotic melanoma.

Figure 11.60 Histology from the specimen shown in Figure 11.59. Postirradiation necrosis, haemorrhage, and exudation have increased the apparent bulk of the tumour. The retina is detached by a haemorrhagic exudate.

Figure 11.61 In a metastatic scirrhous carcinoma of the breast in the choroid, the malignant cells are separated by dense fibrous tissue. The linear pattern of tumour cells is traditionally referred to as "Indian file".

Figure 11.62 The patient was initially diagnosed with what appeared to be a retinal pigment epitheliopathy prior to death due to lung cancer. The globe was removed at autopsy and histology revealed micrometastases in the choroid. The overlying photoreceptors show autolytic change.

Figure 11.63 This is an example of an intraocular B-cell lymphoma involving the retina, which is massively thickened due to haemorrhagic necrosis and tumour infiltration. Tumour nodules are present in the vitreous but the choroid is intact. This patient also suffered from CNS involvement. Previously, this combination was classified as reticulum cell sarcoma of the eye and brain.

2 *Microscopic:* the thickened retina reveals extensive infiltration by malignant lymphoid cells which have large nuclei and scanty cytoplasm – mitotic figures are plentiful. Within the areas of infarcted retina, viable tumour cells are present in the necrotic tissue formed by breakdown of the neural cells (Figures 11.64, 11.65). The retinal pigment epithelium is infiltrated by malignant lymphocytes (Figure 11.65). More detail of the morphology of malignant lymphoid cells is obtained in vitrectomy specimens. The characteristic features of malignant lymphoid cells are scanty cytoplasm, multiple nucleoli, crenated nuclear membranes, and clumps of condensed nuclear chromatin (Figure 11.66).

Secondary

1 *Macroscopic:* in contrast to the retinal involvement in primary intraocular lymphoma, secondary involvement in a patient suffering from systemic disease occurs as nodular infiltrates in any part of the uveal tract (Figure 11.67).
2 *Microscopic:* any part of the uveal tract may be massively thickened by a lymphoid malignant infiltrate which

is intensely basophilic ("if it's blue, it's bad" – Figure 11.68). The cytological features (Figure 11.69) are similar to those described for primary lymphomas (Figure 11.66). In many enucleated eyes, the secondary effects of irradiation, such as cataract, radiation retinopathy, and vitreous exudation, may be present.

Complications

Complications common to both primary and secondary intraocular lymphomas are glaucoma, exudative retinal detachment, and extraocular spread.

Immunohistochemistry

Accurate identification of tumour cell lymphoma subsets by immunohistochemistry has revealed that the infiltrating cells in the primary and the secondary forms are usually of large B-cell type.

A wide variety of lymphocyte markers is available and is constantly expanding. Examples include CD5, which is a T-cell marker, CD20 and CD79, both of which are pan B-cell markers (Figure 11.70).

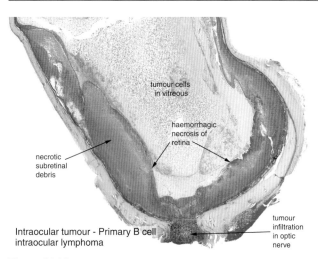

Intraocular tumour - Primary B cell intraocular lymphoma

Figure 11.64

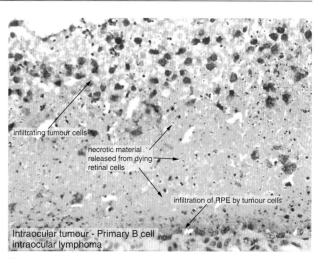

Intraocular tumour - Primary B cell intraocular lymphoma

Figure 11.65

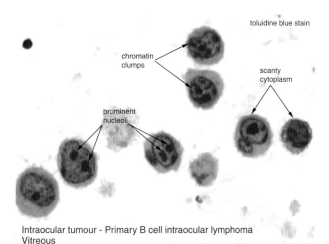

Intraocular tumour - Primary B cell intraocular lymphoma
Vitreous

Figure 11.66

Figure 11.64 Histology from the specimen shown in Figure 11.63 shows the apparent retinal thickening was due to extensive haemorrhagic infarction and subretinal necrotic debris. Malignant cells in the optic nerve are preserved.
Figure 11.65 Detail of the necrotic retina shown in Figures 11.63 and 11.64. Retinal tissue is no longer identifiable and necrosis of the neural cells is seen as a pink amorphous mass within which viable tumour cells can be identified. Tumour cell infiltration of the retinal pigment epithelium (RPE) is characteristic.
Figure 11.66 A plastic section prepared from a vitrectomy specimen provides detail of a malignant B-cell lymphoma: these include multiple nucleoli, chromatin clumping, and a scanty cytoplasm.

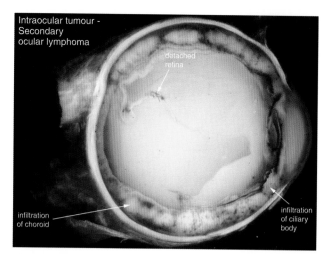

Figure 11.67

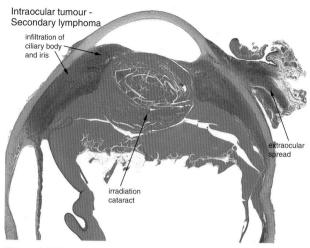

Figure 11.68

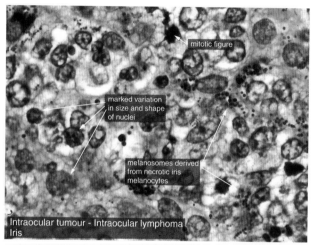

Figure 11.69

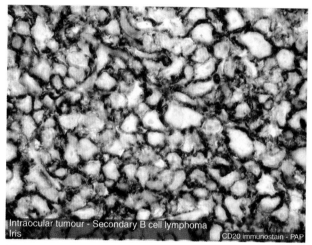

Figure 11.70

Figure 11.67 In this secondary B-cell lymphoma, the tumour infiltration is irregular in thickness and the ciliary body and choroid are extensively involved. The retina is spared but is detached by exudation. Exudates are also present in the vitreous and the anterior chamber.

Figure 11.68 The patient presented with a conjunctival swelling followed by tumour infiltration in the iris after the diagnosis of systemic lymphoma had been made. Enucleation was required to relieve pain. A lymphocytic infiltration is uniformly blue and moulds to the intraocular structures. The patient was irradiated and the lens shows the changes of irradiation cataract.

Figure 11.69 A diagnosis of a malignant lymphoid infiltrate in the iris may be confused by the presence of melanin released from necrotic iris melanocytes. Note the marked variation in nuclear size and shape and the scanty cytoplasm.

Figure 11.70 Immunohistochemical study of an iris lymphoma reveals that the cells are CD20+ which indicates a B-cell lineage (monoclonality).

Index

Note: Page numbers in *italics* refer to figures; those in **bold** refer to tables.